Acquisitions editor: Melanie Tait
Development editor: Myriam Brearley
Production controller: Chris Jarvis
Desk editor: Jane Campbell
Cover designer: Helen Brockway

Total

Total Intravenous Anaesthesia

Nicholas L. Padfield MB BS FRCA
Consultant Anaesthetist, St Thomas' Hospital, London, UK

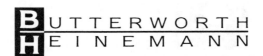

OXFORD   AUCKLAND   BOSTON   JOHANNESBURG   MELBOURNE   NEW DELHI

Butterworth-Heinemann
Linacre House, Jordan Hill, Oxford OX2 8DP
225 Wildwood Avenue, Woburn, MA 01801-2041
A division of Reed Educational and Professional Publishing Ltd

 A member of the Reed Elsevier plc group

First published 2000

British Library Cataloguing in Publication Data
Padfield, Nicholas L.
   Total intravenous anaesthesia
   1. Intravenous anaesthesia
   I. Title
   617.9'62

Library of Congress Cataloguing in Publication Data
Total intravenous anaesthesia/[edited by] Nicholas L. Padfield
   p. cm.
   Includes bibliographical references and index.
   ISBN 0 7506 4171 1
   1. Intravenous anaesthesia.   I. Padfield, Nicholas L.
   [DNLM: 1. Anesthesia, Intravenous.   2. Anesthesia, General.
   WO 285 T7171 2000]
   RD85.I6 T672
   617.9'62–dc21   00–057145

ISBN 0 7506 4171 1

Composition by Genesis Typesetting, Rochester, Kent
Printed and bound in Great Britain by Biddles Ltd, Guildford and Kings Lynn

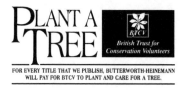

Contents

Foreword   vii
List of contributors   ix

PART 1:   GENERAL CONSIDERATIONS

1   Introduction, history and development   3
    N. L. Padfield

2   Drugs and pharmacology   13
    S. J. Dolin

3   Drug interactions   36
    S. J. Dolin

4   Pharmacokinetics of infusion   44
    F. Engbers

5   Administration of intravenous anaesthesia/total intravenous
    anaesthesia   66
    N. L. Padfield

PART 2: SPECIFIC ISSUES

6   Awareness and total intravenous anaesthesia   87
    J. G. Jones and T. Leary

7   Postoperative nausea, vomiting and recovery   116
    J. M. Millar

PART 3: TYPES OF ANAESTHESIA

8   Day case surgery   147
    W. L. Rowe

9   Cardiac surgery   158
    J. D. Kneeshaw and R. Mills

10   Thoracic surgery   176
    R. Feneck

11   Neurosurgery   203
    C. R. Bailey and M. Sinden

12   Maxillofacial, plastic and ear, nose & throat (ENT) surgery   220
    N. L. Padfield

13 Anaesthesia for the elderly   233
    J. Peacock

14 Sedation for regional anaesthesia   249
    N. L. Padfield

15 Endocrine surgery   263
    N. L. Padfield

16 Ophthalmic surgery   276
    N. Sutcliffe

17 Future developments   285
    S. E. Milne and G. N. C. Kenny

Index   299

Foreword

When propofol was introduced into anaesthetic practice in the 1980s, it became apparent that this was a drug that was suitable not only for induction of general anaesthesia, but that it could be infused to maintain anaesthesia. Furthermore, it was clear that if anaesthetists could be provided with drug delivery systems that were capable of delivering the drug conveniently and accurately, patients would be able to experience the superior recovery characteristics associated with propofol based anaesthesia.

Since then, major technological advances have led to the development of reliable and robust infusion pumps, and increased knowledge of pharmacokinetics resulted in the introduction of 'Diprifusor' target-controlled infusion devices into routine anaesthetic practice in the United Kingdom in 1996. These TCI systems for propofol are now becoming more widely available elsewhere in the world. While fentanyl, sufentanil, alfentanil and ketamine have long been available as the analgesic supplement to propofol, the launch of remifentanil has resulted in an explosion of interest in the art and science of intravenous anaesthesia. Specialist intravenous anaesthesia societies have been formed in the UK (SIVA UK) and Europe (EuroSIVA), and their scientific meetings are attended by growing numbers of anaesthetists. The websites of both societies provide forums for education, information and debate, and are accessed by individuals from all corners of the world.

The editor of this book has assembled an impressive list of authors, all of whom have contributed in some way to this growing interest in intravenous anaesthesia. It is hoped that colleagues will find contained within this publication the practical advice that they require to improve their own anaesthetic practice, and provide their patients with the benefits of total intravenous anaesthesia.

D. Russell FRCA
Consultant Anaesthetist
South Glasgow University NHS Trust, Glasgow, UK

Honorary Secretary
The UK Society for Intravenous Anaesthesia

Contributors

Craig Bailey MB BS FRCA
Consultant Anaesthetist, Department of Anaesthesia, Guys and Thomas' NHS Trust, London, UK

Simon Dolin FRCA PhD
Consultant in Anaesthetics and Pain Relief, St Richard's Hospital, Chichester, UK

Frank Engbers MD
Department of Anaesthesiology, Leiden University Medical Center, The Netherlands

Robert Feneck MB BS FRCA
Consultant Anaesthetist, St Thomas' Hospital, London, UK

Gareth Jones MD FRCP FRCA
Professor of Anaesthesia, Addenbrookes Hospital, Cambridge, UK

Gavin Kenny BSc(Hons) MD FRCA FANZCA
Professor and Head of Department, University Department of Anaesthesia, Glasgow Royal Infirmary, Glasgow, UK

John Kneeshaw MB ChB
Consultant Cardiothoracic Anaesthetist, Papworth Hospital, Cambridge, UK

T Leary ChB FRCA
Specialist Registrar, Department of Anaesthesia, Addenbrookes Hospital, Cambridge, UK

Jean Millar MB ChB FRCA
Consultant Anaesthetist, Nuffield Department of Anaesthetics, Oxford; Honorary Senior Clinical Lecturer, Oxford University, Oxford, UK

R Mills MA MB Bchir
Specialist Registrar, Department of Anaesthesia, Papworth Hospital, Cambridge, UK

E Stewart Milne BSc(Hons) MB ChB FRCA
Lecturer, University Department of Anaesthesia, Glasgow Royal Infirmary, Glasgow, UK

John Peacock MB ChB FRCA
Consultant Anaesthetist, Royal Hallamshire Hospital, Sheffield, UK

Lawrence Rowe MB ChB FRCA DRCOG
Consultant Anaesthetist, Norfolk and Norwich Hospital, Norwich, UK

Mark Sinden MB BS FRCA DCH DA
Consultant Anaesthetist, Kent and Sussex NHS Weald Trust, UK

Nicholas Sutcliffe MRCP FRCA
Consultant in Anaesthetics and Intensive Care, Health Care International, Clydebank, Glasgow, UK

PART 1

GENERAL CONSIDERATIONS

1

Introduction, history and development

N. L. Padfield

- Impediments to the practice
- Changes in drugs and technology
- Merits and limitations of total intravenous anaesthesia
- Nitrous oxide and pollution in perspective

Introduction

The choice of anaesthetic technique not only depends on the nature of the operation and the health of the patient, but also on the personal preference of the particular anaesthetist. The resulting choice may be the result of previous experience with a familiar and favoured technique or a slight modification of it to fit the particular case in question.

Impediments to the practice of intravenous (IV) anaesthesia are due largely to:

- Lack of suitable equipment
- Lack of experience
- Lack of confidence in the technique
- Lack of suitable drugs
- Lack of funds

Unfamiliarity with the technique of IV anaesthesia has probably delayed acceptance and dissemination into general anaesthetic practice. In one survey by Zeneca, 9.8% of anaesthetists questioned said they used total IV anaesthesia (TIVA) for maintenance, and in one other by Glaxo, out of 1300 anaesthetists questioned, 10% said they used TIVA for maintenance. A common fear is that there is an increased risk of awareness when muscles relaxants are employed. A paper published before the widespread availability of target and effect-site analog displays showed that awareness was uncommon, and in the five cases out of approximately 2500 where awareness was reported, each time it was probably the result of the inexperience of the anaesthetist (1). Thus with training and further experience this incidence of awareness is not a problem.

Good practice in anaesthesia is not the result of accident or good luck. It is the result of carefully acquired detailed knowledge of pharmacology, physiology and physics. Armed with this knowledge it is then scientifically applied to the individual requirement of the patient, which includes their preoperative condition, the proposed surgery and their postoperative requirements.

At present we administer drugs and fluids IV, inhalational agents and gases through sophisticated gas conduits, vaporizers and circle systems with facilities to moisturize, warm and remove CO_2. We can measure, display and record almost simultaneously breath by breath variations in gas and vapour composition of inspired and expired gases. We can measure beat to beat variation in blood pressure, ejection fraction and cardiac output by non-invasive methods. We can monitor electrophysiological signals like the electrocardiogram, the electromyogram, evoked potentials and the electroencephalogram (EEG). All this sophisticated application of physics enables us to minutely monitor more and more physiological variables, which allows us to administer anaesthesia safely in more and more complex situations.

However, the basic requirements for anaesthesia have not changed from Lundy's 'Analgesia, anaesthesia and muscle relaxation' (2). In order to achieve this, the minimum requirements remain a faultless airway, a faultless IV access and faultless physiological monitoring, which must be appropriately matched to the complexity of the proposed procedure. Only then is the anaesthetist in the position to look after their perioperative patient properly.

It is interesting to see how TIVA has progressed in 10 years from 1983 when propofol was still solubilized in Cremafor, and consequently quite problematic, to 1994 when not only are the IV agents much improved with the release of new short-acting opiates but also much better infusion syringe pumps tailored for bolus and infusion techniques were available (3,4).

One of the earliest studies using manually adjusted propofol regimes was undertaken in patients with effective regional blockade who had been heavily premedicated (5). However, in another study published the same year where patients were premedicated with pethidine and promethazine but did not have regional anaesthesia, the doses found to be necessary to provide clinically acceptable anaesthesia were much higher (6). These studies are interesting historically as they show (i) how important it is to match patients, techniques and surgery in order to make valid comparisons, and (ii) that the use of heavy premedication has been largely discontinued these days, which also has a bearing on the amount of propofol required for anaesthesia.

At the start of the development of computer-controlled target-controlled infusions (TCI) an early paper where the new system was assessed by TCI 'naive' consultants described how 27 out of 30 consultants reported that the TCI system had changed their use of propofol for maintenance. Whilst some of the consultants had previous experience of TIVA with manually adjusted infusion, most consultants expressed reluctance to use the TCI system in paralysed patients (7). One study published 2 years later describes the comparison of manually administered propofol TIVA with a newly developed TCI system. Whilst more propofol was used in the TCI group, the induction time and time to insertion of a laryngeal mask was quicker, and the anaesthetic associated with less surgery-inspired movement than the manually adjusted group (8). In a recent study involving 29 European anaesthetists (9), all of whom had previous experience with manually adjusted infusions of propofol, the majority expressed a preference for the TCI system compared with a manually adjusted infusion regime. It was also noted that the dose for induction was lower in the TCI group, although it took longer and mean propofol administration was greater in the TCI, similar to the findings of the previous study (5), which resulted in a deeper, more appropriate anaesthetic depth confirmed by a reduced incidence of movement during surgery. The employment of effect-site concentration and plasma target concentrations has now become commonplace.

British Society for Intravenous Anaesthesia

The inception of the British Society for Intravenous Anaesthesia (SIVA) proceeded from the inaugural meeting at the Royal Society of Medicine on 1 July 1997.

The aims of the British SIVA (see p. 12) are to further:

- Education
- Pharmacology
- Training
- Acceptance
- Discussion

The Royal College of Anaesthetists also requires teaching on IV anaesthesia in its syllabus as of March 1997. Candidates are required to know about:

- Methods for achieving specified plasma concentrations
- Bolus, infusion and profiled administration

In fact, such has the interest been amongst anaesthetists internationally in TIVA that many countries have formed their own TIVA societies.

Development of drugs of use in total intravenous anaesthesia

It has only relatively recently in the history of anaesthesia become possible to perform TIVA due to the advances in the drugs available and the equipment used to administer them.

The early days

The first recorded IV injection of opium was recorded by Sir Christopher Wren in 1665 when he used a pig's bladder and a quill to inject it into a dog. The first use of an IV agent was the experiment by Pierre Oré, in Lyons in 1874, using IV chloral hydrate; however, this technique was rapidly abandoned because of side effects.

Induction agents

It is, however, the development of IV induction agents that made the concept of TIVA a reality. Thiopentone was first released into clinical practice in the 1930s and by 1941 Halford, commenting on its use amongst the casualties of the Japanese attack on Pearl Harbour, observed 'that it provided an ideal form of euthanasia'! (10). Clearly work needed to be done to improve the safety of administration. Methohexitone was synthesized in 1957, followed by propranidid and althesin in 1960s, etomidate in 1972, and finally diisopropyl phenol in 1970s, which had to wait until 1986 to be released into clinical practice in its current form as an emulsion in soybean oil and egg lecithin. As will be seen in Chapter 3, drugs that are good induction agents do not necessarily continue to be good maintenance agents because of accumulation, toxicity and cardior-espiratory depression.

The benzodiazepines have been used for sedation or as adjuncts with induction agents for TIVA. Diazepam was synthesized in 1959, reformulated as diazemuls in the 1970s and finally midazolam in 1976, which is currently the most frequently used IV sedative because of its short duration of action.

Ketamine was synthesized in 1959. It occupies an interesting position in that its initial clinical use was directed at dissociative anaesthesia and analgesia. In the high doses required for this type of anaesthesia it was regularly accompanied by dysphoria on recovery. Whilst this could be attenuated by benzodiazepines and minimal stimulation in recovery, this dysphoria curtailed its use as an anaesthetic agent in hospital-based practice, although it remains a popular choice in the 'field'. It does though have desirable properties and with the increase in the sophistication of our knowledge in neurophysiology regarding N-methyl-D-aspartate (NMDA) receptors it is having a resurgence of use. However, as will be explained in Chapter 5, there is now good evidence that the concomitant administration of ketamine will reduce receptor field recruitment and may reduce the development of secondary hyperalgesia postoperatively.

Opiates and non-steroidal anti-inflammatory drugs

Since pain relief and anaesthesia are now an integral part of perioperative care, the development of suitable opiates for IV infusions was equally important. It is only in the 19th century that morphine was synthesized from opium by Saturnier in 1803. Later on diamorphine was synthesized in 1875. Pethidine was synthesized in 1939, followed by methadone in 1945. The relatively new opioid fentanyl was synthesized in 1960, sufentanil in 1974 and alfentanil 1976. Remifentanil, the first esterase-degraded opioid, has only recently been just released (1997). As will be seen in Chapter 4, it is the last two opioids, alfentanil and remifentanil, that are so far the most suitable to combine with induction agents for TIVA. As will also be seen, there is an important synergism between the two opioids and propofol that allows a significant reduction in their dosage when administered simultaneously in order to provide satisfactory anaesthesia for surgery.

Since non-steroidal anti-inflammatory drugs (NSAIDs) are now also an integral part of modern anaesthesia, their development merits a brief mention. Aspirin was applied as tincture of willow bark in herbal medicine and is well documented in mediaeval manuscripts, but acetyl salicylic was only synthesized in 1899 by Hoffman of Bayer. The only NSAIDs to have a product license for IV use are tenoxicam (first licensed in 1988) and ketorolac (released onto the market in 1990). The NSAIDs have a well-documented morphine sparing effect and by their pharmacological action extend the analgesia from the perioperative to the postoperative period and thus into the realm of acute pain management. The newer COX2-specific drugs rofecoxib and celecoxib are not yet licensed for IV use but may be in the future.

Development of new drugs

By the time the induction agents were being developed the scientific community required much more rigorous investigation into the pharmacology, a now rapidly expanding and ever more important science, of these agents, and the time between discovery and release into clinical practice would span several years. The relative costs of research and development have escalated, and sadly this has impacted on the future of producing new drugs. Thus effort has been concentrated on routes and methods of the administration of existing drugs. Improvements in high-performance liquid chromatography and mass spectrometry have increased our knowledge of pharmacokinetics. As a result, our detailed knowledge of elimination half-lives, volume of distribution and clearance of drugs has enabled us to not only select the most appropriate drug on pharmacokinetic grounds but also how to administer the drug itself in terms of boluses and infusion rates. Advances in computer science have enabled us to produce analog pharmacokinetic models that make allowances for patient variables such as age and weight, which have led to the development of software that will instruct a syringe driver to deliver drugs to selected plasma target values.

Equipment

Apart from the famous injection of opium into the dog by Sir Christopher Wren, medical science had to wait until 1853 for the invention of the hypodermic syringe and needle by Wood. As has already been shown, it took nearly 100 years before the first IV induction agent was produced. Modern disposable syringes and needles only became widely available in the 1960s.

Airways were first controlled for means of resuscitation of the newborn and for the relief of airway obstruction due to diphtheria. The early red rubber reusable endotracheal airways were developed by McGill following the development of muscle relaxants. Disposable airways only became available in the 1960s. Laryngeal masks were developed in the 1980s, and have greatly reduced the need for intubation and therefore muscle relaxants.

Syringe drivers started with fixed-rate clockwork ones. The early electrically driven ones could only manage fixed rates up to 100 ml/h or less. They did not have any bolus facility and were wholly unsuitable for TIVA. The first syringe driver that had any potential for TIVA was the Ohmeda 9000 (11), which had a bolus facility as well as a pump whose infusion rate could vary from 1200 to 0.1 ml/h. It has bolus infusion rates of 1200/600 and 300 ml/h.

As will be shown, the infusion rate during induction for manually controlled TIVA is optimal at 400 ml/h. Graseby developed the 3100, which has no bolus facility and a maximum infusion rate of 200 ml/h. The 3400 has a bolus facility at 1200 ml/h and an infusion rate of 999 ml/h, and is thus at present the most suitable syringe driver for manually adjusted TIVA.

After research into pharmacokinetics, target-controlled analog programs have been developed for a number of commonly used IV agents such as propofol, ketamine, etomidate and alfentanil, to name just a few. Graseby have developed the 3500 with the 'Diprifusor' chip which permits target-controlled anaesthesia. A 'Diprifusor' chip is also available for the Fresnius and Alaris pump which display effect-site and plasma concentration. In fact, the preset targets and the actual measured values become separated with time. The target values tend to underestimate the actual values, thus the importance of the continuous presence of the anaesthetist and their ability to read clinical signs of anaesthesia depth/requirement cannot be overemphasized in the absence of a reliable, valid and foolproof method of assessment of anaesthetic depth.

There has been work on computer-simulated effect-site concentration which has become closest to being what we require as anaesthetists to being confident about the depth of anaesthesia without the means for its direct measurement. As will be shown in Chapter 6, measuring/estimating the depth of anaesthesia by measurement of EEG signals is problematic because of delay in the signal acquisition–processing–display and because of hysteresis within the EEG signal itself. We have not yet ascertained the perfect biological signal to analyse in order to give us reliable depth of anaesthesia. However, a recent paper suggests that in addition to using the estimated effect-site concentration to titrate the required level of anaesthesia along with clinical signs, the simultaneous employment of the bispectral index (BIS) may be better for titrating the propofol target effect-site concentration to ensure a more consistent level of sedation and reduce the incidence of implicit memory (12). The same group went on to publish a report of 10 patients undergoing orthopaedic procedures under spinal anaesthesia and propofol TIVA. The bispectral analysis, a newly derived parameter of the processed EEG, was used as the control variable in a closed-loop feedback system to alter the target value of propofol to maintain a constant level of anaesthesia (13). This needs further evaluation but must be the way forward, although depth of anaesthesia is not an easy calculation, as will be shown in Chapter 6.

Before selecting a total IV anaesthetic technique, the merits and limitations need to be considered.

The merits of TIVA include:

♦ Pleasant induction since patients need have no fear of masks or suffocation, which is often exacerbated by the smell of volatile agents. The patient may feel less invasion of their 'space' and thus find the loss of control as they go to sleep less threatening by the IV route.
♦ With TCI systems such as the 'Diprifusor', the transition from induction to maintenance is seamless and, because the syringe drivers used are powered by battery as well as by the mains, anaesthesia continues as the patient is transported from one room to another.
♦ Rapid and predictable recovery. Patients report better quality of recovery than by inhalational methods and report less depression of mood; propofol TIVA compared with propofol or thiopentone induction and isoflurane (14).
♦ Anaesthesia can be deepened quickly. A bolus injection will achieve a new level in about 20 s.
♦ TIVA does not require nitrous oxide (N_2O) with the resultant advantages of (i) no diffusion hypoxia at the completion of anaesthesia; (ii) no diffusion into closed body cavities; and (iii) no bone marrow depression, no increase in pulmonary vascular resistance, no further increase in intracranial pressure in patients with reduced intracranial compliance and raised intracranial pressure; it should be noted that anaesthetic pollution is most likely to arise from equipment problems like spillage when filling vaporizers, leaks around face masks and loose-fitting connections in the anaesthetic circuit which are not prevented by costly scavenging equipment (15).
♦ There has as yet been no reported incidence of terato-, carcino- or mutagenicity as a result of propofol administration.
♦ It has been shown to be perfectly safe, if indeed not the technique of choice, in patients with malignant hyperthermia susceptibility, porphyria, asthma and other allergic conditions.

- There is evidence that TIVA with propofol compared with isoflurane causes less rise in cortisol levels, and that the rise in glucose, lactate and free fatty acids is also lower.
- It has been shown to significantly reduce postoperative nausea and vomiting. While this is not only more agreeable to the patient, it has the sound financial advantages of the reduction of the postoperative stay in hospital and the reduction in unplanned admission because of intractable nausea and vomiting.
- There is evidence that the concurrent administration of opiates and ketamine by infusion will beneficially change the quality, area and intensity of postoperative pain.

The limitations of TIVA include:

- At present the best all-purpose IV induction and maintenance agent is propofol. This is, at present, a very expensive alternative to volatile agents used economically with low flow systems and vapour concentration analysis for operations lasting longer than 30 min.
- There is a wide variety in response to a standard dosage because of numerous factors such as age, sex, obesity, anxiety, hepatic enzyme activity and haemodynamic state. Also there is wide divergence from predicted plasma values when TIVA is administered to computer-controlled target values. As plasma propofol concentration increases, the measured level becomes significantly higher than the predicted value.
- The administered drug cannot be recovered, unlike inhalational agents which can be 'blown off' by increasing alveolar ventilation. It has to be redistributed and metabolized by the patient for its effect to wear off.
- There is no standard monitoring for anaesthetic depth or real-time drug concentration, compared with end-tidal vapour concentrations, for example.
- There is always a threat of awareness in paralysed patients.
- There is no self-regulatory deepening of anaesthesia by increasing minute ventilation and therefore vapour uptake by the patient in response to increased surgical stimulus.
- As with any new technique, the equipment is often unsatisfactory; there are often only inappropriate syringe drivers available.
- A lot of hospitals do not yet have anaesthetic machines that will deliver oxygen and air mixtures – it is only possible to do IV anaesthesia in such circumstances.
- Staff are not sufficiently familiar with the technique, thus training and education with the drawing up of standardized protocols can be necessary, which has resource implications.
- External opthalmoplegia has been reported after TIVA in ENT patients.

There will be much more detailed information in subsequent chapters, illustrated with clinical examples, on the applicability after weighing the merits and limitations of TIVA.

Nitrous oxide, volatile agents and ozone

There has been debate about atmospheric pollution and depletion of the ozone layer by anaesthetic agents. The halogenated hydrocarbons (HCFCs) halothane, enflurane and isoflurane are on balance considered to be 'ozone friendly' when compared with the major chlorofluorocarbons (CFCs). This is because their lifetime in the troposphere is of the order of 5–6 years as opposed to 75–150 years for CFCs. They are broken down to HCl, HBr and CO_2, and returned to Earth as acid rain. By contrast, CFCs break down by photolysis much higher up in the atmosphere, thus releasing free chlorine atoms which enter the ozone layer to destroy by catalysis 100 000 atoms of ozone for each atom of free chlorine. It has been estimated that volatile anaesthetic agents contribute less than 0.01% of the yearly global release of more than 1×10^6 tonnes of CFCs and HCFCs. However, N_2O is remarkably stable in the atmosphere with a life-time of 150 years. It can photo-dissociate in the stratosphere to form nitric oxide (NO), which significantly contributes to the stratospheric destruction of ozone. It is also a 'greenhouse' gas reflecting heat energy back to the earth. The tropospheric N_2O concentration was reported in 1975 to be increasing by 0.25% per annum. However, the major contributor to this was the microbial breakdown of agricultural nitrates. To put it into perspective, compared to the estimated use of 1×10^9 l of N_2O by anaesthetists in the UK during 1988, $8–30 \times 10^9$ l were released from agricultural nitrates.

TIVA therefore only offers a small (though still worthwhile) contribution to preventing global warming by the destruction of the ozone layer and by reducing the release of the greenhouse gas N_2O to the stratosphere!

New combinations of drugs are being tested as we understand more about the genesis of neuropathic pain states in relation to trauma and surgery. This is a rich and dynamic field for further research. Progress in this will be demonstrated in succeeding chapters. As our knowledge of neurophysiology of anaesthesia and pain progresses, the development of total IV anaesthesia will become a bridge between the traditionally separate areas of anaesthesia, i.e. acute and chronic pain management.

The subsequent chapters will show that whatever preference the individual anaesthetist may hold for inhalational or IV methods, any comparison of the two techniques will emphasize their different qualities rather than innate superiority; one over the other.

References

1. Sandin R, Norstrom O. Awareness during total i.v. anaesthesia. *Br J Anaesth* 1993; **71**: 782–7.
2. Lundy JS. Analgesia, anaesthesia and muscle relaxation. *Minnesota Med* 1926; **9**: 399. (Reprinted in 'Classical File'. *Surv Anaesthesiol* 1981; **25**: 272.)
3. Morgan M. Total intravenous anaesthesia [review]. *Anaesthesia* 1983; **38** (suppl): 1–9.

4. Miller DR. CME intravenous infusion anaesthesia and delivery devices. *Can J Anaesth* 1994; **41**: 639–52.
5. O'Callaghan AC, Normandale JP, Grundy EM, Lumley J, Morgan M. Continuous intravenous infusion of disoprofol (ICI 35868, Diprivan). Comparison with althesin to cover surgery under local analgesia. *Anaesthesia* 1982; **37**: 295–300.
6. Major E, Verniquet AJ, Yate PM, Waddell TK. Disoprofol and fentanyl for total intravenous anaesthesia. *Anaesthesia* 1982; **37**: 541–7.
7. Taylor I, White M, Kenny GNC. Assessment of the value and pattern of use of a target controlled propofol infusion system. *Int J Clin Monit Comput* 1993; **10**: 175–80.
8. Russell D, Wilkes MP, Hunter SC, Glen JB, Hutton P, Kenny GNC. Manual compared with target-controlled infusion of propofol. *Br J Anaesth* 1995; **75**: 562–66.
9. Servin F. TCI compared with a manually controlled infusion of propofol: a multi-centre study. *Anaesthesia* 1998; **53** (suppl 1): 82–6.
10. Halford FJ. A critique of intravenous anaesthesia in war surgery. *Anaesthesiology* 1943; **4**: 67–9.
11. Stokes DN, Peacock JE, Lewis R, Hutton P. The Ohmeda 9000 syringe pump. The first of a new generation of syringe drivers. *Anaesthesia* 1990; **45**: 1062–6.
12. Struys M, Versichelen L, Byttebier G, Mortier E, Moerman A, Rolly G. Clinical usefulness of the bispectral index for titrating propofol target effect-site concentration. *Anaesthesia* 1998; **53**: 4–12.
13. Mortier E, Struys M, De Smet T, Versichelen L, Rolly G. Closed-loop controlled administration of propofol using bispectral analysis. *Anaesthesia* 1998; **53**: 749–54.
14. Brandner B, Blagrove M, McCallum G, Bromley LM. Dreams, images and emotions associated with propofol anaesthesia. *Anaesthesia* 1997; **52**: 750–5.
15. Barker JP, Abdelatti MO. Anaesthetic pollution: potential sources, their identification and control. *Anaesthesia* 1997; **52**: 1077–83.

SIVA UK

The UK Society for Intravenous Anaesthesia
Honorary Secretary: Dr Douglas Russell FRCA
Consultant Anaesthetist
South Glasgow University Hospitals Trust
Southern General Hospital
Glasgow G51 4TG
Website: http://www.sivauk.org

2

Drugs and pharmacology

S. J. Dolin

- Anaesthetic mechanism of action
- Basic pharmacokinetics
- Individual drug groups

Introduction

What anaesthetists want to know when they are administering anaesthetic drugs is how much drug is present at the site of action, i.e. the brain. This has been made relatively simple for volatile anaesthetics by the use of real-time measurement of end-tidal drug concentrations and the concept of MAC. However, when using intravenous (IV) agents there is currently no real-time measurement of drug concentrations. Consequently anaesthetists need a thorough understanding of pharmacology of IV drugs to make an informed best estimate of dose requirements in order to maintain anaesthesia and guarantee a rapid recovery. This chapter will cover the basic pharmacology of each of the commonly used IV anaesthetic agents, including mechanism of action, pharmacokinetics, metabolism and side effects.

Anaesthetic mechanism of action

The traditional understanding of anaesthetic drug action is based on the close correlation between anaesthetic potency and lipid solubility (Meyer–Overton rule). This rule has been applied to inhaled anaesthetic drugs, rather than IV agents. Lipid solubility is important in getting a drug to its site of action but still does not explain how anaesthetics work, at least in terms of which neurotransmission systems are involved.

Several anaesthetics including isoflurane, barbiturates, etomidate and steroids act in a diastereo- and enantio-selective manner, indicating a protein site of action. A number of protein sites have now been identified as sites of anaesthetic action. Transmitter-gated ion channels in particular seem to be sensitive targets of anaesthetic action.

Inhibitory neurotransmission is predominantly by GABA and glycine. At anaesthetic concentrations all IV anaesthetic drugs potentiate GABAa receptor-mediated responses. Many anaesthetic drugs exert a similar effect at strychnine-sensitive glycine receptors. A few anaesthetic drugs have been shown to inhibit excitatory responses mediated by nicotinic acetylcholine and ionotropic glutamate receptor subtypes. Moreover, recent work has demonstrated that anaesthetic drugs discriminate not only between transmitter-gated ion channel classes, but also between receptor isoforms of the same class that are differentially distributed within the central nervous system. In short, enhancement of inhibitory and depression of excitatory fast synaptic transmission provides a logical, if perhaps simplistic, explanation of anaesthetic action, and there is increasing evidence that mechanism of action of anaesthetic drugs can be described in these terms (1,2).

Basic pharmacokinetics

Basic pharmacokinetics describes what happens when a drug is administered as a single IV bolus. The pharmacokinetics of repeated doses or infusions are more complex and involve additional concepts which are covered in Chapter 4. The basis of pharmacokinetics is the plasma concentration (log)–time curve (Figure 2.1). The concentration declines initially rapidly then more slowly. The initial rapid decline is due to redistribution of the drug from the plasma into vessel-rich viscera (brain, liver, kidney, heart), then to lean tissue (muscle) and finally into vessel-poor adipose tissue. The order of redistribution to different tissues is determined by their blood flow. The flatter and later part of the curve is due to elimination of the drug from the plasma. This occurs as the drug is cleared by metabolism, predominantly by the liver. During the elimination phase drug is removed directly from the plasma and indirectly via the plasma from the tissues into which it has redistributed.

The plasma drug concentration–time curve of IV anaesthetic drugs can be best explained by fitting either a bi-exponential (most drugs) or tri-exponential curve (most opioids), depending on which best fits the measured curve. The bi-exponential curve assumes a two-compartment model (central and peripheral). The tri-exponential curve assumes a three-compartment model, with a central compartment, a shallow compartment and a remoter deep compartment (adipose tissue). These must be viewed only as mathematical models to help describe the measured curve.

From the plasma concentration–time curve the following pieces of information can be obtained:

◆ Half-times. This is defined as the time taken for the concentration to fall by half. As the models fit a series of straight lines to the curve, the half-time can readily be calculated anywhere on the fitted lines. There will of course be more than one half-time, i.e. the redistribution half-time $t_{1/2\alpha}$ and the elimination half-time $t_{1/2\beta}$, for the fitted

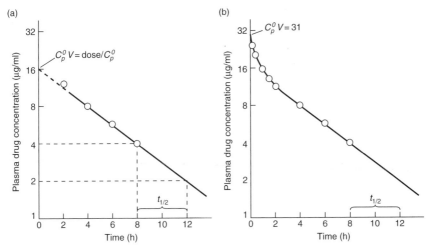

Figure 2.1   Plasma concentration–time curves for IV administration of a drug. The plot is semilogarithmic. In example A drug concentration is measured every 2 h and it appears that the drug is eliminated from a single compartment with a $t_{1/2}$ of 4 h. The volume of distribution (V_d) can be determined from the value of C^0 which is obtained by extrapolation of the line to $t = 0$. Volume of distribution = dose/C^0. Clearance (Cl) of the drug = $V_d \times k$, where $k = 0.693/t_{1/2}$. In example B, sampling occurs before 2 h and it is apparent that the drug follows multiexponential kinetics, and at least two curves can be fitted each with its own $t_{1/2}$, V_d and Cl. From Goodman Gilman A, Rall T, Nies A, Taylor P, eds. *Goodman and Gilman: The pharmacological basis of therapeutics*, 8th edn. Oxford: Pergamon 1990.

bi-exponential curve. For the tri-exponential fitted curve there are two redistribution half-times, a fast curve with $t_{1/2\pi}$ and a slower curve with $t_{1/2\alpha}$, as well as an elimination curve with $t_{1/2\beta}$. As recovery from most anaesthetics occurs by virtue of redistribution, the redistribution half-lives predict to some extent the duration of a single bolus. The elimination half-lives become more important for larger or repeated doses and for full recovery from anaesthetic infusions.

♦ Volume of distribution is defined a dose/concentration at time zero (C^0). The dose is of course known to us, but C^0 needs to be calculated by back extrapolation of the elimination line to the log concentration axis. The volume of distribution is related to lipid solubility, and gives an indication as to how much of the drug is in the central compartment and available for elimination. Large volumes of distribution (more lipid-soluble drugs) have relatively small amounts of the drug in the plasma. Volume of distribution is only important by virtue of its inverse relationship to clearance.

As stated, the elimination half-time is a key concept in defining recovery of anaesthetic drugs, but may not necessarily be helpful for defining the effect-site concentration (i.e. in the brain). The discrepancy between elimination half-times after single bolus and after continuous infusion of many IV anaesthetic drugs lead to the concept of context-sensitive half-time (the time for the plasma concentration to fall by half after continuous infusion).

The great problem for pharmacokinetics of IV anaesthetic drugs is that there are often large differences (up to 2–5 times) in individual drug requirements due to variation in dose–plasma and plasma–effect relationships. This is in marked contrast to volatile anaesthetics where drug–effect relationships are much more predictable and importantly where real-time measurements of drug concentrations have been available for years.

Barbiturates

Barbiturates have been in clinical use as IV anaesthetic agents since 1934 when thiopentone was first used. This marked the advent of IV anaesthesia. Their continued popularity is due to their rapid but short action and good safety record when administered properly. The most widely used barbiturate is thiopentone, while methohexitone is used less widely. The clinical effect of an IV bolus of thiopentone is terminated by redistribution away from the site of action (the brain), rather than by metabolism (3). Barbiturates have been used as prolonged infusions, but resulted in profound falls in blood pressure and prolonged sleeping times. The reason for this was that with prolonged infusion redistribution of the drug becomes less effective as the alternative sites of redistribution approach saturation.

Barbiturates can exist in a water-soluble enol form. This is the form in which they are dissolved for injection, at pH 10–11 in 6% sodium carbonate. Once in circulation the enol form changes to the lipid-soluble keto form. Barbiturates exist as stereoisomers and the *l*-isomer is more potent than the *d*-isomer, indicating a receptor site of action. They are, however, marketed as racemic mixtures. There is a barbiturate recognition site on the GABAa receptor. Barbiturates both enhance GABA transmission and act directly to increase conductance via the receptor-mediated chloride channel. This results in further neuronal hyper-polarization and decreased excitability.

Barbiturate pharmacokinetics

Following an IV bolus, thiopentone mixes rapidly with blood, and is taken up into different tissues and organs according to rate of perfusion, their affinity for the drug and the thiopentone concentration gradient between the tissue and the blood. The log concentration–time curve shows a high initial plasma concentration which falls rapidly as thiopentone enters the tissues (4). The well-perfused but relatively low-volume tissues such as brain equilibrate very rapidly with blood, resulting in rapid onset of anaesthesia. There is also rapid decline in drug concentrations in well-perfused tissues, such as brain, in favour of large-volume less well-perfused lean tissues, such as muscle. This results in relatively rapid recovery from thiopentone-induced anaesthesia. Uptake into fat is very slow and makes only a minor contribution to the pharmacokinetics of a bolus dose. Removal of thiopentone, via hepatic metabolism, is so slow relative to uptake of drug by lean tissues that it makes little contribution to recovery from a bolus dose.

When thiopentone is administered in repeated doses or by continuous infusion (such as for cerebral resuscitation or treatment of refractory seizures) the capacity of the lean tissues such as muscle to absorb the drug is reduced progressively as the tissue approaches equilibrium with blood. In this situation termination of drug effect depends increasingly on uptake into fat tissue and elimination clearance by hepatic metabolism. Thiopentone has a relatively low hepatic extraction ratio (0.15), which is in part due to extensive protein binding. This leads to a low clearance (Cl) of 3.4 ± 0.5 ml/kg/min.

With repeated doses or infusions drug metabolism can become saturated leading to non-linear elimination, and prolonged and unpredictable recovery. This can be compared to some other anaesthetic drugs by comparison of the context-sensitive half-time. This is defined as the time it takes for the drug in the central compartment to decrease by 50% or, more simply, the time it takes for the plasma level to drop to 50% after cessation of an infusion, which is much more predictive of recovery following continuous infusion (Figure 2.2) (5).

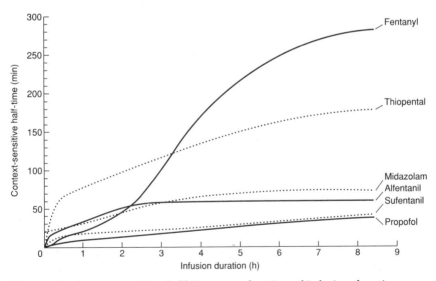

Figure 2.2 Context-sensitive half-times as a function of infusion duration. Thiopentone and fentanyl have progressively longer half-times compared to propofol and sufentanil and alfentanil (see 5).

Organ function effects

- *Central nervous system.* Barbiturates may be hyperalgesic, especially in subanaesthetic concentrations. There is a dose-dependent depression of cerebral metabolism of oxygen (CMR_{O_2}), and a parallel reduction in cerebral blood flow (CBF) and intracranial pressure (ICP). The magnitude of these changes are relevant for neurosurgical anaesthesia. Methohexitone has, unlike thiopentone, been associated with post-operative seizures. Barbiturates also reduce intraocular pressure (IOP), up to 40% after an induction dose.
- *Respiratory.* Central respiratory depression occurs which can lead to apnea on induction. Ventilatory response to hypercarbia and hypoxia are depressed, and are sensitive to even low doses of barbiturates. Laryngeal reflexes remain relatively intact and may contribute to laryngospasm with laryngeal masks (6).
- *Cardiovascular.* The predominant effect is venodilatation, with a fall in cardiac output. There is a mild degree of myocardial depression, but heart rate is increased, increasing myocardial oxygen consumption. Barbiturates should be used with caution in situations where an increased heart rate and decreased preload could be detrimental, such as hypovolaemia, congestive heart failure, ischaemic heart disease and heart block. Hypotension is also more marked in hypertensive patients, both treated and untreated.
- *Other effects.* Urine output can be decreased because of reduced renal blood flow. Heat loss can be aggravated by vasodilation and can result in increased postoperative shivering. Thiopentone decreases plasma cortisol concentrations but does not prevent adrenocortical stimulation from surgical stress, unlike etomidate. Venous thrombosis has been reported as high as 3–4% after thiopentone. Nausea and vomiting is not made worse by barbiturates. Barbiturates can precipitate life-threatening attacks of porphyria due to induction of aminolevulinic acid sythetase, which is the rate-limiting step in the synthesis of porphyrins.

The barbiturates are not ideal IV anaesthetic agents. The produce hypnosis but not other desirable qualities such as analgesia and amnesia. Thiopentone has, however, had a long-standing position as a standard anaesthetic induction agent, largely from its lack of major disadvantages.

Benzodiazepines

Benzodiazepines are sedative, anxiolytic, hypnotic, amnesic, anticonvulsant and produce muscle relaxation via a central mechanism. Chlordiazepoxide was the first benzodiazepine and was introduced in 1953. Diazepem was introduced in 1959. In 1976 the water-soluble midazolam was produced primarily for anaesthetic practice.

The benzodiazepines work via a receptor associated with GABAa which operates a chloride channel. Binding is high affinity, stereospecific and saturable. Enhanced GABA transmission results in neuronal hyper-polarization and decreased excitability. Twenty percent receptor occupancy produces anxiolysis, 30–50% occupancy results in sedation and greater than 60% occupancy results in unconsciousness (7). Highest density of benzodiazepine receptors is in cerebral cortex, cerebellum, hippocampus, brain stem and spinal cord. The benzodiazepine receptor is unique in that some ligands can enhance GABA transmission (agonists), while others can decrease GABA transmission (inverse agonists). Tolerance can also occur at the receptor by down-regulation (decreased numbers) or decreased affinity and there is some evidence that rapid tolerance can occur.

Diazepam is dissolved in propylene glycol, ethanol, benzyl alcohol and sodium benzoate/benzoic acid in water (pH 6.2–6.9). It has also been formulated in a lipid medium as diazemuls. Midazolam is dissolved in 0.8% sodium chloride, disodium edetate and benzyl alcohol. It is made to pH 3 with hydrochloric acid/sodium hydroxide, as it displays pH-dependent water solubility. The imidazole ring accounts for stability in solution and rapid metabolism. Midazolam becomes very lipid soluble at pH 7.4 after injection as the previously open imidazole ring closes. The lipid solubility accounts for its rapid central nervous system effect.

Benzodiazepine pharmacokinetics

Metabolism is via hepatic microsomal oxidation (phase I) or glucuronide conjugation (phase II). Rapid oxidation of the imidazole ring accounts for the high hepatic clearance of midazolam. Diazepam produces active metabolites (oxazepam and desmethyldiazepam). Midazolam has no active metabolites.

Midazolam is short acting (elimination half-time 1.7–2.6 h), while diazepam is long-acting (elimination half-time 20–50 h) (Table 2.1). While duration is related to lipid solubility, rapid redistribution accounts for the short action of a single bolus of midazolam. Recovery is due to redistribution from brain to other less well-perfused tissues. Recovery after 10 mg midazolam is about 15 min and recovery is more prolonged than after thiopentone and propofol. Protein binding and volume of distribution are similar but midazolam has a high clearance (6–11 ml/kg/min), while diazepam has a very low clearance (0.2–0.5 ml/kg/min). Context-sensitive half-times also differ markedly. Termination of action is via redistribution; however, after repeated or prolonged administration midazolam blood levels will fall much more rapidly than diazepam because of high hepatic clearance, but can still result in prolonged recovery.

Organ function effects

◆ *Central nervous system.* Benzodiazepines reduce CMR_{O_2} and also CBF, while maintaining normal ratio CBF/CMR_{O_2}. Benzodiazepines are protective against cerebral hypoxia and are anticonvulsant against local anaesthetic-induced seizures.

Table 2.1　Pharmacokinetics of IV anaesthetic drugs

Drug	Elimination $t_{1/2}$ (h)	Clearance (ml/kg/min)
Thiopentone	11.6 ± 6	3.4 ± 0.5
Methohexitone	3.9 ± 2.1	10.9 ± 3
Diazepam	20–50	0.2–0.5
Midazolam	1.7–2.6	6.4–11
Ketamine	2.5–2.8	12–17
Etomidate	2.9–5.3	18–25
Propofol	4–7	20–30
Droperidol	1.7–2.2	14
Morphine	1.7–4.2	15–39
Pethidine	3–5	18
Fentanyl	2–4	10–20
Alfentanil	1–2	4–9
Sufentanil	2.7 ± 0.3	12.7 ± 0.8
Remifentanil	0.2–0.3	34.2 ± 8

- ◆ *Respiratory.* Benzodiazepines produce central respiratory depression. Ventilation response curve to hypercarbia is flatter than controls but not shifted to the right like opioids. Increasing plasma concentration of midazolam results in increased resting P_aCO_2. Peak onset of respiratory depression with midazolam (0.1–0.2 mg/kg) is rapid (about 3 min), duration 60–120 min (8). Opioids and benzodiazepines produce synergistic effects on respiratory depression.
- ◆ *Cardiovascular.* Benzodiazepines produce only modest changes, with slight decrease in systolic blood pressure due to decreased systemic vascular resistance (SVR). There is preservation of homeostatic reflex mechanisms, but baroreflexes may be somewhat impaired. Heart rate, ventricular filling pressure and cardiac output are generally well maintained. Benzodiazepines are safe even with severe aortic stenosis. All cardiovascular effects are increased dramatically when benzodiazepines are combined with opioids, probably related to reduction in sympathetic tone when given together.
- ◆ *Other.* The stress response to surgery is not altered by benzodiazepines. Venous irritation and thrombophlebitis are problems with diazepam, but reformulation as diazemuls has limited this.

Midazolam gives better amnesia and smoother cardiovascular effects than thiopentone. It also reduces opioid requirements and reduces inhalational anaesthetic requirements, but respiratory depression remains a problem.

Flumazenil

Flumazenil is a high-affinity, specific competitive benzodiazepine antagonist with minimal intrinsic activity. It produces rapid reversal of unconsciousness, respiratory depression, sedation and amnesia when due to benzodiazepine action.

The half-time of the receptor–ligand interaction is milliseconds to seconds. The dynamic situation depends on the law of mass action, affinities, and concentrations of agonist and antagonist. Flumazenil has a similar structure to other benzodiazepines, with a carbonyl group replacing a phenyl group. It is available in an aqueous solution, but has moderate lipid solubility at pH 7.4. Flumazenil is rapidly metabolized in liver. There are several metabolites with minimal intrinsic activity. It has the highest clearance and shortest half-life of the benzodiazepines (elimination half-time 0.7–1.3 h). Clearance is aided by a high proportion of unbound, free drug (54–64%).

Because flumazenil is cleared rapidly there is potential for resedation, especially with diazepam due to its long elimination half-life, but not so much with midazolam. There may be a need for repeated doses of flumazenil or continuous infusion (0.5–1 µg/kg/min). It is free of cardiovascular effects, both alone and after reversing the effects of benzodiazepines (unlike opioid reversal with naloxone). It produces differential reversal, having relatively more effect on sedation and respiratory depression than amnesic effects. Doses are 0.1–0.2 up to 1 mg. There is a high safety margin with flumazenil.

Ketamine

Ketamine is a phencyclidine first used in 1959. It has proved to be a useful anaesthetic, with significant analgesic effects and minimal cardiovascular or respiratory effects, but with a high incidence of hallucinations and delirium.

Ketamine contains a chiral centre, and has two optical isomers S-(+) and R-(–). It is used as a racemic mixture. The S-(+) form is more potent and has faster onset of action. Site of anaesthetic action is thought to be the thalamo-neocortical projection. Ketamine depresses cortex and thalamus while stimulating the limbic system such as the hippocampus, and produces a functional disorganization of pathways of midbrain and thalamic areas. There is some occupation of opioid receptors in brain and spinal cord, especially by the S-(+) form. Inhibition of the NMDA subtype of glutamate receptor effect may mediate the analgesic effect. There is no known antagonist to ketamine.

Ketamine has a pK_a of 7.5 and is partially water soluble. It is 5–10 times more lipid soluble than thiopentone. It is prepared in an acid solution (pH 3.5–5.5) in sodium chloride and the preservative is benzathonium chloride.

Ketamine pharmacokinetics

Metabolism is via hepatic microsomal enzymes involving methylation and hydroxylation rather than glucuronidation. The major metabolite is norketamine (methylation) with 20–30% activity.

A two-compartment model best describes the ketamine plasma concentration–time curve. With high lipid solubility ketamine enters the brain rapidly with a rapid onset of action. There is rapid redistribution ($t_{1/2\alpha}$ 11–16 min), and recovery is probably due to redistribution from brain and other tissues of the vessel-rich group. Onset of action after IV bolus of 2 mg/kg is 30–60 s, with a duration of action of 10–15 min, with full orientation in 15–30 min. There is a large volume of distribution due to high lipid solubility, but also high clearance (12–17 ml/kg/min) leading to a short elimination half-time of 2.5–2.8 h. Clearance is equal to liver blood flow, so any drug that decreases hepatic blood flow (e.g. halothane) will reduce ketamine clearance. Ketamine can be given by infusion at a rate of 30–90 µg/kg/min and this can be reduced when given with nitrous oxide (N_2O) or a benzodiazepine.

Organ function effects

♦ *Central nervous system.* Ketamine produces a state that is different to other IV anaesthetic drugs. This state is called dissociative anaesthesia as patients appear to be in a cataleptic state with profound analgesia, but eyes open and many reflexes intact, including corneal, cough and swallow reflexes. Whether or not these reflexes are sufficient to be protective is not certain. There is no recall of surgery but amnesia is not as profound as with benzodiazepines. Induction is associated with pupillary dilatation, nystagmus, lacrimation, salivation, and increased muscle tone with movements of arms, legs, trunk and head. Analgesia occurs at lower concentrations (0.1 µg/ml) than required for anaesthesia (0.7–2.2 µg/ml), so analgesia can be prolonged after anaesthesia and subanaesthetic doses can be analgesic.

Ketamine increases cerebral metabolism, CBF and ICP, and produces a generalized excitatory effect on electroencephalogram (EEG). Autoregulation of cerebral circulation is preserved, so reduction in P_aCO_2 will attenuate the rise in CBF and ICP.

Psychological reactions after ketamine are called emergence reactions, and are characterized by vivid dreams, out of body experiences and illusions, and are associated with excitement, confusion, euphoria and fear. They can last 1–3 h, with an incidence of 10–30%

♦ *Respiratory.* Ketamine produces minimal respiratory effects. The ventilatory response to CO_2 is unaltered. Blood gases are also unaltered. When other drugs are added, however, respiratory depression can occur. Ketamine acts to relax bronchial smooth muscle. This action may be sympathomimetic but there are also thought to be some direct effects. In children salivation can result in laryngospasm; in spite of reflexes being intact some aspiration may occur.

◆ *Cardiovascular.* Ketamine increases blood pressure, cardiac output and heart rate, in contrast to most other anaesthetics. This results in increased myocardial oxygen consumption. In patients with congenital heart disease shunt direction or fraction remains unaltered, but ketamine may elevate pulmonary pressure selectively in pulmonary hypertension (9). There is central attenuation of baroreceptor function and central sympathetic stimulation, as ketamine has been shown to inhibit neuronal reuptake of catecholamines. These stimulatory cardiovascular actions can be attenuated by benzodiazepines, barbiturates, droperidol, adrenergic antagonists and clonidine.

Etomidate

Etomidate was introduced in 1972, and was developed because of its haemodynamic stability, minimal respiratory depression and cerebral protective effects. Its pharmacokinetics favoured rapid recovery, with a wider margin of safety than thiopentone. However, a number of problems became apparent including inhibition of steroid synthesis, pain on injection, thrombophlebitis, myoclonus, and increased nausea and vomiting, which lead to its decreased use.

Etomidate is an imadazole derivate. There are two stereoisomers and only the +-isomer is active. Etomidate is water insoluble and is prepared in propylene glycol 35% at a pH 6.9.

Etomidate pharmacokinetics

Metabolism is by ester hydrolysis and *N*-dealkylation, producing an inactive metabolite which is excreted via kidney and bile.

Etomidate pharmacokinetics are best described by a three-compartment model. This gives a rapid redistribution half-time of 2.7 min, a slower redistribution half-time of 29 min and an elimination half-time of 2.9–5.3 h. There is a high clearance with an hepatic extraction ratio of 0.5–0.9. The short elimination half-time and rapid clearance are ideal for repeated doses and continuous infusion. There is a high volume of distribution and protein binding is about 75%.

Onset of action after IV injection occurs in one arm–brain circulation time. Doses for infusion are 10 µg/kg/min, which is best used in combination with an opioid. Maintenance of anaesthesia occurs between 300 and 500 ng/ml, and awakening occurs at 150–250 ng/ml. Rapid recovery occurs after infusions.

Organ function effects

◆ *Central nervous system.* While etomidate produces hypnosis, it has no analgesic properties. Its actions are in part GABA mediated. CBF is decreased and CMR_{O_2} is also decreased without altering mean arterial pressure, resulting in a net increase in cerebral oxygen supply/demand ratio. ICP is lowered in conditions where it is raised (e.g.

space-occupying lesions). Reduction of ICP and EEG burst suppression are not associated with falls in systemic arterial pressure. However, cerebral vascular reactivity is still maintained so further reduction in ICP can be obtained by P_aCO_2 reduction. Etomidate has been shown to have neuroprotective effects in animal studies. IOP is reduced for up to 5 min following a bolus and this can be maintained by an infusion. EEG studies show increased activity in epileptogenic foci and grand mal seizures have been reported. There is a high incidence of myoclonic movement without EEG activity, probably due to activity in the brain stem.

♦ *Respiratory.* Etomidate produces minimal respiratory effects. There is no histamine release. The ventilatory response to CO_2 is depressed. There is a brief increase in ventilation on induction, often followed by apnea. Hiccoughs and coughing commonly occur on induction.

♦ *Cardiovascular.* The minimal cardiovascular effects, even in patients with ischaemic or valvular heart disease, of etomidate set it apart from other induction agents. On induction, myocardial blood flow and oxygen consumption are decreased, so myocardial oxygen supply/demand ratio is maintained. There is a lack of effect on sympathetic and baroreceptor function. Etomidate alone may not ablate the effects of intubation as it has no analgesic properties, so an opioid such as fentanyl is often added.

♦ *Endocrine.* Etomidate inhibits production of cortisol via a dose-dependent reversible inhibition of two enzymes involved in producing cortisol from cholesterol: 11-β-hydroxylase (major site) and 17-α-hydroxylase (minor site). The free imadazole radical of etomidate binds to cytochrome P450, on which the hydroxylase enzymes are dependent. This action is also linked to inhibition of ascorbic acid resynthesis and vitamin C supplementation can restore cortisol production. There is also decreased mineralcorticoid production via the same hydroxylase enzymes. There is temporary adrenocortical suppression even following single induction doses, without any apparent adverse outcome. However, when etomidate was used for sedation in intensive care by prolonged continuous infusion, profound adrenocortical suppression and increased mortality occurred.

♦ *Other effects.* Nausea and vomiting are increased by etomidate, probably to a greater extent than other induction agents. This effect is worsened by opioids, and etomidate is best avoided in those with history of postoperative nausea and vomiting. Pain occurs on injection and thrombophlebitis has been reported in up to 20%. Preinjection of lignocaine prevents pain on induction.

Propofol

2,6-Di-isopropofol, a substituted derivate of phenol, was first used in 1977. Where cost allows, it has rapidly become the most popular anaesthetic induction agent and has many of the properties of the ideal agent for continuous IV infusion for maintenance of anaesthesia, with rapid recovery even after prolonged infusion. Propofol has depressant effects on blood pressure and ventilation, but these are only modest at doses used for continuous infusion.

Anaesthetic action is thought to be via enhancement of GABA neurotransmission.

Propofol is highly lipid soluble, and is available in an emulsion of 10% soybean oil, 2.25% glycerol and 1.2% purified egg phosphatide at pH 7.

Propofol pharmacokinetics

Propofol is rapidly metabolized to inactive metabolites by conjugation to glucuronide and sulphate, which are then excreted via the kidneys. Clearance exceeds hepatic blood flow, so extrahepatic metabolism must occur.

Pharmacokinetics of an IV bolus are best described by a two-compartment model, with a redistribution half-time of 2–8 min and an elimination half-time of 1–3 h. A three-compartment model has also been described, with a longer elimination half-time of 4–23.5 h, due to a theoretical deep compartment with limited perfusion, with slow return of propofol to the circulation. In practice propofol demonstrates a stable context-sensitive half-time of 40 min, even after 8 h of continuous infusion. The volume of distribution is 20–40 l, which increases to 150–700 l at equilibrium.

Propofol is rapid in onset and anaesthesia occurs in one arm–brain circulation. Anaesthesia lasts 5–10 min after 2–2.5 mg/kg and recovery is rapid. Propofol can also be used for sedation and amnesia at infusions of 2 mg/kg/h.

Organ function effects

♦ *Central nervous system.* Propofol has a complex relationship to neuronal excitability. It has been shown to have anticonvulsant properties against a number of convulsant stimuli and to result in shorter EEG seizure activity following electroconvulsant therapy, compared to methohexitone. There have been a number of clinical reports of grand mal seizures after anaesthesia. Propofol decreases ICP by a greater amount than it reduces cerebral perfusion pressure. CMR_{O_2} is also reduced. Propofol has been shown to be neuroprotective when given to burst suppression in animal models. Normal cerebral autoregulation is maintained during propofol infusion. It can ablate the rise in ICP with intubation, especially when fentanyl is added. ICP is reduced and propofol can prevent the rise due to intubation or suxamethonium. Propofol is not antianalgesic, but can result in hallucinations, sexual fantasies and opisthotonus.

♦ *Respiratory.* Apnea commonly occurs (25–30%) on induction, and is dependent on dose, speed of injection and other drugs. Apnea can be prolonged and last over 30 s, an effect which is increased by opioids. It is usually preceeded by tidal volume reduction and tachypnea. Respiratory rate and minute ventilation may remain decreased for several minutes after induction. Infusions of propofol decrease tidal volume and respiratory rate, as well as the ventilatory response to CO_2 and hypoxia. Bronchdilatation occurs even with chronic obstructive pulmonary disease, but the effect is not as marked as with halothane.

- *Cardiovascular.* Induction doses decrease mean arterial pressure by 25–40%, and there is associated reduction in cardiac output. This effect is due to both vasodilation and myocardial depression. Vasodilation is due to reduced sympathetic activity and a direct effect on smooth muscle calcium mobilization. Propofol affects baroreceptor function and can reduce tachycardia in response to hypotension. With infusion of propofol, blood pressure remains 20–30% below preinduction values, but cardiac output is unaltered. However, if an opioid or N_2O is used with propofol infusions then reduction in cardiac output can occur. Infusion results in significant reduction in myocardial blood flow and oxygen consumption, but the oxygen supply/demand ratio is preserved.
- *Other effects.* Propofol is free of effects on the neuromuscular function, does not precipitate malignant hyperpyrexia nor does it affect corticosteroid synthesis. The emulsion does not affect hepatic, haematological or fibrinolytic function. Some anaphylactoid reactions have been reported and it should be used with caution in patients with a history of allergic responses. There is no histamine release. Propofol is antiemetic at low doses. Prolonged infusion of propofol appears to be safe. Tolerance probably occurs but is not great. Pain on injection commonly occurs and can be reduced by adding lignocaine.

Opioids

Opioids are ideal IV anaesthetic agents and are key elements in balanced anaesthesia, although they probably are not capable of producing anaesthesia alone. Morphine was introduced in 1803, pethidine in 1939 and fentanyl in 1963. Subsequent fentanyl derivatives are alfentanil, sufentanil and remifentanil.

Opioids produce analgesia, but have a variety of side effects. Morphine alone produces incomplete amnesia, histamine release, prolonged respiratory depression, marked venodilatation possibly requiring additional transfusion, hypotension and hypertension. Fentanyl produces less cardiovascular depression, no histamine release and no venodilatation, but postoperative respiratory depression remains a problem. More rapid decline in plasma concentrations with sufentanil and alfentanil results in much faster recovery than fentanyl, especially after termination of IV infusions. Rapid recovery is even more marked with remifentanil, which is so short acting that it needs to be administered as a continuous infusion. This drug is increasingly widely used for IV anaesthesia and has the advantage of easy titration to effect, enabling rapid response to changes in intraoperative analgesic requirements.

Opioids work as agonists at opioid receptors in the brain and spinal cord. Opioids occur as optical isomers, and usually the levo-rotatory isomer is the more active. The predominant receptor type for opioid clinical effect is the μ opioid receptor, but actions at κ and δ receptors may also play a part. Opioid receptors have recently been reclassified as OP1 (δ), OP2 (κ) and OP3 (μ) (13). Major sites of action include medulla, spinal cord, the spinal trigeminal nucleus and the periaquaductal grey which modulates transmission from peripheral nerves to the central neuraxis. Peripheral opioid receptors exist in many tissues, including the cardio-vascular system. Opioids act via G proteins, resulting in changes in membrane ionic conduction (increased potassium and decreased calcium conductance), which result in neuronal inhibition. In the spinal cord opioids work by decreasing calcium entry and decreasing potassium efflux reducing cyclic AMP levels which have presynaptic inhibitory effects on release of neurotransmitters involved in pain transmission (glutamate and Substance P).

Opioid pharmacokinetics

Morphine

Morphine pharmacokinetics after a bolus dose are best described by a tri-exponential equation, with redistribution half-times of 1–2.5 and 10–20 min, and an elimination half-time of 1.7–4.5 h. Morphine has low lipid solubility (about 1/40 that of fentanyl). It has a pK_a of 8, so normally only 10–20% is unionized, which combined with low lipid solubility limits the availability to tissues. There is excessive uptake by skeletal muscle. High clearance (15–39 ml/kg/min) suggests some extrahepatic metabo-lism, most likely renal. Morphine-3-glucuronide is the major metabolite and is probably inactive, although it has been proposed that it may act as an antagonistic. Morphine-6-glucuronide is more potent than morphine with similar duration, but only accounts for about 10% metabolism. There is a relatively slow onset of central nervous system effect of about 15–30 min after an IV bolus. Thus brain morphine concentration and effects are not reflected in plasma concentrations, and elimination from brain is greater than plasma elimination half-time would predict.

Pethidine

Pethidine pharmacokinetics are best described by a bi-exponential equation, with a redistribution half-time of 5–15 min. There is an initial high first-pass uptake into lungs, which is later released slowly. There is high plasma protein binding (70%) and less than 10% of pethidine is in the unionized form. However, it is much more lipid soluble than morphine, so plasma concentration is more highly correlated with analgesia. Clearance (18 ml/kg/min) is high and similar to morphine.

The high hepatic extraction ratio results in biotransformation that is dependent on hepatic blood flow. Norpethidine, the major metabolite, has some intrinsic action but is twice as neurotoxic as pethidine. There is a low therapeutic index because of norpethidine. The elimination half-time of pethidine is 3–5 h, while that of norpethidine is much longer so it can accumulate with renal failure. Adequate analgesia with pethidine may be short-lived owing to the rapid decrease in plasma concentrations.

Fentanyl

Fentanyl pharmacokinetics are best described by a three-compartment model. There is rapid elimination, with up to 98% of a bolus dose removed from the plasma within 1 h. Redistribution half-times are 1–2 and 10–30 min. Redistribution occurs predominantly to lungs and muscle. Elimination half-time is 2–4 h. Brain levels parallel plasma with a lag time of about 5 min, as assessed by spectral edge analysis (11). Variability in plasma concentrations are due in part to surges in muscle blood flow producing second peaks. At steady state clearance is 10–20 ml/kg/min, which approaches hepatic blood flow. Fentanyl is rapidly metabolized and metabolites, which are inactive, appear as early as 1.5 min and can still be detected up to 48 h later. Fentanyl is highly bound to plasma protein and also taken up by red blood cells. It has pK_a 8.4 which means less than 10% exists in the unionized form. This combined with high lipid solubility contributes to a highly variable pharmacokinetic profile.

Sufentanil

Sufentanil pharmacokinetics are best described by a three-compartment model. It has rapid onset, with 98% of a bolus dose removed within 30 min. Redistribution half-times are 1.4 and 17.7 min. Elimination half-time is 2.7 ± 0.3 h. There is high clearance (12.7 ± 0.8 ml/kg/min) which is hepatic blood flow dependent. Sufentanil has a shorter duration of action and 5–10 times the potency of fentanyl. This is due to greater lipid solubility and higher receptor affinity. Also sufentanil pK_a is 8, so it is about 20% unionized, although it is also highly protein bound.

Alfentanil

Alfentanil pharmacokinetics fit either a two- or three-compartment model. There is rapid distribution with half-times in the range of 4–17 min. Elimination is also rapid with half-times in the range of 70–112 min. Clearance by liver metabolism is 4–9 ml/kg/min, which is lower than fentanyl. Noralfentanil is one of many metabolites which are all inactive. Relatively low lipid solubility of alfentanil accounts in part for its rapid onset and decline. The pK_a is 6.5, so about 90% is in the unionized form. This leads to rapid brain penetration. High plasma protein binding does not seem to be rate limiting. A bolus dose produces a rapid effect within 1–2 min; however, without a subsequent infusion a subtherapeutic effect may occur within a few minutes.

Remifentanil

Remifentanil pharmacokinetics have been described by either two- or three-compartment models, the latter describing prolonged administration. Remifentanil is less soluble than other opioids, which results in a rapid onset of action due to a rapid blood–brain equilibration time. Redistribution half-times are 0.5–0.9 and 5.8–9.5 min assuming a three-compartment model. There is, however, minimal redistribution of remifentanil into other tissues. The short duration and rapid offset of remifentanil result from its rapid hydrolysis by non-specific esterases in blood and tissue. These enzymes are distinct from plasma cholinesterases that are involved in the metabolism of suxamethonium. Rapid enzyme degradation allows higher dosing without the risk of accumulation and prolonged duration of action. Rapid and predictable recovery from remifentanil occurs irrespective of duration of infusion and independent of renal or hepatic function. Elimination half-time is 10–25 min which is substantially less than any other IV agent. The major metabolite has minimal activity. Plasma protein binding (70%) is generally less than other opioids.

Central nervous system effects of opioids

Opioids produce a selective depression of the central nervous system. Modest decreases (10–25%) occur in cerebral metabolic rate and ICP. The effect on CBF is variable but reductions in the region of 40–50% have been reported in some animal models with fentanyl, alfentanil and remifentanil. Autoregulation is generally preserved. However, opioid-induced neuroexcitation can result in regional increases in brain metabolism, while producing a mild to moderate overall decrease. On balance opioids are not neuroprotective. They do, however, offer cardiovascular and cerebrovascular stability, which may be a great advantage during threatened brain insult.

Muscle rigidity, especially of thoracic and abdominal muscles, is an occasional and potentially dangerous problem with opioids. It appears to be related to dose and speed of administration. Rigidity can impair both spontaneous and controlled ventilation, and can occur either during induction or recovery. Rigidity can result in hypoxia, hypercarbia and increased ICP. It can be treated by suxamethonium. The mechanism is unclear and may be due to stimulation of GABAergic interneurons in central nuclei.

Neuroexcitation with tonic–clonic movements, but no evidence of EEG seizure activity or morbidity has been described with opioids.

Norpethidine with its long elimination half-time (15–40 h) has been implicated in some cases. A variety of possible mechanisms have been proposed, some involving enhancement of excitatory neurotransmission via subcortical opioid receptors.

Opioids result in constriction of the pupil, partly through inhibition of the Edinger–Westphal nucleus, and also sympathetic inhibition. Opioids decrease the thermoregulatory threshold which can result in post-operative shivering, which may have undesirable consequences. Itching occurs commonly with opioids, but the mechanism is not understood.

Cardiovascular effects of opioids

Opioid receptors occur in the cardiovascular regulatory centres, sympathetic nervous system, vagal nuclei and adrenal medulla. Opioids blunt significant haemodynamic responses to noxious stimuli. Alone they produce minimal cardiac depression with modest if any decrease in pre- and afterload, minimal depression of baroreceptors, and no effect on coronary vessels. They are effective in reducing heart rate and can be helpful in patients with ischaemic heart disease. Despite an apparently ideal cardiovascular profile, problems are: hypertension due to inadequate block of response to surgery, hypotension and bradycardia.

Hypertension is generally related to intubation and surgery. Patients with good left ventricular function are more likely to develop hypertension. Other possible contributing factors are the degree of β-adrenergic blockade, calcium channel antagonism, volume status and awareness. The hyperdynamic cardiovascular responses that occur with high-dose fentanyl can occur via central sympathetic activation or stimulation of the renin–angiotensin system.

Opioid-induced hypotension is due to reduced sympathetic and enhanced parasympathetic tone, especially if not accompanied by surgical stimulation or an anticholinergic. Those patients dependent on sympathetic drive are most at risk. Morphine results in a marked increase in plasma histamine, which leads to decreased blood pressure and SVR, and increased cardiac output. There is both arteriolar and venodilatation, the latter resulting in increased blood requirements during and after surgery. These effects can be blocked by H_1 and H_2 antagonists. Pethidine also releases histamine and may also have some direct depressant action on myocardium. In spite of inhibition of central sympathetic outflow fentanyl and alfentanil tend to maintain blood pressure, even with poor left ventricular function. Hypotension can still occur, however, when sympathetic drive is needed, such as hypovolaemia. Sufentanil causes more hypotension, due to decreased sympathetic drive and vagally induced bradycardia. Hypotension and bradycardia can also be problems with remifentanil Care must be exercised in patients dependent on sympathetic drive and with poor left ventricular function.

All opioids except pethidine reduce heart rate due to stimulation of central vagal nuclei and decreased central sympathetic drive. Anticholinergic drugs can attenuate opioid-induced bradycardia. Patients with a history of vasovagal attacks may be more susceptible, as may those taking β-adrenergic and calcium channel antagonists. Pethidine can cause tachycardia through atropine-like actions. Severe bradycardia and asystole can occur during intubation, especially with sufentanil and alfentanil. Fentanyl and other opioids can slow atrio-ventricular conduction, increase the nodal refractory period and prolong the action potential duration. Opioids do not generally promote other arrhythmias. Bradycardia also occurs with infusions of opioids.

Respiratory effects of opioids

Opioid receptors occur in brain stem respiratory centres. Following opioid administration the ventilatory response to CO_2 is shifted to the right and the slope is decreased. Resting P_aCO_2 is also increased and apnea threshold (CO_2 concentration below which spontaneous ventilation is not initiated without hypoxia) is lowered. Decreased hypoxic respiratory drive occurs via effects on carotid body chemoreceptors. Opioids alter the pattern of respiration with increased respiratory pauses, irregular and periodic breathing. The rate rather than tidal volume is affected. Rib cage responses are diminished but diaphragmatic motion tends to be preserved. With high-dose opioids it is possible to lose respiratory drive without loosing consciousness and patients can breathe on request. Postoperative safety is a concern with opioids as desaturation, slow respiratory rate and obstruction can occur, and these effects can outlast the analgesic effects. With higher dose opioids ventilation may need supporting for a number of hours. While alfentanil and sufentanil have more rapid recovery than fentanyl, delayed or recurrent of respiratory depression can occur. Secondary peaks occur in plasma opioid concentration, where large peripheral compartments especially muscle may release stored drug following muscle movement or shivering. The stomach can also sequester fentanyl in its acid environment. Remifentanil appears to be without risk of recurrent respiratory depression because of its rapid elimination.

Opioids can overcome hyperventilation from pain and anxiety. They also possess antitussive effects, which can be of help in tolerating tracheal tubes without bucking which can lead to hypoxia. Some opioids, such as fentanyl, decrease airway smooth muscle tone and can be used for acute asthma.

Endocrine effects of opioids

The stress response to surgery is characterized by increases in growth hormone, renin, antidiuretic hormone, and catabolic hormones including catecholamines, cortisol, glucagon and thyroxine. There are also decreases in anabolic hormones (insulin and testosterone). Opioids in large doses can attenuate the stress response by decreasing nociceptive input and influence centrally mediated neuroendocrine responses. Endogenous opioids are involved in the stress response and can be inhibited via negative feedback by exogenous opioids. Fentanyl is more effective than morphine in attenuating the stress response, but high doses are required. Sufentanil, alfentanil and remifentanil are also effective. The stress response may be harmful by affecting haemodynamic stability and immune function.

Gastrointestinal effects of opioids

Opioids delay gastric emptying via vagal stimulation. There is also a direct effect on opioid receptors in cholinergic nerve terminals in the myenteric plexuses, resulting in decreased release of acetylcholine. This results in decreased gastric motility, increased sphincter tone and decreased propulsive activity. There is also increased biliary duct pressure and sphincter of Oddi tone, especially with morphine, although this is probably not a major effect. Postoperative nausea and vomiting is a persistent major problem with opioids. Opioids stimulate the chemoreceptor trigger zone in the area postrema of medulla. They also increase gastrointestinal secretions and decrease gastrointestinal tract activity which further promotes nausea and vomiting. Factors affecting postoperative nausea and vomiting include age, gender, type of surgery, time of menstrual cycle, obesity, history of motion sickness, anxiety, duration of surgery and ambulation. Opioid premedication, pain, gastric distention, etomidate and N_2O may promote postoperative nausea and vomiting, while propofol and TIVA may reduce the incidence

Naloxone

Naloxone is a neutral opioid antagonist, devoid of any intrinsic activity. It has affinity for all opioid receptors, but greatest affinity for the μ receptor. It was first used in the late 1960s and a number of serious complications have been reported with its use, including hypertension, ventricular tachycardia, cardiac arrest and pulmonary oedema. When given to reverse opioid action it may result in pain, rapid awakening, sympathetic activation, increased coronary blood flow and increased minute ventilation. Naloxone alone does not alter cardiovascular parameters or plasma catecholamines in normotensive or hypertensive patients (except those treated with clonidine) who have been anaesthetized without an opioid. Naloxone may have some non-specific analeptic effects through central nervous system stimulation, and is best avoided in patients with pheochromocytomas, carcinoid syndrome, central nervous system problems and ischaemic heart disease. Onset of action is 1–2 min and duration of action is 30–60 min. Recurrence of respiratory depression may occur due to the short half-life of naloxone and reuptake of opioid from peripheral stores, especially after longer-acting opioids.

Antiemetics

Antiemetics can be divided into four classes:

- Anticholinergics: scopolamine and atropine
- Butyrophenones: droperidol (due to antidopaminergic properties)
- Dopamine antagonists: metoclopramide (acts at chemoreceptor trigger zone and peripherally on gastrointestinal tract)
- Serotoninergic antagonists: ondansetron

Droperidol

Droperidol is a butyophenone (fluorinated derivative of phenothiazine) and was first used in 1959. It produces a state characterized by marked apparent tranquillity and cataleptic immobility. Droperidol can be used with fentanyl to create neuroleptanaesthesia.

Droperidol has potent antiemetic properties; it affects dopaminergic, noradrenergic and serotoninergic neurotransmission. Action is via occupation of GABA receptors in the chemoreceptor trigger zone which inhibits neurotransmission of dopamine

Droperidol pharmacokinetics

Droperidol is metabolized in the liver and there are two inactive metabolites. Pharmacokinetics of an IV bolus dose is best described by a two-compartment model. Clearance is large and there is a short elimination half-time of 103–134 ms.

Organ function effects

- *Central nervous system.* Droperidol produces potent cerebral vasoconstriction, with reduced CBF, but no change in cerebral metabolic rate. Extrapyramidal effects can occur (dyskinesia, especially of the face and neck, speech and swallowing difficulties, oculogyric spasms and torticollis). Malignant neuroleptic syndrome (hyperthermia, muscular rigidity, autonomic instability) is a rare but serious complication.
- *Respiratory.* There are minimal effect on respiratory rate or tidal volume.
- *Cardiovascular.* Droperidol produces moderate α-adrenergic blockade, resulting in vasodilatation with decreased blood pressure. There is no effect on dopamine-induced renal blood flow and no effect on myocardial contractility.

Ondansetron

Ondansetron is a selective serotonin 5-hydroxytriptamine receptor antagonist. It has central sites of action in several midbrain and brain stem structures, including the area postrema (chemoreceptor trigger zone/vomiting centre). It may also result in blocking of dopamine release and cell firing in the nucleus accumbens. Peripheral actions include inhibition of vagal and myenteric neurons.

Ondansetron pharmacokinetics

Elimination half-time is 3.5–5.5 h. Clearance is high (40–50 ml/kg/min). There is extensive metabolism via multiple forms of cytochrome P450, which limits the likelihood of interactions with other drugs. Metabolites are inactive.

Organ function effects

Alone ondansetron seems to be free of major effects on most systems, but some gastrointestinal actions and some neurological effects including anxiolysis and analgesia have been described. In contrast to other antiemetics ondansetron is generally well tolerated with a low incidence of sedation and minimal extrapyramidal effects (12). Some cases of anaphylactoid/anaphylactic reactions have been reported following IV administration of ondansetron. No adverse effects have been reported on cardiovascular and respiratory systems.

References

1. Lambert JJ, Belilli D, Hill-Venning C, Peter JA. Neurosteroids and GABAa receptor function. *Trends Pharmacol Sci* 1995; **16**: 295.
2. Sigal E, Buhr A. The benzodiazepine binding site of GABAa receptors. *Trends Pharmacol Sci* 1997; **18**: 425.
3. Price HL. A dynamic concept of the distribution of thiopentone in the human body. *Anaesthesiology* 1960; **21**: 40.
4. Henthorn TK, Avram MJ, Krejcie TC. Intravascular mixing and drug distribution: the concurrent disposition of thiopental and indocyanine green. *Clin Pharmacol Ther* 1989; **45**: 56.
5. Hughes MA, Glass PSA, Jacobs JR. Context-sensitive half-time in multi-compartment pharmacokinetic models for intravenous anesthetic drugs. *Anesthesiology* 1992; **76**: 334.
6. Barker P, Langston JA, Wilson IG, Smith GS. Movements of the vocal cords on induction of anaesthesia with thiopentone or propofol. *Br J Anaesth* 1992; **69**: 23.
7. Amrein R, Hetzel W, Harmann D, Lorscheid T. Clinical pharmacology of flumazenil. *Eur J Anaesthesiol* 1988; **2**: 65.
8. Gross JB, Zebrowski ME, Carel WD, *et al.* Time course of ventilatory depression after thiopental and midazolam in normal subjects and in patients with chronic obstructive pulmonary disease. *Anesthesiology* 1983; **58**: 540.
9. Spotoft H, Korshin JD, Sorensen MB, *et al.* The cardiovascular effects of ketamine used for induction of anaesthesia in patients with valvular heart disease. *Can J Anaesth* 1979; **26**: 463.

10. Ledingham IM, Finlay WEI, Watt I, McKee JI. Etomidate and adrenocortical function. *Lancet* 1983: **i**; 1434.
11. Scott JC, Ponganikis KV, Stanski DR. EEG quantitation of narcotic effect: the comparative pharmacodynamics of fentanyl and alfentanil. *Anesthesiology* 1985; **62**: 234.
12. Joslyn AF. Ondansetron, clinical development for postoperative nausea and vomiting: current studies and future directions. *Anaesthesia* 1994: **49**: suppl 34.
13. Dhawan BN, Raghubir CR, Reisine T, Bradley PB, Portoghese PS, Hamon M. International Union of Pharmacology. XII. Classification of opioid receptors. *Pharmacol Rev* 1997: **48**: 567.

3

Drug interactions

S. J. Dolin

- Factors influencing pharmacokinetics
- Factors influencing pharmacokinetics of individual drugs

The previous chapter described in detail the basic pharmacology of intravenous (IV) anaesthetic drugs. This chapter examines how drugs may interact with each other and, importantly, how disease processes may interfere or enhance anaesthetic drug action. Many issues will be dealt with in greater detail in specific chapters and the reader will be directed to them.

Factors influencing pharmacokinetics

Dose

IV anaesthetic drugs at clinically relevant doses are generally eliminated by first-order (drug concentration dependent) kinetics. However, repeated doses or prolonged infusions can alter pharmacokinetics. For example, after a 2 h infusion of fentanyl the plasma elimination half-time is quadrupled compared to a 1 h infusion (1). Other opioids such as sufentanil, alfentanil and remifentanil are much less affected by repeated or continuous dosing. With higher or repeated doses elimination with its longer half-time becomes more important than redistribution, as plasma level at higher doses remains in the clinical range even after redistribution has occurred. The pharmacokinetics of infusion are discussed in detail in Chapter 4.

pH

Most IV anaesthetic drugs are either weak bases or weak acids, and exist in both ionized and unionized forms, at a ratio dependent on their pK_a and ambient pH. In the unionized form brain penetration and plasma protein binding is favoured, which reduces availability for metabolism. However, the effects of changes in pH are complex. For example, acidosis increases ionization of fentanyl (pK_a = 8.4) and decreases plasma protein binding, which leaves more ionized drug at the receptor site and enhances opioid effect. Alfentanil with pK_a of 6.5 will not be as affected by acidosis. Alkalosis favours the unionized form of morphine (pK_a = 8) and may enhance brain penetration in spite of decreased cerebral blood flow and increased plasma protein binding.

Plasma protein binding

Basic drugs bind to α_1-acid glycoprotein, albumin and other lipoproteins which limit drug availability at the receptor site. Examples of high plasma protein binding are fentanyl (84%), sufentanil (93%) and alfentanil (92%). Only half or less of the binding of these drugs is to albumen and the rest predominantly to α_1-acid glycoprotein. A number of disease states such as inflammatory diseases, myocardial infarction, renal failure, recent surgery, rheumatoid arthritis, advanced cancer and pneumonia can lead to an increase in α_1-acid glycoprotein and to an increase in opioid binding. Increased binding results in a decreased volume of distribution and also decreased clearance, so the elimination half-time may remain unaltered. Pregnancy and the oral contraceptive pill can decrease α_1-acid glycoprotein. Dilution of plasma proteins increases the free fraction of bound drugs.

Age

At the extremes of age (see Chapter 13) there is increased central nervous system sensitivity to IV anaesthetic drugs (Figure 3.1). With aging various factors affect drug pharmacokinetics such as increased body fat, decreased plasma protein binding, decreased liver blood flow and hepatic enzyme function. At the other extreme, premature babies and term neonates have decreased drug clearance and increased elimination half-times due to decreased hepatic blood flow, immature hepatic enzymes and open ductus venosus. Enhanced drug effects may be due to better brain penetration due to a poorly developed blood–brain barrier. Lower levels of α_1-acid glycoprotein in newborns and infants results in enhanced anaesthetic drug effects, increased volume of distribution and prolonged elimination. By 28 days cytochrome oxidase and hepatic blood flow reach adult values.

Hepatic blood flow

Normal liver blood flow is about 20 ml/kg/min. Table 2.1 in Chapter 2 shows the clearance of IV anaesthetic drugs. Drugs with low clearance (below 10 ml/kg/min) such as thiopentone, diazepam and alfentanil tend to be less affected by changes in liver blood flow. Drugs with clearances approaching liver blood flow, such as propofol, etomidate and morphine,

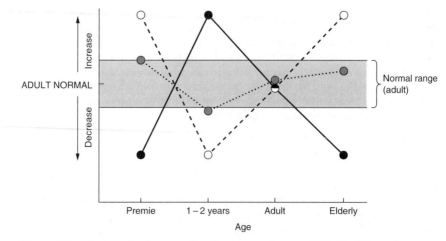

Figure 3.1   The effects of age on the clearance, volume of distribution and elimination half-times of opioids. Clearance is significantly reduced at the extremes of age. Open circles, clearance; filled circles, elimination half-life; open squares, steady-state volume of distribution (V_{dss}). From Bailey PL, Stanley TH. Intravenous opioid anaesthesia. In: Miller RD, ed. *Anesthesia*. New York: Churchill Livingstone 1994. (Published by permission of the publishers).

are sensitive to reduced liver blood flow. The exception to this is remifentanil, where clearance remains independent of liver blood flow because of its unique clearance by plasma and tissue esterases. Major abdominal surgery can reduce hepatic blood flow and reduce clearance, resulting in prolonged elimination half-times. Many IV anaesthetic drugs can produce dose-dependent hypotension which may contribute with lowered hepatic blood flow.

Liver disease

Liver disease may affect pharmacokinetics by several mechanisms. Plasma proteins can be reduced and total body water increased in liver disease. Viral hepatitis and cirrhosis affect pericentral regions of hepatic lobes and affect drugs metabolized by oxidative processes. Chronic active hepatitis and primary biliary cirrhosis affect periportal regions, and have relatively little effect on drug metabolism. A number of drugs have been shown to undergo extrahepatic metabolism, such as morphine, which may diminish the impact of liver disease on drug handling. In seriously ill patients, elevated bilirubin and hypoalbuminaemia may increase the sensitivity to many IV anaesthetic drugs, particularly the opioids with high plasma protein binding. Bilirubin competes for binding sites on albumin and leads to high free fraction of drug which can result in augmented and prolonged effects in cirrhosis. Heavy drinkers may require higher doses of anaesthetic drugs and this effect may also be in part pharmacodynamic.

Cardiopulmonary bypass

Cardiopulmonary bypass (CPB) has many pharmacokinetic consequences (2) (see Chapter 9). Haemodilution produces a dramatic reduction in plasma concentration of many drugs. It results in lower plasma protein concentrations, resulting in relatively more free drug. The result of these contrasting effects will depend on the volume of distribution and degree of plasma protein binding. Hypotension decreases hepatic blood flow and clearance, and increases elimination half-times. For example, fentanyl elimination half-times increase 2- to 4-fold on CPB. Uptake of drugs onto membrane oxygenators adds to the decline of plasma drug concentrations. However, most drug will have already left plasma and be in tissue stores. After the initial decrease, plasma drug concentrations are likely to remain steady due to decreased clearance. Inadequate anaesthesia is a possible consequence of these pharmacokinetic changes. Hypothermia decreases hepatic enzyme function and also decreases the need for anaesthesia. Termination of CPB may result in a return to previous or even enhanced drug concentrations, due to reperfusion of organs with sequestered drug (lungs, muscles).

Renal disease

As IV anaesthetic drugs are generally lipid soluble they are not directly dependent on renal function. However, their metabolites which are generally water soluble can be very sensitive to deterioration in renal function. Accumulation of morphine metabolites, especially morphine-6-glucuronide, can result in enhanced opioid effects. The metabolite is more potent than morphine and has a longer elimination half-time (3). Renal metabolism of morphine also appears to be important. Norpethidine, the major metabolite of pethidine, can accumulate in renal failure. This situation can be aggravated by enhanced pethidine metabolism, e.g. chlorpromazine, which enhances N-demethylation, or previous and prolonged pethidine consumption as may occur with patient-controlled analgesia resulting in enzyme induction. Norpethidine accumulation can result in seizures. Renal failure is less of a problem with most other IV induction agents as metabolites are generally inactive and non-toxic.

Obesity

As IV anaesthetic drugs are generally lipophilic they will accumulate in obese patients who have increased volumes of distribution, reduced clearance and prolonged elimination half-times. Drugs are probably best administered on a lean weight basis.

Factors influencing pharmacokinetics of individual drugs

Barbiturates

Following a bolus of thiopentone uptake into brain is so rapid that brain and blood effectively form a single central compartment. In the presence of hypovolaemia the fraction of the dose received by the brain is increased, resulting in an increased effect. Also, removal of thiopentone from the brain will be diminished because of reduced blood flow, which will result in delayed recovery. There is also an age-related decrease in dose requirement (4). This appears to be related to a decreased proportion of lean body mass with increasing age. Patients with severe anaemia, burns, malnutrition, advanced cancer, uraemia, ulcerative colitis, intestinal obstruction or shock require lower doses of barbiturates. Hypothermia and circulatory failure slow circulation and prolong induction. Hypoproteinaemia in patients with hepatic or renal disease leads to a greater fraction of unbound thiopentone.

Induction of hepatic microsomal enzymes by chronic barbiturate use will accelerate metabolism. Other drugs with sedative effects such as ethanol, antihistamines, isoniazid and monoamine oxidase inhibitors cause greater central nervous system depression when used with barbiturates.

Benzodiazepines

Clearance of benzodiazepines is substantially reduced with advancing age, especially diazepam. This may be in part due to pharmacodynamic changes in elderly patients. Benzodiazepine pharmacokinetics are also affected by gender, race, enzyme induction, hepatic and renal disease. Obesity results in an increased volume of distribution and prolonged elimination half-time. Use of lean body weight in obese patients is recommended because benzodiazepine clearance remains unaltered.

Co-induction is the synergistic interaction between benzodiazepines and other IV anaesthetic drugs, including opioids (5). Anaesthetic induction can be achieved by using subanaesthetic doses of two or more anaesthetic drugs. This effect is synergistic rather than simply additive. Apnea occurs on induction in about 20% of patients with midazolam. Apnea is more common when benzodiazepines are administered with opioids, in the elderly, in the presence of debilitating disease and other sedative drugs. Respiratory depression appears to be more pronounced and of longer duration with chronic obstructive airways disease. Metabolism of benzodiazepines is impaired by aging (diazepam only), disease states (cirrhosis) and other drugs that can impair oxidation (cimetidine). Chronic ethanol consumption increase metabolism of midazolam.

Ketamine

Ketamine is contraindicated in a number of conditions including raised intracranial pressure, open eye injury or other ophthalmic pathology, ischaemic heart disease (due to increased myocardial oxygen consumption), vascular aneurysm and psychiatric disorders such as schizophrenia. Ketamine should also be avoided when other possible causes of postoperative delirium are present, e.g. alcohol or drug withdrawal and head trauma. Ketamine-induced emergence reaction is affected by dose, age (tends not to occur in children), gender (women more susceptible), psychological susceptibility and the presence of other drugs (benzodiazepines reduce the incidence). The doses of ketamine should probably be reduced in the elderly and seriously ill. Seriously ill patients may have depleted circulating catecholamines and may have cardiovascular depression with ketamine.

Ketamine potentiates non-depolarizing neuromuscular blockers, by a mechanism which is unclear. As ketamine clearance is equal to liver blood flow any drug that decreases hepatic blood flow (e.g. halothane) will reduce ketamine clearance. The duration of action is dose dependent, but is also influenced by other anaesthetic drugs which will prolong recovery.

Etomidate

Conditions that alter protein binding (hepatic or renal disease) vary the amount of free etomidate and can produce exaggerated effects. Patients with cirrhosis have larger volumes of distribution, while clearance remains unaltered, resulting in elimination half-times that can be greatly increased. Increasing age results in smaller volumes of distribution and decreased clearance of etomidate.

Etomidate reduces the potency of pancuronium. Etomidate also inhibits aminolevulinic acid synthetase but has been used in patients with porphyria without precipitating an attack.

Propofol

A number of factors affect propofol pharmacokinetics including gender, weight, pre-existing disease, age and medication. Women have higher clearance but also a higher volume of distribution, so elimination half-time is unaltered. Elderly patients have decreased clearance but a lower central volume of distribution, so elimination half-time is unaltered. Dose requirements are less in the elderly. Children have a larger central volume of distribution and more rapid clearance, and have higher dose requirements than adults, both for induction and continuous infusions. Patients with hepatic disease have larger steady-state and central-compartment volumes, with unaltered clearance but elimination half-time may be prolonged.

Opioids including fentanyl may reduce propofol clearance. Propofol doses should be reduced in the presence of opioids, and in aged patients and those with systemic illness.

Opioids

A number of factors and drugs may alter opioid pharmacokinetics. Renal function is important, especially for elimination of morphine-6-glucuronide, which is an active metabolite. Neonates are more sensitive to respiratory depressant effects of opioids with more frequent apnea, periodic breathing and obstruction. Morphine and fentanyl pharmacokinetics are generally similar between children and adults, but alfentanil elimination half-time is decreased in children. Sufentanil clearance is faster in children. Children generally have faster clearance of opioids, with a lower initial volume of distribution. Sensitivity to opioids increases in older patients who experience higher blood and brain concentrations of opioids, and require lower doses. Elderly patients generally have decreased cardiac output and vascular volume, which leads to more drug delivery to brain. Decreased plasma protein (especially albumin) in the elderly results in increased free drug fraction. The smaller initial volume of distribution leads to transiently increased plasma concentrations after bolus administration. Also, steady-state volume of distribution can also be smaller in the elderly and even when combined with reduced clearance can result in shorter elimination half-times. However, central nervous system effects of opioids, especially morphine, do not always parallel plasma concentrations and, in general, opioids in the elderly have a prolonged effect. In the elderly, fentanyl has elevated plasma concentrations and also decreased clearance resulting in prolonged elimination half-time. Reductions in fentanyl and alfentanil dose requirements of up to 50% in the elderly have been demonstrated using power spectral analysis (6). Clearance of many opioids, e.g. fentanyl, approaches hepatic blood flow, so anything that decreases hepatic flow decreases clearance and will prolong opioid effects. Cimetidine decreases hepatic blood flow and diminishes hepatic metabolism via the cytochrome P450 system, thereby potentiating opioid effects.

Many drugs interact with opioids to alter their pharmacodynamics. Opioids are generally noted for their cardiovascular stability, but addition of volatile anaesthetic agents and nitrous oxide may result in significant depression of the cardiovascular system. Changes may include a decrease in mean arterial pressure and reduced coronary blood flow with myocardial ischaemia. Benzodiazepines when added to opioids produce a synergistic effect for sedation and loss of consciousness, as well as occasional profound drops in blood pressure and cardiac output, due to a sustained decrease in sympathetic tone and negative inotropic effects. Propofol combined with opioids can produce hypotension due to direct depression of the myocardium and decreased sympathetic drive. Etomidate in combination with opioids can also produce hypotension.

β-Adrenergic blockade (esmolol) can further improve opioid cardiovascular stability at the time of surgery or intubation, and can decrease myocardial ischaemia. α_2-Adrenergic agonists (clonidine and dexmedetomidine) reduce opioid requirements, but bradycardia and hypotension can be problems. Pancuronium attenuates opioid-induced bradycardia but may increase heart rate and ischaemia. Vecuronium alone is without cardiovascular effects but with high-dose opioids can produce negative inotropic and chronotropic effects, and vagal stimulation can enhance the bradycardia. Tricyclic antidepressants and phenothiazines increase the magnitude and duration of all opioid actions. Monoamine oxidase inhibitors and pethidine can result in excitatory agitation, headache, haemodynamic instability, fever, rigidity, convulsions and coma due to excessive central serotinergic activity as pethidine blocks neuronal uptake of serotonin. Also, respiratory depression, hypotension and coma can occur due to monoamine oxidase inhibition of metabolism of pethidine. Respiratory effects of opioids are increased and prolonged with other sedative drugs (volatile and IV anaesthetic agents) which affect brain stem response to hypercarbia and hypoxia. Respiratory depressant effects are not enhanced by α_2-adrenergic agonists or droperidol.

References

1. Shafer SL, Varvel JR. Pharmacokinetics, pharmacodynamics and rational opioid selection. *Anesthesiology* 1991; **74**: 53.
2. Holley FO, Ponganis KV, Stanski DR. Effects of cardiopulmonary bypass on the pharmacokinetics of drugs. *Clin Pharmacokinet* 1982; **7**: 234.
3. Sear JW, Hand CW, Moore RA, McQuay HJ. Studies on morphine disposition: influence of renal failure on the kinetics of morphine and its metabolites. *Br J Anaesth* 1989; **62**: 28.
4. Macleod SM, Giles HG, Bengert B. Age and gender related differences in diazepam pharmacokinetics. *J Clin Pharmacol* 1979; **19**: 15.
5. Vinik HR, Bradley EL, Kissin I. Preopofol–midazolam–alfentanil combination: is hypnotic synergism present? *Anesth Analg* 1993; **76**: S450.
6. Scott JC, Stanski DR. Decreased fentanyl and alfentanil dose requirements with age. A simultaneous pharmacokinetic and pharmacocdynamic evaluation. *J Pharmacol Exp Ther* 1987; **240**: 159.

4

Pharmacokinetics of infusion

F. Engbers

- Pharmacokinetics
- Age
- Body mass index
- Bolus
- Target-controlled infusions
- Distribution and elimination
- Plasma levels

Pharmacokinetics of infusion

Pharmacokinetics is the science that describes the way a biological system, e.g. the human body, handles a drug by distribution and elimination, whereas pharmacodynamics describe the effects of the drug on this system. In other words, the relationship in time between dose and blood or plasma concentration is described by the pharmacokinetics, and the concentration–effect relationship is described by the pharmacodynamics. It is important to realize that these definitions are valuable for research in circumstances where concentrations and effect can be measured and described. In clinical situations like anaesthesia no real-time blood concentrations are available and the measured effect is highly dependent on an uncontrollable stimulus such as ongoing surgery. In these clinical situations the endpoint is not to create a predictable blood or plasma concentration, but to create and change the required effect in a predictable manner. Onset of action after bolus delivery or infusion change, effect overshoot and effect wear-off are important in controlling the anaesthetic process. This is different than, for example, the oral administration of an antibiotic that usually has a much wider therapeutic window and works on a different time scale. Dosage principles for this type of administration are useless for the anaesthetist who has to titrate his drugs in a rapidly changing situation. Rather than applying pharmacokinetic and dynamic principles, the anaesthesiologist uses his 'feel' for the drug and the effect on the patient to adjust the administration. Nevertheless, new insights in pharmacokinetics, pharmacodynamics, drug interaction and the emergence of computer-controlled systems such as target-controlled infusion (TCI) make it worthwhile to re-assess some of the pharmacological principles and their usability for anaesthesia.

Parameters used for calculating a constant blood concentration: finding the right dose

As stated above the aim of [intravenous (IV)] drug administration in anaesthesia is usually not to create a fixed blood concentration. The principles of the creation of a steady blood concentration are, however, a starting point for many drug regimens. A steady blood concentration is also important to create a stable condition for assessing the drug effect.

When at steady state, no drug is being distributed through the body and in this case input by infusion equals drug loss from the central compartment: the clearance. For most drugs the clearance is a first-order process. This means that the amount of drug eliminated in time is a fraction of the amount of drug available. This in contrast to a zero-order process, where the amount of drug eliminated in time is fixed and therefore independent of the amount of drug available. In the case of a first-order process, the elimination path of a drug still has the capacity to increase, whereas in a zero-order elimination process the breakdown or excretion system becomes saturated. A first-order elimination process can become a zero-order process at high concentrations (1). An example of limited excretion is the case of thiopentone. Real accumulation exists when the drug input exceeds this maximum excretion. This phenomena is seldom. What usually is called accumulation is nothing else than the distribution process whereby the body compartments are filled. This type of accumulation is actually explained by the context-sensitive half-live principle (see later in this chapter).

If an infusion is started that equals the clearance of the drug, then the concentration will increase until this steady state is achieved.

The patient parameters used in the following examples are given in Table 4.1.

Example: propofol (Figure 4.1)

Cl = 1893 ml/min
C_{SS} = 3 µg/ml
Drug loss = infusion = 1893 × 3 = 5680 µg/min * 60 = 340 mg/h

When simulated this infusion scheme will achieve the desired blood concentration (C_{SS}) only in hours. About 10–15 h is required to achieve more than 95% of the C_{SS}. The time required to achieve this concentration *and the shape of the curve* is dependent on the distribution volume and half-live of the distribution process. Drugs with smaller distribution volumes and half-lives will reach this steady state much more quickly. An example

Table 4.1 Patient parameters used in the examples

Patient data	Pharmacokinetic data	Units	Propofol	Remifentanil
Weight: 70 kg	K_{10}^{*}	/min	0.119	0.508781
Age: 40 years	K_{12}^{*}	/min	0.112	0.400279
Gender: male	K_{21}^{*}	/min	0.055	0.208077
Height: 170 cm	K_{13}^{*}	/min	0.0419	0.01484
LBM:[a] 55.3 kg	K_{31}^{*}	/min	0.0033	0.014022
BSA:[b] 1.81 m²	$V_c^{*,\dagger}$	l	15.911	5.121
	$V_2\ (= V_c * K_{12}/K_{21})$	l	32.401	9.852
	$V_3\ (= V_c * K_{13}/K_{31})$	l	202.021	5.420
	$Cl\ (= V_c * K_{10})$	l/min	1.893	2.605684
	$Cl_2\ (= K_{12} * V_c)$	l/min	1.78	2.05
	$Cl_3\ (= K_{13} * V_c)$	l/min	0.67	0.077
Pharmacokinetic/ dynamic link	$t_{1/2}k_{eo}$	min	2.6	1.1

[a]Lean body mass.
[b]Body surface area.

Parameters marked by different superscripts (*,†) are different notations, both give a full model description.

Simulations in this publication performed with simulation software: TivaTrainer©; Gutta BV, Aerdenhout, The Netherlands (1999).

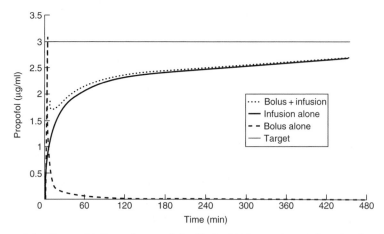

Figure 4.1 Concentration of propofol: effect of infusion to reach a steady state of 3 µg/ml ('Infusion alone'), effect of bolus to fill the central compartment ('Bolus alone') to 3 µg/ml , and effect of bolus and infusion when administered together ('Bolus+infusion'). See text for calculations.

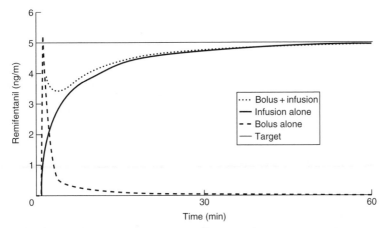

Figure 4.2   Concentration of remifentanil: effect of infusion to reach a steady state of 5 ng/ml ('infusion alone'), effect of bolus to fill the central compartment ('Bolus alone') to 5 ng/ml, and effect of bolus and infusion when administered together ('Bolus+infusion'). See text for calculations.

of such a drug is remifentanil. Notice the differences in the volumes of the compartments and the high clearance.

Example: remifentanil (Figure 4.2)

$Cl = 2606 \, \text{ml/min}$
$C_{SS} = 5 \, \text{ng/ml}$
Drug loss = infusion = $0.005 \times 2606 = 13.03 \, \mu\text{g/min} * 60 = 0.78 \, \text{mg/h}$

In contrast to propofol, remifentanil requires only 30 min to reach steady state with a continuous infusion. For anaesthetic purposes this is still too long. It is clear that a loading dose is necessary to decrease the time to achieve the C_{SS}. There are two approaches possible: (A) calculate the dose to fill the central compartment (2) or (B) calculate the dose to fill the total distribution volume (3).

Approach A: Loading the central volume

Propofol
$V_c = 15 \, 911 \, \text{ml}$
$C_{SS} = 3 \, \mu\text{g/ml}$
Bolus = $3 * 15 \, 911 = 477 \, 333 \, \mu\text{g} = 47.733 \, \text{mg}$

Remifentanil
$V_c = 5121 \, \text{ml}$
$C_{SS} = 5 \, \text{ng/ml}$
Bolus = $5 * 5121 = 25 \, 605 \, \text{ng} = 0.0256 \, \text{mg}$

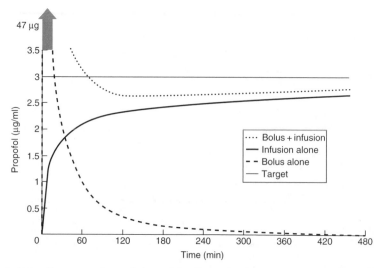

Figure 4.3 Concentration of propofol: effect of infusion to reach a steady state of 3 μg/ml ('Infusion alone'), effect of bolus to fill the distribution volume ('Bolus alone') to 3 μg/ml, and effect of bolus and infusion when administered together ('Bolus+infusion'). See text for calculations.

Approach B: Loading the central + distribution volume

Propofol (Figure 4.3)

$V_{ss} = V_c + V_2 + V_3 = 15\ 911 + 32\ 401 + 202\ 021 = 250\ 333$ ml
$C_{SS} = 3\ \mu g/ml$
Bolus $= 750\ 999\ \mu g = 750$ mg
Resulting initial peak blood concentration $=$ bolus$/V_c = 750\ 999/15\ 911 \approx$ 47 μg/ml

Remifentanil (Figure 4.4)

$V_{ss} = 5121 + 9852 + 5420 = 20\ 393$ ml
$C_{SS} = 5$ ng/ml
Bolus $= 101\ 965$ ng $= 0.1$ mg
Resulting initial peak blood concentration $=$ bolus$/V_c = 101\ 965/5121 \approx 20$ ng/ml

If kinetics are assumed to be linear (see below) then the effects of the different dosages can be added. Therefore the blood concentrations that are the result of the bolus dose may be superimposed on the blood concentration that is the result of the infusion. It is clear from the simulation that both loading dose approaches will fail in the case

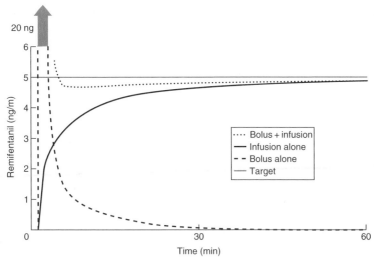

Figure 4.4 Concentration of remifentanil: effect of infusion to reach a steady state of 5 ng/ml ('Infusion alone'), effect of bolus to fill the distribution volume ('Bolus alone') to 5 ng/ml, and effect of bolus and infusion when administered together ('Bolus+infusion'). See text for calculations

of propofol. Method A will fail because of too long a period where the concentration is below the desired concentration; method B will fail because of the side effects that this massive dose will cause.

In the case of remifentanil, method A looks clinically effective at a first glance and method B again will most likely cause side effects. Notice that there is a difference between the two drugs in the amount of overshoot in the central compartment. In the case of propofol, the overshoot is about 15 times the wanted C_{SS}. For remifentanil, the overshoot is 'only' 4 times. Apart from the fact that obtaining a blood concentration is not the goal of the anaesthetist, the conclusion must be that these 'classical' approaches of applied pharmacokinetics are less suitable for anaesthesia. More complex infusion strategies are necessary to achieve the desired initial blood concentration. Many of these infusion schemes that have been published in the past are designed with the help of a computer (4). Computer programs and computers that can help in pharmacokinetic calculations are becoming more and more generally available. It is important to have some idea how these programs work to understand their suitability and limitations.

The computer algorithms that perform these simulations are based on a pharmacokinetic model to calculate the required dosing schemes.

Computer simulations and pharmacokinetic models

Pharmacokinetic models were initially used in pharmacology to explain the drug concentration after a given bolus and or infusion in a specific person or group of persons over a specific period of time. Predicting the blood concentration and calculating the required drug dosing using the same models means reversing this modelling process. Care must be taken when pharmacokinetic parameters derived from a study are used for these calculations. For example, pharmacokinetic parameters derived from bolus studies are not very usable for predicting the infusion rates necessary to maintain a constant blood concentration. When predictions are made for a specific subject, this subject may not belong to the population in which the pharmacokinetic parameters have described. Blood concentration measurements may differ between study centres based on the way the measurements are performed or the site where the sample is taken from: venous, at different locations or arterial (5). The pharmacokinetic property of a subject may change because of concomitant delivery of other anaesthetic drugs and applied techniques. Physiologic parameters like cardiac output have been shown to influence the drug distribution and thereby the pharmacokinetic behaviour. Even when a pharmacokinetic model is derived for an individual at one time, it may not describe the same individual accurately a second time (6).

It is very unlikely that a set of pharmacokinetic parameters derived from healthy volunteers will be able to describe accurately the pharmacokinetic behaviour of the sick patient in theatre. This is not an argument against the use of pharmacokinetic models. Even if we do not use an applied mathematical pharmacokinetic model like in TCI, we use a model in our brain that is based on our experience with the drug.

There are several models that can be used for computer simulations. The most commonly used is the open two- or three-compartment model. It is a purely mathematical model. There is no assumption on what these compartments are. Although it is tempting to translate the three compartments to physiological compartments like central blood volume, richly perfused tissues such as muscles and poorly perfused tissues such as fat, the volumes are merely calculated on the concentration–time curve from the only compartment where samples are taken: the central compartment.

We can consider this model with a sink to which two other compartments are connected. Water is lost from the central compartment but not from the other compartments. If we want to regulate the input in such a way that the level in the central compartment stays constant, then we first have to fill it, i.e. the initial bolus, and then quickly reduce the flow once the level has been reached. From then on at a certain point in time the input has to equal the loss by elimination to the outside plus the distribution to the other compartments. As the other compartments fill up, the input flow has to be slowly reduced until the level in the other compartments equals the level in the central compartment and there is no change necessary in the input to maintain a constant concentration in the central compartment. This is the steady-state situation. In Figure 4.5 the models of the two example drugs propofol and remifentanil are drawn on scale according to this concept. The widths of the columns V_1, V_2 and V_3 represent the compartmental volumes, the widths of the connecting tubes represent the magnitude of the intercompartmental clearances Cl_1 and Cl_2 and the clearance of the drug to the outside Cl_0. Drug input is assumed into the central compartment. The effect compartment is a virtual compartment inside V_1. Figure 4.6 shows the model with hypothetical filling of a drug.

In TCI, the period during which the input slowly decreases to maintain the constant blood concentration is often called the *pseudo steady state*.

The model in a sense is static and linear. Linear means that doubling the input will double the concentration. Static means that the model assumes immediate mixing from drug in the central compartment. From studies with fast sampling techniques it is known this is not the case. From the point of injection the drug is moved through the body as a concentration front by the force of the blood circulation and passes the

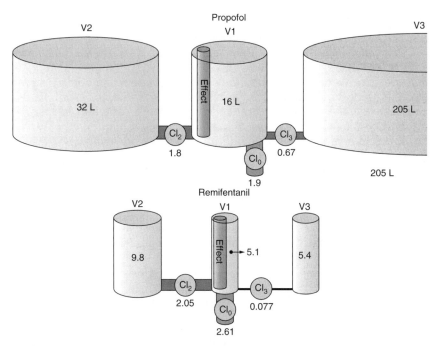

Figure 4.5   Representation of the open three-compartment model. Drug input is assumed to occur into the central compartment (V_c). Drug disposition from the central compartment to the peripheral compartments is represented by the intercompartmental clearances Cl_1 and Cl_2. Drug loss is described by Cl_0. All items are drawn to scale, apart from the effect compartment that has an infinitely small volume.

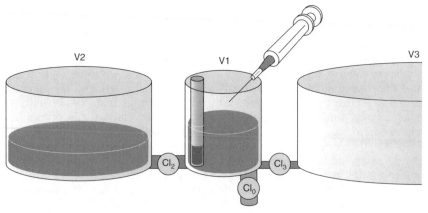

Figure 4.6 Model with hypothetical filling of a drug.

lungs in which some drugs may be absorbed or possibly even metabolized before it reaches the sample site (7). These kinds of phenomena cannot be modelled with the relatively simple three-compartment model. There are of course many other possible models to describe the concentration–time relationship. The most interesting models for anaesthesia are pure physiology-based models, and models that are a mixture of physiologic and compartmental models (hybrid models). With these models it is possible to incorporate, for example, the influence of the cardiac output on the drug distribution of the compartmental model (8) or the change of going on and off bypass during cardiovascular procedure. Although physiologic models have theoretical advantages and may have a smaller prediction error under many circumstances, their main disadvantage is that the model parameters, e.g. regional flow and tissue uptake, are very difficult to assess in the individual patient and that the validation of these models is difficult. The open two- or three-compartment, however, is robust, computer algorithms can easily be verified and at this moment there is a lot of experience with the validation of these models. Most computer-controlled infusion or TCI systems use this type of model.

The pharmacokinetic–pharmacodynamic link parameter: $t_{1/2}k_{eo}$

Apart from the difficulties in calculating the dosage scheme to obtain a constant blood concentration (see above), the problem still exists that in daily practice, this blood concentration is most times not the anaesthetist's target. Anaesthetics do not have their intended effect in the blood. The target organ for hypnotics, for example, is the brain. Also, studies done with the analgesics show that there is a considerable lag time before an increase in the blood concentration results in an increase in effect (9). This lag time is drug dependent, and exists for both IV anaesthetics and inhalation anaesthetics. However, for most non-anaesthetic drugs a short delay between starting dosing and the maximum effect may not be so important. This lag time is very important for anaesthetic drugs that are used to control a dynamic process and will have consequences for the drug-dosing strategy.

The delay between change in blood and brain concentration can be incorporated into the open two- or three-compartment model by means of an effect compartment. The lag time can be expressed as the half-life of the equilibration process between blood and the target organ: the brain. Usually this half-life is called $t_{1/2}k_{eo}$. It is important to understand that this delay is most important both for research and for clinical practice. Suppose we are inducing two patients with propofol with a constant infusion. Suppose that both patients are exactly the same in terms of pharmacokinetics and pharmacodynamics, and that the observed effect occurs once the concentration in their brain is exactly $4\,\mu g/ml$. The only difference in induction technique is a difference in infusion rate of 1200 versus 100 ml/h. The simulations in Figure 4.7 show what is to be expected. The faster the infusion rate, the faster the patient will show the effect; however, after the infusion rate has been stopped, the concentration at the effect site will continue to increase. When a lower infusion rate is selected the blood and brain are equilibrated and no overshoot occurs, but it will take more time before the effect occurs. Up to a certain point less drug is required when the infusion rate is reduced. This phenomena has already been demonstrated in research. If blood samples would have been taken to measure the concentration at the moment of desired effect, an incorrect high concentration would have been found in the case of the high infusion rate. Thus two research protocols that only differ in the rate of infusion will come up with completely different blood concentrations that are related to the same effect. The difference may also be clear in daily practice. For example, if two anaesthetists try to find the minimal infusion rates for successful laryngeal mask insertion and the only difference is that anaesthetist A waits 1 min longer than anaesthetist B, A will find lower infusion rates than B. Given the fact that other drugs influence each other's requirements, like opioids and propofol (10), and that every single drug has its own $t_{1/2}k_{eo}$, it is no wonder that one technique is successful in one place but may fail somewhere else. It also explains why bolus techniques, despite the theoretical disadvantages of high peaking blood concentration, are still not totally abandoned in practice. Figure 4.8 shows the simulated blood concentration of a 1 h anaesthesia with a bolus technique of fentanyl, and the corresponding blood and effect concentration. The high peaks in the blood concentration are less prominent in the effect-site concentration. Note that the interval times at which the boluses are given slowly increase because of the loading of the system or, in other words, the increasing context-sensitive half-life.

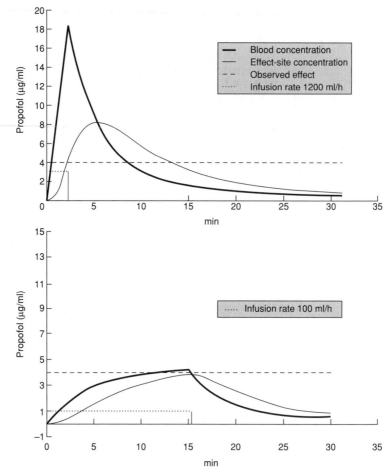

Figure 4.7   Simulations of the blood and effect compartment concentration with a fast infusion (1200 ml/h) and a slow infusion (100 ml/h) of propofol continued until the theoretical effect compartment concentration equals 4 µg/ml.

It has been stated that the high blood concentrations are responsible for the side effects. However, this is questionable. Side effects most likely have their own lag times and therefore peak blood concentrations do not create equally high concentrations at the site where the side effect occurs.

Depending mainly on the speed of distribution and the $t_{1/2}k_{eo}$, the theoretical ideal initial bolus will be large enough to create a required *effect* concentration without overshoot. Best examples of drugs with different properties in this respect are the opioids fentanyl, sufentanil, alfentanil and remifentanil. Figure 4.9 shows the initial bolus and the

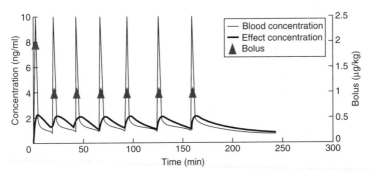

Figure 4.8 Bolus doses of fentanyl (loading 2 µg/kg and thereafter 1 µg/kg). Note the increase in interval time (from 22 to 35 min) between administrations.

resulting effect. Notice the limited overshoot of alfentanil which is mainly caused by the slower initial decay and relative short $t_{1/2}k_{eo}$. A drug like sufentanil, however, has a much faster decay initially and its longer $t_{1/2}k_{eo}$ requires a much higher overshoot of the blood concentration. Unfortunately the calculations necessary to develop the dosing schemes to control the effect compartment are impossible without the help of advanced computer algorithms. The most advanced IV dosing system that is available for every day clinical use in most parts of the world at the time of writing, i.e. the 'Diprifusor', does not have these calculations implemented yet. Therefore the same kind of overshoot in the blood target must be selected by the user to obtain an adequate effect concentration in an reasonable amount of time (see below). The target for maintenance that is selected after the induction target is lower. A good starting point for the target at maintenance is the effect concentration at which a successful induction was achieved. The big advantage of TCI is that it is able to show this theoretical effect-site concentration.

There are several hypotheses about what causes this delay. It could be the diffusion of the drug from the blood through a membrane-type barrier to reach the receptor. The other possibility is that the brain itself has a large distribution volume causing the drug concentration after entrance of the brain to drop because of distribution. There also may be a delay in the actual response itself or the measurement or clinical evidence of the response or there may be two responses that counteract like initial agitation before sedation occurs. Although as stated above the delay is important for anaesthetic drugs, the data on the actual $t_{1/2}k_{eo}$'s of our anaesthetics are sparse. One of the reasons for this is that the measurement is difficult. The most common way of measurement is creating a hysteresis loop between the measured drug concentration and a continuous measurement of the effect. The $t_{1/2}k_{eo}$ of the drug can be estimated by collapsing this loop. If a $t_{1/2}k_{eo}$ is used in relation to a compartmental model then the hysteresis loop of that particular model should be used, because as stated above the simple compartmental models are very

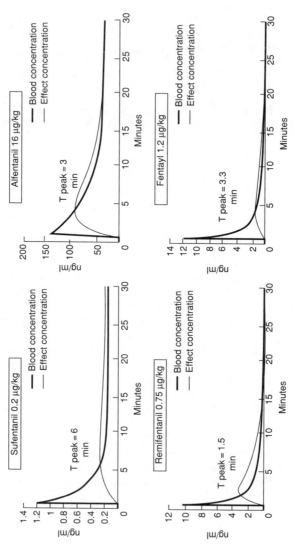

Figure 4.9 The opioids most used intraoperatively: the blood concentration, the effect concentration and the time until the maximum effect occurs after a bolus dose.

inaccurate in predicting fast changes of blood concentrations and therefore a part of the delay could be caused by the implemented pharmacokinetic parameters (11). At this moment there are only a very few studies that take into account that a $t_{1/2}k_{eo}$ when used in conjunction with a pharmacokinetic model it *belongs* to that specific model and cannot be separated. A good example is a study on the pharmacokinetic–pharmacodynamic properties of remifentanil (12), where it has been shown that the $t_{1/2}k_{eo}$ in that model is age dependent.

Population characteristics and pharmacokinetics

IV dosing schemes are usually made dependent on the weight of the patient. Although it is clear that one cannot give the same dose to a child of 10 kg as to an adult of 100 kg, there is not so much hard evidence that weight is the most important co-variable that influences the dose requirements of a patient when looking at blood concentrations. For some drugs the body surface area (BSA) appears to be the factor influencing the model parameters together with the age (remifentanil). When the central volume of the two- or three-compartment model is adjusted for weight, as is the case with the 'Diprifusor', the volumes of the other compartments are also changed in a linear fashion. The effect of this is that the dosage changes proportionally. Thus a target of 2.5 µg/ml in a patient weighting 100 kg will produce the same infusion scheme as a target of 5 µg/ml in a 50 kg patient. Apparently adjusting for weight in obese patients is appropriate for propofol (13). Children are, however, a different problem. The problem with the determination of pharmacokinetic parameters in children is that there are no volunteer studies with sufficiently long sample times, so that the only data available is from patient studies. Population analyses on the data available show that there is at least a difference in clearance between children and adults (Schüttler and White, personal communications). Even when corrections for pharmacokinetic parameters are made there might be a difference in pharmacodynamic differences or, for example, there could be a difference in protein binding. As samples are determined in whole blood or plasma and only the free fraction of the drug is available for receptor binding, differences in protein binding may appear as differences in the pharmacodynamics. Although there is limited information available, model-based infusion systems like TCI could make delivery of drugs in children much easier and safer as the system will handle implementation of the influence of body surface area and age on drug dosing without complicated calculations by the anaesthetist.

The context-sensitive half-life

Anaesthetists are unlike other medical specialists in that they are interested in the time required for a drug to wear off. The elimination half-life is seemingly a sound parameter to compare the duration of drugs. Again, for anaesthesia this is not the case. As long as no real steady state is achieved, decay in the central compartment is dependant on both distribution and elimination. This makes duration of action dependent on the time the drug has been delivered: the context. The time necessary for a drug to halve its concentration will increase while drug delivery goes on. To make the context-sensitive half-life even more usable for anaesthesia, the creators defined the half-life related to the *effect compartment* instead of the blood compartment. Furthermore, a pseudo steady state is assumed in the definition of context-sensitive half-life. This is necessary because this is the only way the amount of drug available for (re) distribution and elimination can be calculated. The context-sensitive half-life in itself is not concentration dependent. If a pseudo steady state is maintained for a concentration x and a concentration $2x$ for the same amount of time, the time to halve this concentration will be the same. However, if a concentration x is maintained for time T and for time $2T$, the time required for the concentration to decay to half x is now dependent on the balance between distribution and elimination, or the 'filling state' of the compartments; in other words, on what happened with the drug before it was switched of: the context. Figure 4.10 shows the graphical representation of the context-sensitive half-life of the opioids. Notice that the context-sensitive half-life of fentanyl seems to increase indefinitely. This is not true. After reaching a steady state the context-sensitive half-life equals the elimination half-life (if the context-sensitive half-life was related to blood concentration). This can be observed with alfentanil that reaches steady state after 3 h and remifentanil that reaches a steady state after 15–20 min. The big distribution volume of the drugs sufentanil and fentanyl means that the context-sensitive half-life increases for a far

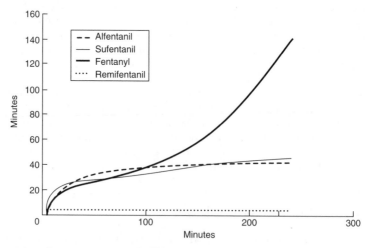

Figure 4.10   Context-sensitive half-live (CSH) of the four opioids.

longer period. The observation that sufentanil up to 3 h has a shorter context-sensitive half-life than alfentanil is interesting, and also that fentanyl with the smallest clearance is even shorter then both alfentanil and sufentanil during the first hour of administration shows that 'classical' elimination half-lives do not characterize the drugs in clinical anaesthesiology practice. However, before translating these findings in clinical practice one should realize that the context-sensitive half-life gives information on the drug, not the pharmacodynamic action in the patient. For example, if one was able to keep the fentanyl concentration just above the required level for adequate anaesthesia so that only a reduction of 5% was necessary, it might appear to work shorter than alfentanil if that was dosed in such away that 50% reduction was required. The predictability of drug effect is therefore also important together with the skills of the anaesthesiologist. This predictability is influenced by the variation in the concentration–response relationship in the population. If all our patients would be asleep at 2.5 µg/ml and awake at 2.4 µg/ml propofol concentration, independent of stimulus and concomitant administration of drugs, it would not matter if our drug was short or long acting, provided that the pharmacokinetic variability was low. We would even not need TCI to achieve a steady 'level of anaesthesia'. Indeed the fact that drug effect is less predictable and the pharmacodynamic variability exceeds the kinetic variability makes tools like TCI useful to 'calibrate' the drug effect to the individual patient, the surgical stimulus and the interaction with other drugs.

Practical applications of pharmacokinetics

Target-controlled infusion

TCI emerged a number of years ago. Research protocols often require a more or less predictable and stable blood concentration of the drug being investigated. TCI can also be used in clinical situations to control other drugs that may influence the drug effect measurements (10). In 1983, Schüttler et al. (14) described the use of a computer programme for calculating the loading dose and the required exponentially decaying infusion rate to obtain a theoretical stable blood concentration: the bolus elimination transfer scheme (BET). Since then many research groups have built their own system. The first systems where bulky, due to the big computers and infusion pumps. Miniaturization of computers and the availability of infusion pumps that allow remote control have stimulated the development of flexible systems usable in daily clinical practice. Most systems available for research these days allow the user to select a blood concentration and change that predicted blood concentration depending on the patient's response to surgical stimulation or side effects. The required changes in the infusion rate are calculated by a computer and sent to a commercially available infusion pump. These systems became known as titration of IV anaesthesia by computer (TIAC), computer-aided continuous infusion (CACI), computer-controlled infusion (CCI) and, more recently, TCI systems. Although the technique involved in TCI is more simple than many of the other hardware and software systems that surround the anaesthetist in the operating theatre, it took a long time before such a system for one drug became available for every day use: the 'Diprifusor'. The main reasons for this delay were safety issues. Software that controls and automates the delivery of a drug must conform to very high standards. For example, automated syringe recognition is necessary to prevent a drug being delivered with the wrong pharmacokinetic parameters. As no computer chip manufacturer or software designer can guarantee fault-free operation, double-processor control is useful. On top of this, the model parameters have to be proven applicable to the patient population where the TCI system is used (15).

Although TCI systems take care of the pharmacokinetic calculations, some aspects of how they operate must be understood.

After selecting a target concentration, the TCI system begins with a small bolus. This bolus-loading dose is just enough to fill the theoretical central volume. Usually the loading dose is less than one would give when the drug is delivered manually. The loading dose is followed by a exponentially decreasing infusion rate that initially is higher than when delivered manually. Decreasing the target is accomplished by stopping the infusion and then dependent on how much drug has already been distributed, an increasing or decreasing infusion scheme. If the model predicts drug redistributing from the peripheral compartment(s) to the central compartment, then the infusion will increase, otherwise the drug will decrease. Increase of the target will cause a new loading dose to be given, followed by a slowly decreasing infusion. During this process the computer sometimes has to correct inaccuracies from the pump. From time to time larger infusion rates can be seen on the display than actually necessary from a pharmacokinetic point of view.

Apart from taking away the complexity of applied pharmacokinetics in continuous drug delivery, TCI systems can also be used for calculating the appropriate pharmacokinetic parameters depending on the co-variables. In the commercially available 'Diprifusor' systems, only the weight of the patient has been taken into the initial model-determining factors. For other drugs the dependency on patient characteristics may be more complex. If experimental TCI is used for remifentanil (see above), then age, weight and length will have to be provided at start-up. Based on these co-variables the proper pharmacokinetic model parameters will be calculated and used. Although the anaesthesiologist will always have to titrate the drug to effect, reducing the bandwidth in which he has to operate and increasing the reproducibility of his actions in individual patients will ameliorate the control of anaesthesia.

Pharmacokinetic model-driven systems have been tried in other areas. Target-controlled sedation, possibly even controlled by the patient him/herself, is under investigation at the moment of writing (see Chapter 14).

Another field is postoperative pain control. By letting the patient control the delivery device, pain control can be individualized. Patient-controlled analgesia (PCA) is normally used with morphine. From a pharmacokinetic point of view morphine is not the most ideal drug. It has a long onset of action and an active metabolite. Alfentanil is theoretically more appropriate. However, if we try to set-up the bolus dose and lockout period for alfentanil PCA, simulations show that if we want to use the fast onset we need appropriate bolus doses and short lock-out intervals, which will possibly lead to too high concentrations after a while because of the decreasing drug distribution. If we plan our dosing strategy on a safe drug delivery after distribution occurs, we will lose the fast onset property. Indeed, straightforward PCA with alfentanil has not proven to be very successful. With TCI, however, it is possible to develop a PCA system that is controlled by the patients. A button push will increase the target concentration instead of a fixed bolus. There have been a few of these systems described in the literature (16). In contrast to the conventional PCA with alfentanil, they appear to be save and successful.

One would expect that model-driven infusion would also be useful for non-anaesthetic drugs that require accurate titration because they have a narrow therapeutic window. This area still has to be investigated. There are a only few studies showing the success of this approach (16).

Target-controlled infusion and blood–brain equilibration

Although the relationship between blood concentration and effect is more tight and less time dependent than between infusion rate and effect, the predicted blood concentration target is not the objective of a given anaesthetic. The blood–brain equilibration time influences the selected target in the clinical use of TCI systems. Suppose that for a hypothetical patient the blood concentration window required to accomplish anaesthesia in conjunction with an opioid is $3 \pm 0.2\,\mu g/ml$. With a theoretical $t_{1/2}k_{eo}$ of 2.6 min ($t_{1/2}k_{eo}$ used in the 'Diprifusor', Ian Glenn personal communication) it would take $4 \times 2.6\,min = 10.4\,min$ to achieve 93.75% (50 + 25 + 12.5 + 6.25) of that concentration. The effective window will then be entered. If an initial target of $6\,\mu g/ml$ is selected, the same concentration will be reached in about 2.5 min. In this case doubling the initial target reduces the time to the effective window to 25%. Further doubling of the initial target to $12\,\mu g/ml$ does not decrease this time as much: the window will be entered in about 1.75 min, i.e. a decrease to 17% of the time required with $3\,\mu g/ml$. Therefore, up to a certain point, an increase of the initial target will decrease the induction time significantly; however, a further decrease requires a non-linear increase of the initial target. This phenomenon is known from the use of muscle relaxants where a decrease in time of onset is achieved by 'priming' with a small dose rather than an unlimited increase of the initial bolus (17). It will be clear that these high initial targets may cause considerable side effects. However, one should realize that the side effects have their own equilibration constant and are also only indirectly influenced by the blood concentration. For example, in contrast to what could be expected for the hemodynamic effects of propofol, they appear to be slower than the main 'central' effect (1).

The consequences of the blood–brain equilibration delay for TCI are:

♦ Usually, the induction target must be reduced after induction and during maintenance
♦ When longer induction times are acceptable, lower targets for induction can be selected and reduction for maintenance is less necessary
♦ With appropriate analgesic medication the difference between induction target and maintenance will decrease, thereby providing more information on the patient requirements already at induction
♦ Increase of the target (or initial dose) will decrease the onset time of action, although only until a certain limit
♦ There is a theoretical optimum between induction time and effect overshoot

In theory the computer could manage the predicted blood concentration in such a way that the effect concentration becomes the target of TCI. Some experimental systems are capable of controlling the effect compartment. The next generation of TCI systems might be implemented with this capability. At the moment, information on the effect compartment is already perceived by experienced anaesthetists as a valuable parameter in IV anaesthesia.

Target-controlled infusion and prediction of the awakening time

The pharmacokinetic model in the TCI system makes it possible to predict on-line the time required for achieving a lower concentration if the system would be shut down. This time is displayed on the 'Diprifusor'. There are a few precautions to be taken into consideration when this time is interpreted as an awakening time.

The decay curve of the drug is exponential. Predicting the time to another lower concentration becomes increasingly inaccurate at lower concentrations, when the decay curve is flatter. Furthermore, the average awakening concentration cannot simply be related to the average awakening time because of the non-normal distribution of the awakening time caused by the exponential behaviour of the decay curve.

Recent research has shown that, analogous to the blood–brain delay at induction, the awakening concentration is more related to the predicted effect concentration than to the measured blood concentration. Thus the measured concentration at which the patient wakes is dependent on the duration of the anaesthesia (18).

From a pharmacodynamic point of view, the awakening concentration is not a fixed point but is influenced by the concentration of other drugs (19) like opioids and premedication (20), and the amount of stimulation and pain. All these factors make the time at which the patient will wake up as unpredictable as the winning number in the national lottery!

Conclusions

Without model-driven drug delivery systems or computers to simulate blood and effect-site concentrations, pharmacokinetics are of limited added value for the practising anaesthetist because:

◆ The blood concentration is not really the goal of the drug administration in anaesthesia
◆ Calculations available to obtain a blood concentration are not usable for anaesthetic practice
◆ The dosing scheme of (IV) drugs is highly influenced by the blood–brain equilibrium delay
◆ Advanced pharmacokinetics that incorporate dependency on covariates like age and lean body mass are to complex to use

References

1. Stanski DR, Mihm FG, Rosenthal MH, Kalman SM. Pharmacokinetics of high-dose thiopental used in cerebral resuscitation. *Anesthesiology* 1980; **53**: 169–71.
2. Boyes RN, Scott DB, Jebson PJ, Godman MJ, Julian DG. Pharmacokinetics of lidocaine in man. *Clin Pharmacol Ther* 1971; **12**: 105–15.
3. Mitenko PO, Olgilvie RI. Rapidly achieved plasma concentrations plateaus with observations on theophyline kinetics. *Clin Pharmacol Ther* 1971; **13**: 329–35.
4. Roberts FL, Dixon J, Lewis GTR, Tackley RM, Prys-Roberts C. Induction and maintenance of propofol anaesthesia. A manual infusion scheme. *Anaesthesia* 1988; **43** (suppl): 14–7.
5. Chiou WL. The phenomenon and rationale of marked dependence of drug concentration on blood sampling site: implications in pharmacokinetics, pharmacodynamics, toxicology and therapeutics (part I). *Clin Pharmacokinet* 1989; **17**: 175–99.
6. Hill HF. Pharmacokinetic tailoring of computer-controlled alfentanil infusions. In: Kroboth PD, Smith RB, Juhl RP, eds. *Pharmacokinetics and pharmacodynamics. Volume 2: Current problems, potential solutions.* Cincinnati, OH: Harvey Whitney 1988: 158–66.
7. Boer F, Hoeft A, Scholz M, Bovill JG, Burm AGL, Hak A. Pulmonary distribution of alfentanil and sufentanil studied with system dynamics analysis. *J Pharmacokinet Biopharm* 1996; **24**: 197–218
8. Henthorn TK, Krejcie TC, Avram MJ. The relationship between alfentanil distribution kinetics and cardiac output. *Clin Pharmacol Ther* 1992; **52**: 190–6.

9. Scott JC, Ponganis KV, Stanski DR. EEG quantitation of narcotic effect: the comparative pharmacodynamics of fentanyl and alfentanil. *Anesthesiology* 1985; **62**: 234–41.
10. Vuyk J, Lim T, Engbers FHM, Burm AGL, Vletter AA, Bovill JG. The pharmacodynamic interaction of propofol and alfentanil during lower abdominal surgery in female patients. *Anesthesiology* 1995; **83**: 8–22.
11. White M, Schenkels MJ, Engbers FH, *et al*. Effect-site modelling of propofol using auditory evoked potentials. *Br J Anaesth* 1999, **82**: 333–9.
12. Minto CF, Schnider ThW, Egan TD, *et al*. Influence of age and gender on the pharmacokinetics and pharmacodynamics of remifentanil: I. Model development. *Anesthesiology* 1997; **86**: 10–23.
13. Servin F, Farinotti R, Haberer JP, *et al*. Propofol infusion for maintenance of anesthesia in morbidly obese patients receiving nitrous oxide. A clinical and pharmacokinetic study. *Anesthesiology* 1993; **78**: 657–65.
14. Schüttler J, Schwilden H, Stoeckel H. Pharmacokinetics as supplied to total intravenous anaesthesia: theoretical considerations. *Anaesthesia* 1983; **38**: S51–2.
15. Vuyk J, Engbers FH, Burm AG, *et al*. Performance of computer-controlled infusion of propofol: an evaluation of five pharmacokinetic parameter sets. *Anesth Analg* 1995; **81**: 1275–82.
16. van den Nieuwenhuyzen MC, Engbers FH, Burm AG, *et al*. Computer-controlled infusion of alfentanil for postoperative analgesia. A pharmacokinetic and pharmacodynamic evaluation. *Anesthesiology* 1993; **79**: 481–92.
17. Silverman DG, Swift CA, Dubow HD, *et al*. Variability of onset times within and among relaxant regimens. *J Clin Anesth* 1992; **4**: 28–33.
18. Kazama T, Ikeda K, Morita K, *et al*. Comparison of the effect-site k(eO)s of propofol for blood pressure and EEG bispectral index in elderly and younger patients. *Anesthesiology* 1999; **90**: 1517–27.
19. Vuyk J, Lim T, Engbers FH, *et al*. The pharmacodynamic interaction of propofol and alfentanil during lower abdominal surgery in women [see comments]. *Anesthesiology* 1995; **83**: 8–22.
20. Vuyk J, Mertens MJ, Olofsen E, *et al*. Propofol anesthesia and rational opioid selection: determination of optimal EC_{50}–EC_{95} propofol–opioid concentrations that assure adequate anesthesia and a rapid return of consciousness. *Anesthesiology* 1997; **87**: 1549–62.

Nomenclature

C_{pT}	target plasma concentration
C_{eT}	target effect-site concentration
C_{pM}	measured plasma concentration
C_{pCALC}	calculated plasma concentration
C_{eCALC}	calculated effect-site concentration
C_{SS}	concentration at steady state
Cl	clearance
V_c	volume of the central compartment
V_d	distribution volume
K_{10}	rate constant for drug disposition from V_c to outside

$K_{12}, K_{21}, K_{13}, K_{31}$ rate constants for intercompartmental drug disposition

$t_{1/2}k_{eo}$ half-life of transport process of drug to the effect compartment (actually the transport process from the effect compartment to the outside, a mathematical consequence of the fact that the effect compartment is not a compartment as the other compartments but has an infinitely small volume)

5

Administration of intravenous anaesthesia/total intravenous anaesthesia

N. L. Padfield

- Intermittent bolus techniques
- Manually adjusted infusion rates
- Target-controlled infusions – analog estimation plasma concentration
- Target-controlled infusions – estimating the effect-site concentration
- Combination of separate infusions
- Combination of drugs – same infusion

Manually adjusted infusion rates

Since this technique requires a change of focus on equipment there are practical aspects that need to be considered. These are well outlined in one paper (1) but the local situation may suggest other aspects that also matter.

Important practical points

Venous access

Since interruption of delivery of anaesthetic agent to the circulation will allow the patient to wake up, reliable intravenous (IV) access is mandatory. This is secured by using a large peripheral vein which ideally can be seen during the operation. The arm should not be bent at an acute angle if the antecubital fossa veins are used but they are better avoided if there are large accessible veins elsewhere. The cannula should be secured preferably with a purpose made IV dressing rather than sticky tape to reduce the risk of displacement during positioning of the patient or during surgery.

The use of IV fluids in day surgery

The administration of 15–20 ml/kg crystalloid solution helps to reduce postoperative nausea and vomiting (PONV) in day case patients. It also helps to flush drugs into the patient's circulation, and helps to provide an indication that the vein is patent and not being compressed proximally. The sudden appearance of a pool of crystalloid on the floor should alert the anaesthetist to the possibility of a disconnection in the system.

Dead space and connectors

Avoid using a large dead space before different infusions reach the IV cannula. Large dead spaces result in wide fluctuations in plasma concentrations as different infusions are stopped and started, e.g. when changing syringes or bags of fluid. An ideal solution is to use a purpose-made double or triple lumen connector. All connectors and taps should be the Luer-lock type to reduce the risk of disconnection.

One-way valves

When more than one infusion is used a one-way valve should used to prevent the risk of one infusion backtracking into another.

Infusion devices

Use an infusion device specifically designed for IV anaesthesia. Check the pump settings very carefully before each case, making sure the units are correct. Some rechargeable batteries can become completely discharged with very little warning resulting in data loss in the middle of an operation, so keep them connected to the mains electricity supply whenever possible and only use the batteries for transferring patients for as short a time as possible.

Summary: practical points to note

- Choose a large peripheral vein wherever possible
- Avoid bending the arm more than 90° (the IV infusion helps to indicate that the vein is not being compressed)
- Fix the IV cannula securely
- Keep the injection site visible
- Avoid a large dead space before the cannula
- Use one-way valves to avoid the possibility of drugs back-tracking another infusion line
- Use an infusion device designed for anaesthetic use
- Keep batteries well charged

Induction

Propofol is now established as the best IV agent for the majority of cases. although etomidate still has a place. In a paper comparing the two agents administered as a bolus then followed by a fixed infusion rate, propofol demonstrated not only a more rapid return of consciousness but also less nausea and vomiting and no mental side effects which still troubled a few patients in the etomidate group at 3 months (2).

One paper looking at the necessary induction doses and comparing 5 s bolus delivery with a variety of infusion speeds noted that the cardiovascular variables depended on dose administered rather than the speed of infusion (3). As has been explained in earlier chapters, because the difference between reaching a plasma target and an effect-site target depends on the rate of infusion and effect-site equilibration half-life, enormous differences in changes in cardiovascular parameters can occur if the induction infusion rate is too rapid. Similarly, in a comparison of different plasma propofol targets of 5, 6, 7 and 8 µg/ml the time from induction to the successful insertion of the laryngeal mask shortens as the target value of propofol rises, but at the cost of more perturbations in cardiovascular parameters (4). Animal studies have looked at various rates of infusion with a view to optimizing the length of time of induction (5), i.e. not too long, with minimizing the cardiovascular perturbations. If the infusion is too fast then too much propofol is administered before clinical signs of anaesthesia are apparent. This causes two problems:

- This 'flash' rate of administration means that the plasma level is much higher than the effect site (which correlates with the level of anaesthesia) so that when equilibration between plasma and brain has subsequently occurred the effect-site concentration is much higher than desired and causes prolonged CNS depression, often resulting in a period of apnoea (6). This apnoea is likely to be particularly pronounced with concomitant administration of opiates.
- This 'flash' rate of administration also means that the plasma concentration reaching the heart and blood vessels is higher than necessary, and will cause significant vasodilatation and possibly bradycardia, mediated through increased vagal tone. This can jeopardize patients with critical myocardial ischaemia who cannot tolerated a reduction in diastolic perfusion pressure. Similarly it can jeopardize patients with critical cerebrovascular insufficiency and in septic patients with critical changes in renal and splanchnic perfusion.

Intermittent bolus

Total IV anaesthesia has been successfully administered by repeat boluses of methohexitone, ketamine and alcuronium after co-induction with diazepam (7).

It is possible to produce continuous anaesthesia using small (20–30 mg) intermittent boluses of propofol following an initial sleep

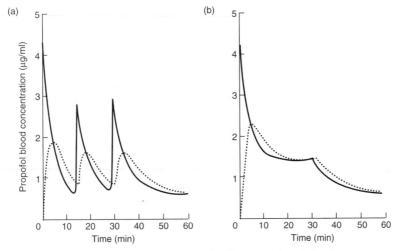

Figure 5.1   Propofol blood (solid line) and effect-site (dotted line) concentrations after a propofol bolus injection of 70 mg followed by (a) two incremental bolus doses of 35 mg each or (b) a continuous infusion of 70 mg over 30 min (2.33 mg/min). Reproduced with permission from Blackwell Science Ltd from Gepts E. Pharmacokinetic concepts. *Anaesthesia* 1998; **53** (suppl 1): 9; figure 7.

dose (2–3 mg/kg). However, this technique cannot be recommended for anything longer than the shortest of cases (5 min) as there is a danger of recovery from anaesthesia in between boluses. Figure 5.1 shows not only the wide swings in plasma concentrations but also those in the 'effect-site' concentrations (8). However, it is important to note that the 'effect-site' concentrations do not swing as widely, thus explaining how we can 'get away with it' by this technique for a short simple procedure.

Figure 5.1 also compares intermittent boluses with a continuous infusion over a similar period of time.

Also it has been shown that infusion techniques can reduce the total drug requirements by 25–30% when compared with repeat boluses (9). Co-induction with a small dose of midazolam reduces the overall requirement for propofol when given 2 min before the start of induction. Small doses of fentanyl (25–50 µg) or alfentanil (250–500 µg) can be given at the same time to achieve a satisfactory respiratory rate. Co-induction with a small amount of propofol, 30 mg, also reduced the induction dose then required of propofol as well as 2 mg of midazolam (10); however, in the abstract the authors then questioned whether midazolam pretreatment by reducing the induction of dose of propofol was cost-effective since propofol pretreatment still enabled satisfactory induction with less than 200 mg, i.e. one ampoule. With the widespread adoption of target-controlled infusion (TCI) with tagged prefilled syringes such a concern has become irrelevant.

Summary: Intermittent bolus techniques

♦ Only suitable for very short procedures
♦ Risk of recovery between bolus doses
♦ Simple technique without the need for complex technology

Bolus plus manual infusion techniques

This technique has been described for etomidate in gynaecological patients in 1981 (12). It was recognized that pharmacokinetic studies were important in being able to predict 'asleep' concentrations that could be maintained (13). However, simplicity in application was also important and a two-stage infusion regime has been described (14). Another paper related the maintenance infusion to the initial bolus (15). Many models have been described for manually adjusted infusion regimes, some with sequential step reductions (16) that provided a degree of stability in plasma concentration.

These techniques require the use of a suitable infusion device. A device which has been specifically designed for giving anaesthetic drugs (e.g. Graseby 3400, Fresenius Pilot or IVAC Alaris) is highly recommended as these devices usually incorporate dose-calculating software which simplifies their use and also helps to reduce dose-calculation errors. These devices can also be used to deliver boluses for induction and, when required, during the maintenance phase.

Summary: Bolus plus manual infusion techniques

♦ Dedicated anaesthetic infusion pumps recommended
♦ Many different dosage regimes are used: not all applicable to young fit day case patients
♦ Be prepared to be flexible due to inter-patient variability

Induction: infusion rates and dosage

The first Ohmeda 9000 syringe drivers (hailed as the great technological advance in infusion anaesthesia at the time) could deliver a bolus of induction agent at 1200, 600 and 300 ml/h. The accompanying advice was to infuse 2.25 mg/kg body weight at 1200 ml/kg body weight/h for 'normal' adults but with the caveat that this should be reduced to 600 ml/kg body weight/h for elderly or 'frail' patients. Such a technique was followed often by long periods of apnoea – especially if the patient had been given 1–1.5 µg/kg body weight of fentanyl as was established practice with induction with thiopentone. This troublesome apnoea was probably responsible for the delay in acceptance of the technique of total IV anaesthesia (TIVA) into general anaesthetic practice, as experienced practitioners used to thiopentone induction found this new technique more troublesome.

The ideal infusion rate for induction for a manual technique is 400 ml/ h, i.e. 1 ml every 8 s. This is much slower than the rate at which most IV drugs were administered. However, when using this rate and titrating the induction dose to the loss of eyelash reflex, it became immediately apparent that a far smaller dose of propofol was required to induce anaesthesia than the traditionally taught 2.25 mg/kg body weight. More importantly, provided the patient had not been given a heavy premedicant or heavy IV opiate analgesia, the period of apnoea following induction could be minimized and even eliminated with experience. It also follows that the perturbations in blood pressure, heart rate and ST segments were also greatly reduced and allowed for the possible safe employment of TIVA in patients where ischaemia by significant reduction in diastolic perfusion pressure was a risk.

By matching the induction dose to the response of the patient, variables such as anxiety, age and body build, i.e. factors known to affect anaesthetic requirements, were automatically taken into account.

Maintenance: infusion rates and dosage

Initially, as TIVA with propofol was being developed as an alternative technique to inhalational anaesthesia, there were various empirical formulae designed to provide a more or less constant plasma level. These varied from 12/9/6 mg/kg body weight/h to the well known 'Bristol' technique of 10/8/6 mg/kg body weight/h where the step-wise reductions were effected at 10 min intervals (16).

These formulae attempted to 'even out' the problems of trying to administer TIVA by repeated IV boluses which often lead to dramatically inappropriate awakening from anaesthesia and unsatisfactory oscillations in the level of consciousness. More rescue boluses were required when using a fixed bolus and fixed maintenance rate of 6 mg/kg/h compared with a fixed bolus and a step wise reduction of 10, 8 and then 6 mg/kg/h at 10 min intervals (17).

However, the Bristol technique was employed for patients (i) heavily premedicated with opiates and (ii) breathing 70% nitrous oxide (N_2O) in oxygen – both of which factors are known to significantly reduce the propofol requirement. Thus the 3 µg/ml plasma target that such a technique reasonably achieves is only acceptable in those circumstances. For patients breathing oxygen-enriched air, i.e. true TIVA, the plasma levels have to be higher.

Propofol has recently been released as a 2% formulation along side the established 1% formulation. In a recent paper where induction was by a bolus of 2 mg/kg over 40 s and anaesthesia was maintained by 15 s repeat boluses for surgery of a moderate duration, no statistically significant differences were found between the two formulations in respect of induction times, total induction doses, fentanyl requirements, cardio-respiratory perturbations or recovery times (18).

Manual Infusion rates: matching clinical circumstances and patient requirements

Early pharmacokinetic studies demonstrate that a constant rate infusion leads to an asymptotic rise and that a series of parallel graphs (Figures 5.2 and 5.3) are achieved when comparing differing infusion rates over time (19).

The combination of a bolus followed by a constant infusion leads to a more rapid achievement of the desired level (Figure 5.4.).

Fairly constant plasma concentrations can be maintained by inducing anaesthesia at a rate of 400 ml/h to the desired anaesthetic end-point immediately followed by a constant infusion rate of 10 times that bolus volume per hour followed by three exponential 20% reductions of the infusion rate at 5 min intervals. For example, if it takes 10 ml to induce anaesthesia, then the infusion rate for the first 5 min is 100 ml/h, for the second 5 min is 80 ml/h, for the third 5 min is 64 ml/h, and 5 min thereafter the rate is reduced and maintained at 51 ml/h. Thus one can observe that the 'steady state' rate is approximately half the initial rate.

This rate-reducing regime is titrated against each individual patient's response and thus automatically takes into account anxiety, age, body build, etc.

When jaw relaxation is adequate an appropriately sized laryngeal mask airway can be inserted and the patient allowed to breathe an air/oxygen mixture spontaneously. The infusion rate can be adjusted to maintain a respiratory rate between 10 and 14 breaths per minute. After 10 min the

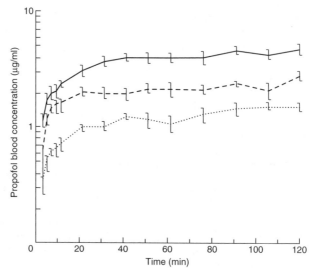

Figure 5.2   Mean propofol blood concentration ± SEM as a function of time during propofol infusions at 3 (dotted line), 6 (dashed line) or 9 (solid line) mg/kg/h.

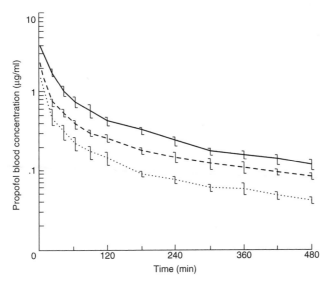

Figure 5.3   Mean propofol blood concentration ± SEM as a function of time after cessation of propofol infusions at 3 (dotted line), 6 (dashed line) or 9 (solid line) mg/kg/h. For clarity SEM of the first 10 data points are omitted.

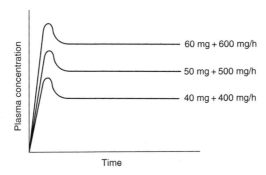

Figure 5.4   Graph showing theoretical combination of bolus + 10× ml/h infusions as parallel lines.

infusion rate should normally reduced to 8 mg/kg/h, but again, inter-patient variability needs to be taken into account. After another 10 min the infusion should be stepped down again, usually to 6 mg/kg/h.

However, anaesthetic requirements vary minute to minute with changes in surgical stimulus. The individual anaesthetist has to decide if such a regime needs to be increased or decreased to match the surgical stimulus. Employment of regional anaesthesia where possible will iron out such surgical perturbations.

Concomitant administration of opiates, non-steroidal anti-inflammatory analgesics and/or prior co-induction with benzodiazepines like midazolam will also affect the level of anaesthesia required (20). However, whilst the induction dose of propofol can be reduced by as much as 50%, it does reduce psychomotor recovery in the immediate postoperative phase following propofol infusion anaesthesia (21) even though it does not appear to have a significant effect on awakening time.

Drug combinations for concomitant infusion with propofol

Alfentanil

- Alfentanil was initially the most popular choice of opiate to administer with propofol because of all the available opioids its pharmacokinetic profile seemed to be the closest match. Since it is pharmaceutically stable as a mixture with propofol it can be simultaneously administered.
- Suggested ratios: for spontaneously breathing patients 1 μg of alfentanil to 400 μg of propofol and for ventilated patients 2 μg of alfentanil to 400 μg of propofol.
- Like propofol the pharmacokinetic profile of alfentanil follows a three-compartment model.
- However, the context-sensitive half-life of alfentanil makes it unsuitable for procedures longer than 1 h as its elimination can then take significantly longer than propofol.
- If it is planned to use alfentanil as the concurrent opiate then it must be administered by a separate infusion so that its administration can be stopped before that of propofol.
- Alfentanil is thus administered as a bolus of 10–15 μg/kg body weight followed by an exponentially decreasing step-wise infusion rate similar to propofol of 100/80/64–50 μg/kg body weight/h It can be very difficult, if not indeed frank guesswork, to decide when to terminate its infusion before that of propofol.
- A recent paper reminds us that recurrent respiratory depression although fortunately rare still can occur with alfentanil and that in day case anaesthesia standards of postoperative surveillance must not be allowed to fall too low (22).

Remifentanil

- Remifentanil with not only its short half-life but far more importantly its zero-order kinetics, because of its degradation by ubiquitous tissue cholinesterases, is the ideal choice for longer anaesthetics as its half-life is not context sensitive.
- For spontaneously breathing patients 1 μg of remifentanil is diluted in 40 ml of normal saline.

- The induction dose is 0.25–0.5 µg/kg body weight. The manufacturers recommendation of the higher 1 µg/kg body weight will result in frequent apnoea! (author's observations). Thus a 75 kg adult has an induction dose of 3–6 ml of this mixture given as a 'flash' bolus. This is then followed by an infusion of 0.25–0.5 µg/kg body weight/h, i.e. 18.75–37.5 ml/h for the 75 kg patient.
- This level will again need varying according to the surgical stimulus, the respiratory rate and the observed sympathetic responses.
- If the patient is breathing 70% N_2O the infusion rates of remifentanil may need to be halved or even quartered to 5–10 ml/h.
- Since it does not accumulate the infusion should not be discontinued until the surgical wound is dressed.
- A postoperative analgesic strategy [i.e. opiate patient-controlled analgesia (PCA), regional anaesthesia, intramuscular opiates, non-steroidal anti-inflammatory drugs (NSAIDs)] must be implemented before the remifentanil infusion is stopped.
- In the ventilated patient very high infusion rates have been employed, especially where the aim is to obtund the sympathetic response such as in anaesthesia for cardiac surgery, safe in the knowledge that such patients can still be expected to breathe spontaneously in recovery provided the infusion has been discontinued for a sufficient time before the end of the procedure.

Ketamine

Before the arrival of propofol, solubilized in soya emulsion and egg lecithin, ketamine had received a lot of attention as an IV anaesthetic. It was combined with flunitrazepam for induction (23) or with Althesin (24). Both techniques had numerous problems from muscular hyper-tonus, spontaneous movement, and a high incidence of postoperative nausea and vomiting. It lost favour but is now being re-examined because of further knowledge about its pharmacology.

- Ketamine is now infused preoperatively as an analgesic adjunct. It is administered in order to decrease secondary wound hyperalgesia postoperatively by its antagonistic action on N-methyl-D-aspartate receptors (25) but the concentration is much lower than previously employed.
- It can be satisfactorily mixed with propofol and alfentanil as the mixture is pharmaceutically stable for the period of anaesthesia; however, the ratio is under scrutiny as earlier papers published reported an unacceptably high incidence of psychotropic reactions (26).
- It has a similar pharmacokinetic profile to both alfentanil and propofol for operations of up to 1 h duration, though it has a slightly longer brain equilibration half-life.
- A dose of 25 mg of ketamine to 500 mg propofol, i.e. a ratio of 1:20, is sufficient to provide analgesia and obtund secondary hyperalgesia. At

this level of administration psychotropic side effects are rare. (Compare the dose of 2 mg/kg body weight as the recommended IV induction bolus, i.e. 150 mg for a 75 kg patient with the 25–50 mg that is administered if only 50–100 ml of the anaesthetic mixture is required for a whole operation.)

♦ It is therefore unnecessary to have the big 'QUIET – KETAMINE ANAESTHESIA' placards over the patient's bed!

♦ This dosage level of ketamine may be modified in the future in the light of the discovery of peripheral ketamine receptors. Combinations of local anaesthesia and ketamine administered regionally may further reduce anaesthetic requirements.

♦ Once the S-(+)-ketamine enantiomer is clinically available, the dose may need further reduction as S-(+)-ketamine is more potent than the racemic ketamine.

Changes in surgical stimulus and alterations in manually adjusted infusion rates

♦ If the increase in stimulus is likely to be short lived then an empirical bolus of 2–5 ml of TIVA mixture without the need to alter the predetermined infusion rates will probably suffice.

♦ However, if it appears that the increase in surgical stimulus is likely to be prolonged, or that the level of anaesthesia previously set is too light, then in addition to the bolus an increase in the infusion rate by 10 times the amount of the bolus is required. For example, if the infusion rate is 80 ml/h and a 4 ml bolus is required, then the new infusion rate should be set at 120 ml/h immediately after the bolus has been given (at 400 ml/h remember).

♦ If this occurs in the middle of the reducing steps, then the reductions must continue at the new higher level until the fourth step has been reached.

♦ Note the converse is also true. If the rate seems too high and the rate is reduced by 20% stat, then the next step reduction goes for the new lower value. For example, if the rate was 100 ml/h and it needs to be reduced to 80 ml/h stat, then the next step reduction, when due and not 5 min from the last stat reduction, must be 20% of the lower value, i.e. to 64 ml, so the rate will have gone from 100 to 64 ml/h in 5 min.

Target-controlled infusion techniques in day surgery

The TCI system (i.e. the 'Diprifusor') has greatly simplified the administration of IV anaesthesia with propofol. The manual infusion techniques are sometimes difficult to control, needing extra boluses and alterations in infusion rates with unpredictable effects on blood pressure, respiratory rate and recovery time. The computer-controlled model helps by maintaining a constant plasma concentration of anaesthetic agent against which the anaesthetist can judge whether depth of anaesthesia is sufficient. If the anaesthetist needs to adjust the depth of anaesthesia either up or down, the TCI system will achieve a new steady state as rapidly as possible. The system has in-built safety features which help prevent the administration of incorrect drugs. Software also takes into account what the pump has actually delivered to adjust for pump mechanism errors. Current 'Diprifusor' software can accommodate patients over 15 years of age and up to 150 kg body weight. It is possible to connect computers running TCI software (e.g. Stan pump) obtained from the Internet to some infusion pumps (e.g. the Graseby 3400). This practice should be strongly discouraged, as this type of software is only intended for use in ethically approved clinical research projects and does not have regulatory approval like the 'Diprifusor' system. Also this type of software does not allow for inaccuracies in what the pump actually delivers to the patient, so at some settings there may be significant under-dosage of anaesthetic.

Effect-site anaesthetic concentration

Newer TCI systems also compute and display effect-site anaesthetic concentration which can help to predict more accurately timing of recovery from anaesthesia. The effect-site concentration display also helps when learning the technique by showing the anaesthetist how long the drug takes to reach its site of action.

The TCI system has important benefits when inducing anaesthesia in elderly patients for whom large rapid boluses can produce profound hypotension and apnoea. There is a tendency for the required target plasma concentration of propofol to decrease with increasing age, but the spread of inter-patient variability makes it impossible to predict what will be required in a given individual. With a TCI system it is possible to induce anaesthesia very gradually, building up the plasma concentration in a stepwise fashion. This avoids peaks in plasma anaesthetic concentration of propofol and gives time for the effect-site concentration to build up slowly in parallel with the plasma concentration. The result is a smooth pleasant induction without large changes in blood pressure or respiratory rate, even when used for elderly patients with poor left ventricular function. Day case surgery is now being offered to increasingly elderly and less fit patients: the TCI system helps to minimize potential anaesthetic complications and achieve a rapid recovery from anaesthesia more reliably.

Advantages of TCI systems

◆ Simplifies IV anaesthesia techniques
◆ Rapid control of depth of anaesthesia
◆ A constant plasma concentration of anaesthetic aids decisions about when to alter depth of anaesthesia
◆ Effect site concentration helps to predict recovery time and induction of anaesthesia
◆ Slower induction techniques reduce hypotension and apnoea in elderly and less fit day case patients

Some examples of TIVA for common general and gynaecological surgical cases

The young fit patient: rapid induction of anaesthesia for day case laparoscopic cholecystectomy [uses: TCI propofol, separate remifentanil infusion, intermittent positive pressure ventilation (IPPV)]

Laparoscopic cholecystectomy can be a successful day case procedure, provided the patient is selected carefully, the procedure is uncomplicated, postoperative analgesia is adequate and there is appropriate support for the patient following discharge.

◆ Establish IV infusion, e.g. 1000 ml Hartmann's solution
◆ Co-induction with 2 mg midazolam given 2 min before induction
◆ Attach propofol and remifentanil infusion lines, as close to the IV cannula as possible, remifentanil nearest the patient
◆ Start remifentanil infusion (20 µg/ml solution or 1 mg in 50 ml saline) at 0.1 µg/kg/min
◆ Start propofol TCI system at 6 µg/ml
◆ Continue verbal contact with patient for as long as possible – a few patients may need a higher target concentration, particularly if young and anxious (but be prepared to wait for effect-site concentration to catch up with plasma concentration)
◆ When you have adequate anaesthesia, with no response to painful stimulus (e.g. pressure behind the angle of mandible), reduce the plasma target concentration to equal the effect-site concentration
◆ Give suitable dose of neuromuscular blocking drug (e.g. 0.5 mg/kg atracurium – it is possible to do laparoscopic cholecystectomy in less than 20 min) and commence manual ventilation until an endotracheal tube has been placed satisfactorily
◆ Nitrous oxide or air can be used for IPPV using this technique
◆ If there are signs of inadequate analgesia give a bolus of remifentanil (0.2 µg/kg) and increase the infusion to 0.2 µg/kg
◆ Keep TCI target unless there is hypotension when it can be reduced by 20%
◆ Postoperative analgesia is vital with remifentanil: consider diclofenac 75 mg by IV infusion or ketorolac 10 mg IV
◆ At the end of the procedure the surgeon can spray 20 ml of 0.5% bupivacaine at the gall bladder bed with the patient slightly head down and tilted to the right
◆ Stop the propofol infusion, reverse any residual neuromuscular blockade if necessary and stop the remifentanil infusion
◆ Spontaneous respiration normally returns within a few minutes followed shortly afterwards by a rapid return of consciousness when the endo-tracheal tube can be removed

Some patients may need further analgesia which can be achieved by a number of means: intermittent IV fentanyl, PCA alfentanil, PCA

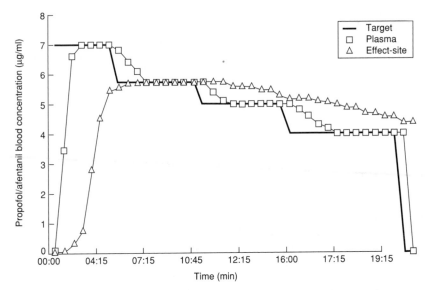

Figure 5.5 Example of rapid induction technique (propofol/alfentanil mixture) (actual recording from a 32-year-old ASA I day case patient for laproscopic sterilization using a Fresenius Master TCI system).

remifentanil or a slow continuous infusion of remifentanil (e.g. 0.02 µg/kg/min) for 2–4 h provided delivery devices, monitoring equipment and trained recovery staff are available. A few patients may initially need small doses of IV morphine titrated to effect. Take-home analgesia: diclofenac 75 mg BD and co-dydramol 2 tablets 6 hourly for 4 days.

Figure 5.5 shows an example of real data from a patient where the rapid TCI induction technique was used.

In this case a mixture of propofol 500 mg and alfentanil 1.25 mg was used and the patient allowed to breathe an air/oxygen mixture spontaneously. Here an initial target of 7 µg/ml was selected for rapid induction and insertion of a laryngeal mask airway (LMA). Once the operation was underway (laparoscopic sterilization) the target concentration was gradually reduced while observing the patients response to surgery. This technique is analogous to the overpressure technique used during induction of patients with volatile anaesthetics.

The elderly day case patient: slow induction of anaesthesia for open repair of inguinal hernia (uses: TCI propofol combined with alfentanil, spontaneous ventilation via LMA)

◆ Establish IV infusion, e.g. 1000 ml Hartmann's solution
◆ Co-induction with 2 mg midazolam given 2 min before induction

- Inject 1.25 mg alfentanil using aseptic precautions into 500 mg propofol pre-filled syringe and mix thoroughly
- Pre-oxygenate with 100% oxygen via face mask
- Start TCI system with an initial target plasma concentration of 1–2 µg/ml
- Increase plasma target concentration by 0.5 µg/ml every 30 s until loss of consciousness and LMA can be inserted
- Adjust target concentration according to surgical stimulus and patient response

For large hernias which are difficult to reduce it may be necessary to give a small dose of neuromuscular blocking drug, e.g. atracurium 0.5 mg/kg, and commence gentle IPPV via the laryngeal mask airway, keeping inflation pressures below 15 cmH$_2$O until recovery of neuromuscular function.

Postoperative analgesia options: ilio-inguinal nerve block, direct infiltration of local anaesthetic by surgeon, diclofenac IV or PR, ketorolac 10 mg IV. Take-home analgesia for 4 days.

Figure 5.6. shows an example of real data from an 83-year-old man with atrial fibrillation having varicose vein surgery using the slow induction technique with a Fresenius Master TCI system. The syringe contained 500 mg propofol and 1.25 mg alfentanil. All parameters were maintained within acceptable limits with no great fluctuations. Ventilation was spontaneous throughout and he awoke within 5 min without complications. Satisfactory postoperative analgesia was achieved using 10 mg of IV ketorolac.

An example technique for day case laparoscopic sterilization using a bolus and manual infusion (uses: combined propofol and alfentanil infusion)

- Insert and secure a suitable indwelling IV cannula
- Start IV infusion of 1000 ml Hartmann's solution or normal saline
- Midazolam 2 mg IV 2 min before induction of anaesthesia
- Co-induction is useful to reduce the overall anaesthetic requirements without increasing the recovery time in day case patients. It also helps in the anaesthetic room or theatre to reduce anxiety, which is often at its highest just before induction in these unpremedicated patients.
- A simple analgesic technique is to mix 1.25 mg alfentanil with each 500 mg of propofol in the same syringe. Taking aseptic precautions, this mixture is stable for up to 6 h

Postoperative pain relief should be started before the end of surgery. Ketorolac 10 mg IV or diclofenac 75 mg by IV infusion can be given in theatre or diclofenac 100 mg orally or rectally can be given preoperatively. The timing should be such that adequate plasma levels are achieved before the patient recovers from anaesthesia. Local anaesthetics can also be used, externally around the access ports, and topically, as gel on the

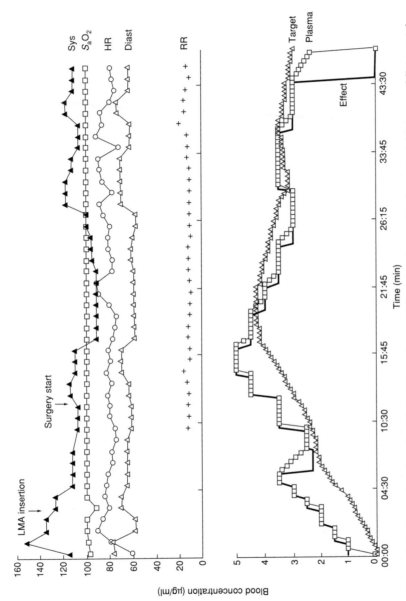

Figure 5.6 Example of gradual induction using a TCI system in an elderly patient (83 years old) in atrial fibrillation with poor left ventricular function (automatic recording of vital signs and recording of infusion data from a Fresenius Master TCI system).

Fallopian clips, or by spraying (e.g. 20 ml 0.5% plain bupivacaine) over the Fallopian tubes with the patient in a slight head-up tilt so that the local anaesthetic collects in the pouch of Douglas.

Some patients may require additional small boluses of fentanyl in the recovery unit, but most should be able to go home within 4 h with adequate take-home analgesia for at least 3 days. Diclofenac 75 mg 12 hourly with co-dydramol 2 tablets 6 hourly is an effective combination if there are no contra-indications to NSAIDs.

References

1. Miller DR. Intravenous infusion anaesthesia and delivery devices. *Can J Anaesth* 1994; **41**: 639–50.
2. Fuergaard K, Jenstrup M, Schierbeck J, Wiberg-Jorgensen F. Total intravenous anaesthesia with propofol or etomidate. *Eur J Anaesth* 1991; **8**: 385–91.
3. Peacock JE, Spiers SP, McLaughlan GA, Edmonson WC, Berhoud M, Reily CS. Infusion of propofol to identify smallest effective doses for induction of anaesthesia in young and elderly patients. *Br J Anaesth* 1993; **70**: 383–4.
4. Taylor IN, Kenny GNC. Requirements for target-controlled infusion of propofol to insert the laryngeal mask airway. *Anaesthesia* 1998; **53**: 222–6.
5. Larsson JE, Wahlstrom. Optimum rate of administration of propofol for induction of anaesthesia in rats. *Br J Anaesth* 1994; **73**: 692–4.
6. Struys M, Versichelen L, Thas O, Herregods L, Rolly G. Comparison of computer-controlled administration of propofol with two manually controlled techniques. *Anaesthesia* 1997; **52**: 41–50.
7. Knell PJ. Total intravenous anaesthesia by an intermittent technique. Use of methohexitone, ketamine and a muscle relaxant. *Anaesthesia* 1983; **38**: 586–7.
8. Gepts E. Pharmacokinetic concepts. *Anaesthesia* 1998; **53** (suppl 1): 9.
9. Bailey JM. A technique for approximately maintaining constant plasma levels of intravenous drugs. *Anaesthesiology* 1993; **78**: 116–23.
10. Anderson L, Robb H. Comparison of Midazolam co-induction with propofol pre dosing for induction of anaesthesia. *Anaesthesia* 1998; **53**: 1117–29.
11. White PF. Use of a continuous infusion versus intermittent bolus administration of fentanyl or ketamine during out patient anaesthesia. *Anaesthesiology* 1983; **59**: 294–300.
12. Rocke DA, Rubin J, Brock-Utne JG, Downing JW. Total intravenous anaesthesia for major gynaecological surgery. *Anaesthesia and Intensive Care* 1981; **9**: 119–23.
13. Fragen RJ, Avram MJ, Henthorn TK, Caldwell NJ. A pharmacokinetically designed etomidate infusion regimen for hypnosis. *Anaesth Analg* 1983; **62**: 654–60.
14. Less NW, Antonios WR. Two-stage infusion of etomidate for the induction and maintenance of anaesthesia. *Br J Anaesth* 1984; **56**: 1239–42.
15. Kay B. Etomidate and alfentanil infusion for major surgery. *Acta Anaesthesiol Belgica* 1984; **35**: 19–24.
16. Tackley RM, Lewis GTR, Prys-Roberts C, Boaden RW, Harvey JR. Open loop control of propofol infusions. *Br J Anaesth* 1987; **59**: 935P
17. Gill SS, Lewis RP, Reilly CS. Maintenance of anaesthesia with propofol – a comparative study of a step down infusion of propofol and a low dose infusion supplemented by a incremental doses. *Eur J Anaesth* 1992; **9**: 203–7.

18. Servin FS, Desmonts JM, Melloni C, Martinelli G. A comparison of 2% and 1% formulations of propofol for the induction and maintenance of anaesthesia in surgery of moderate duration. *Anaesthesia* 1997; **52**: 1212–29.
19. Gepts E, Camu F, Cockshott ID, Douglas EJ. Disposition of propofol administered as constant rate intravenous infusions in humans. *Anaesth Analg* 1987; **66**: 1256–63.
20. Tzabar Y, Brydon C, Gillies GW. Induction of anaesthesia with midazolam and a target-controlled propofol infusion. *Anaesthesia* 1996; **51**: 536–8.
21. Tighe KE, Warner JA. The effect of co-induction with midazolam upon the recovery from propofol infusion anaesthesia. *Anaesthesia* 1997; **52**: 998–1014.
22. Sternlo JEG, Sandin RH. Recurrent respiratory depression after total intravenous anaesthesia with propofol and alfentanil. *Anaesthesia* 1998; **53**: 369–81.
23. Barclay A, Houlton PC, Downing JW. Total intravenous anaesthesia: a technique using flunitrazepam, ketamine, muscle relaxants and controlled ventilation of the lung. *Anaesthesia* 1980; **35**: 287–90.
24. Keith I, Shenoy BJ. Total anaesthesia with low dose ketamine and Althesin. Assessment of a technique for minor surgery in difficult situations. *Anaesthesia* 1981; **36**: 702–4.
25. Guit JB, Koning HM, Corter ML, *et al.* Ketamine analgesia for total intravenous anaesthesia with propofol. *Anaesthesia* 1991; **46**: 24–7.
26. Dunnihoo M, Wuest A, Meyer M, Robinson M. The effects of total intravenous anaesthesia using propofol, ketamine, and vecuronium on cardiovascular response and wake up time. *Am Assoc Nurse Anaesthet J* 1994; **62**: 261–6.

PART 2

SPECIFIC ISSUES

6

Awareness and total intravenous anaesthesia

J. G. Jones and T. Leary

- Consciousness and memory
- Effect of different agents on memory
- Changes in depth of anaesthesia on implicit memory
- Incidence of awareness with differing anaesthetic techniques
- Methods of measuring depth of anaesthesia

Consciousness and memory

Awareness during general anaesthesia implies both *consciousness* and *memory* of a particular intraoperative event. Almost invariably this means a failure to deliver sufficient anaesthetic to the patient. Remember that it is possible for a very lightly anaesthetized patient to be conscious but to have no explicit memory of intraoperative events. While the experience of *consciousness* is familiar to all of us, it has not been feasible to produce a convincing explanation of this state nor has it been possible to explain the effects of general anaesthetics on consciousness and memory.

At a simple level the content of consciousness is provided by four interconnected regions of the brain which sequentially deal with (i) stimulus uptake or perception, (ii) stimulus processing, (iii) stimulus evaluation and (iv) the response to the stimulus. We must distinguish between stimulus uptake or perception by the brain, which is unconscious, and the conscious experience of this stimulus. Positron emission tomography (PET) may be used to produce beautiful pictures showing activation of some of the different regions of the brain which may be involved in these processes. It is easy to imagine how a general anaesthetic, which interrupts synaptic transmission, can thereby interfere with the transmission between these regions and thus ablate consciousness.

An example of a conscious response to a stimulus, implying the operation of all four regions, is the use of language to describe an object perceived by the eye. For example, a subject may see a desk and describe it as 'an untidy desk'. Also one can see an untidy desk and, without uttering a word, think 'what an untidy desk'. Interestingly, whether or not words are spoken, the PET picture of the speech area (Broca 44) shows simultaneous activation. Thus the four functional domains work together – the end result is to activate a response in the speech area with or without the subject actually enunciating any audible words.

Surgical division of the corpus collosum presents an important example of the effects of interrupting access between the visual cortex and the speech centre. If, in such a right-handed person, an object is placed in the right visual field, the left optic cortex is activated and impulses pass to the speech centre on that side. As expected, the subject sees the object and describes it. If, however, an object is placed in the left visual field the impulses cannot pass from the right visual cortex to the speech centre and the subject is unaware of the object. He may, however, make a correct guess but he is nevertheless unconscious of the existence of that object (Figure 6.1).

Description of a more complex scene by normal subjects will need to include the use of other parts of the brain which are involved in *memory*. Memory can be thought of as a mirror of our perceptions, thoughts and experiences (1). We rely on memory when taking part in conversation, preparing a meal, reading, contemplating past events, planning future events, travelling and many other activities. In organic amnesia, e.g. Alzheimer's disease, the first two examples may be preserved but the other activities may be completely disrupted because the ability to learn new information is impaired. Such patients are living only in the present and cannot register or recall any long-term memories. Alzheimer's patients are always meeting new people! The processes underlying the registration of memories which may last a lifetime probably involve long-term potentiation in the hippocampus, then gene expression and new protein synthesis in cells of the frontal cortex. It is not known how this process breaks down during either general anaesthesia or organic amnesia.

Anaesthetic sedation and memory

It is now becoming more widely known that a sedative dose of a general anaesthetic produces a reversible model of organic amnesia and creates a state where the patient can carry on a perfectly normal conversation but within a few seconds has no memory of that particular event. However, unlike organic amnesia such as Alzheimer's disease, there is no disturbance of recall from previously encoded long-term memory.

Implicit memory – the painful handshake

Other comparisons of the effect of organic amnesia and anaesthetic sedation on *explicit* and *implicit* memories are interesting. In organic

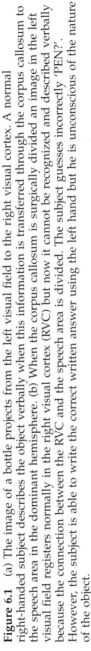

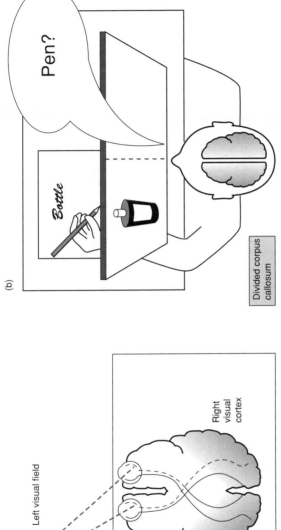

Figure 6.1 (a) The image of a bottle projects from the left visual field to the right visual cortex. A normal right-handed subject describes the object verbally when this information is transferred through the corpus callosum to the speech area in the dominant hemisphere. (b) When the corpus callosum is surgically divided an image in the left visual field registers normally in the right visual cortex (RVC) but now it cannot be recognized and described verbally because the connection between the RVC and the speech area is divided. The subject guesses incorrectly 'PEN?'. However, the subject is able to write the correct written answer using the left hand but he is unconscious of the nature of the object.

amnesia the explicit memory of contemporaneous events is much more disrupted than is the implicit memory of these events. In fact implicit memory in organic amnesia may be unaffected. A classical example of this is as follows. A physician on his rounds sees a patient with an organic amnesia. He shakes hands with the patient but he has previously concealed a pin in his hand which causes the patient to jump away with pain. The next day the doctor sees the patient again and after a chat it is obvious that she has no recollection of seeing him before. Nevertheless, she refuses to shake hands at the end of the consultation. She had no explicit memory of their previous meeting but she did have an *implicit memory* of the painful experience. She cannot recall the memory of the painful experience but the cue of offering to shake hands leads to appropriate avoiding action.

Only a very small fraction of the stream of sensory stimuli which is continually entering the brain is ultimately represented in consciousness. This stream of information may continue during general anaesthesia but in the unconscious patient, while the processes which underlie conscious experience are completely disrupted, there may well be registration of memories of some perioperative events which can be recalled post-operatively but only by the presentation to the patient of relevant cues. These *implicit memories*, unlike *explicit memories*, cannot be retrieved by making an effort to recall some specific information or chronological sequence of events. In contrast, explicit memory describes the effort needed to recall events often in vivid detail and in correct chronological sequence. Implicit memory is the automatic recall in response to a cue of a previous experience (the painful hand shake). We will discuss in more detail below the effects of low-dose general anaesthetics on these two types of memory.

Cognition and memory during general anaesthetic administration

It has frequently been claimed that general anaesthetics cause greater effects on explicit than implicit memory and there are impressive demonstrations in the literature of implicit memories being encoded even in anaesthetized patients. However, recent research suggests that the effect of anaesthetic sedation on both types of memory may be similar in volunteers who are not undergoing surgery (2) but the stress of surgery may facilitate the registration of implicit memory (Andrade, personal communication).

Awareness during anaesthesia is not simply an all or none phenom-enon. A gradual increase in the dose of a general anaesthetic produces a progressive impairment of memory. We (1) divide what is probably a continuous process into four stages of perception and memory of intraoperative events:

1. Conscious perception with explicit memory
2. Conscious perception without explicit memory   INCREASING ↓
3. Subconscious perception with implicit memory   ANAESTHETIC ↓
4. No perception

A paralysed patient in Stage 4 with neither explicit or implicit memory of intraoperative events may awaken fully to Stage 1 during surgery if there is a failure of the anaesthetic delivery system. The patient wakes up, may be in agony, is naturally terrified, particularly if he/she cannot move, and will remember all the explicit details afterwards. The incidence of this is not known with any certainty but may be about 1:10 000 of elective general anaesthetics. A more common problem, about 2:1000 elective general anaesthetics, is that the patient may have an explicit recollection of part of the procedure. This is often elicited only on postoperative questioning and is rarely volunteered by the patient. Stage 2 has been well demonstrated by Russell (see 1) using the isolated arm method in patients with neuromuscular blockade. His lightly anaesthetized but paralysed patients are able to communicate with the anaesthetist using the isolated hand but after the operation they have no explicit memory of intraoperative events. Bethune *et al.* have shown similar results in cardiac surgical patients and they also showed implicit memory of intraoperative events (see 1). As we shall discuss below, there is considerable debate about Stage 3, subconscious perception with implicit memory of intraoperative events.

While implicit memory is a normal process in fully awake subjects it is not yet clear if this may be more resistant to the effects of anaesthetics than the processes involved in registration of explicit memory. *What is not in dispute is that the concentration of general anaesthetic required to abolish consciousness and explicit memory of intraoperative events is much less than that required to abolish movement in response to painful stimulation. Unfortunately this end-point, and the concept of MAC, has underpinned thinking in anaesthesia for 30 years, but it is now time to move on to reconsider other, cognitive, end-points of anaesthetic action.*

Anaesthetic sedation and conscious perception

Relatively few experiments have been carried out to examine cognitive end-points in subjects exposed to gradually increasing doses of general anaesthetic. Artusio (see 1) used small doses of ether alone to provide analgesia during cardiac surgery. He divided the earliest stages of anaesthesia into three planes as shown in Figure 6.2. Plane 1 existed from the start of anaesthetic administration to the start of impaired pain sensation. Cognitive function seemed to be normal at this stage. Partial analgesia in Plane 2 begins as Plane 1 ends. During Plane 2 there is only partial pain relief but there was a considerable impairment of memory for contemporary events. There was absent memory for these events during Plane 3, the patient seemed comfortable, had

	Plane 1	Plane 2	Plane 3
Response to spoken voice	Normal	Normal	Slowing → nil
Cerebration	Normal	Normal	Slowing → nil
Memory for contemporary events	Normal	Considerably impaired	Absent
Memory for past events	Normal	Normal	Normal → nil
Focus of eyes	Normal	Normal	Impaired → nil
Analgesia	None	Partial	Profound

Figure 6.2 Cerebration and sensory perception during stage 1 of anaesthesia after Artusio (see 1).

difficulty in focussing the eyes, colour perception was dimmed, there was a confused response to questions, then consciousness was lost. Artusio felt that this was the ideal state for surgery, in fact at this stage cardiac surgery was carried out in the majority of his patients and intra-abdominal surgery on the remainder. *More than 40 years ago Artusio felt that the use of larger doses of general anaesthetics associated with the surgical stage of anaesthesia would become a thing of the past.* This has recently been endorsed in an editorial in the *British Journal of Anaesthesia* by Andrade and Jones (2).

Tomlin *et al.* (3) studied subjective and objective sensory responses to inhalation of either nitrous oxide (N_2O) or methoxyflurane in 11 subjects and made the following observations:

- Hearing: objective testing indicated that hearing remained unchanged almost to the point of unresponsiveness but failure of response to sound occurred before the subject appeared unconscious as judged by two observing anaesthetists
- Vision: no changes in field of vision or colour vision were detected in any subject up to the point of loss of responsiveness
- Pain: sharp pain was felt only as touch very early during methoxyflurane inhalation
- Peripheral sensation and vibration sense did not change until consciousness was lost

Tomlin *et al.* reported flights of ideas and delusions of grandeur during experiments breathing N_2O, and that 'During the second or third gaseous experience there is a regretful awareness that it will be difficult to recall these thoughts later'. There was also an intense feeling of *déjà vu*. Tomlin describes dealing brilliantly with some problem but 'couldn't remember what the problem was'. He mentioned that previously Humphrey Davy had reported that 'Vivid ideas poured rapidly through my mind. I existed in a world of newly connected and newly modified ideas. I imagined that I had made discoveries. I endeavoured to recall the ideas, they were feeble and indistinct'. The author (J. G. J.) has consistently noted similar experiences when breathing low concentrations of N_2O but has never experienced such flights of ideas with low doses of either halothane, isoflurane, enflurane, sevoflurane or propofol. This suggests that N_2O has unique properties on cognitive function at these doses which may be mediated through an opioid system. It would be interesting to see if naloxone prevented this effect.

Effects of isoflurane alone on memory

Artusio's study using ether has been confirmed in two studies with low doses of isoflurane, 0.2 MAC end-tidal concentration. At Northwick Park, Newton *et al.* (see 1) showed that this concentration produced amnesia for words presented to volunteers when they were equilibrated at this anaesthetic concentration although they were able to respond normally to commands and carry on conversations at this concentration. Here in Cambridge we (see 1) have carried out more detailed studies of the effects of isoflurane on working memory. This was assessed by the within-list recognition (WLR) test where memory of a word is tested within a few seconds of presentation. Performance on this task depends on a combination of working memory, attention and longer-term recognition memory. A number of word lists are read out to the subject, each list comprising 16 relatively infrequent and abstract nouns; seven of these words being repeated, giving a total of 23 words per list (Figure 6.3a). Words were repeated either immediately or after one, two, four, eight or 16 intervening words. The position of the repeated words varied from list to list, with the proviso that one immediate repeat came near the start of the list and the other came near the end. The subject has to identify the repeated word as soon as it is presented.

A typical list is shown in Figure 6.3(a) and the mean values of the results are given for a group of subjects breathing low-dose isoflurane following a baseline run breathing air (Figure 6.3b). With 0.2% end-tidal isoflurane there was a fall in WLR for repeat word intervals of four or greater. With 0.4% end-tidal isoflurane there was considerable inaccuracy in identifying even words which were immediately repeated. However, a painful (electrical) nerve stimulation produced sufficient arousal to improve the accuracy of WLR particularly for repeats with fewer than four intervening words. After such experiments, although the subjects looked fully conscious at the time, they had no recollection of performing the WLR test.

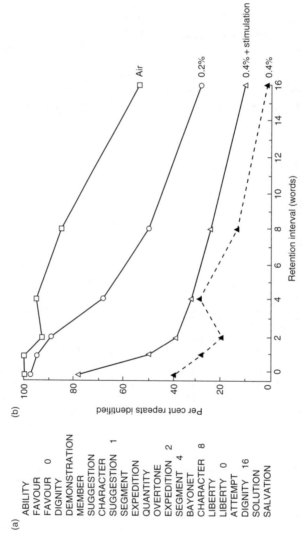

Figure 6.3 (a) A WLR test was used to test working memory in volunteers breathing air or low concentrations of isoflurane. Some words are repeated at different word intervals, shown by the number written after the words, and the subject must identify these repeated words. Two sets of direct repeats are included to confirm that subjects' attention was maintained throughout the list. (b) The right panel shows that the control subject has an accurate recall of words presented with few intervening words (see text) but performance declines with increasing word interval. Performance at different end-tidal concentrations of isoflurane is indicated. A painful stimulus, applied at a constant end-tidal concentration, improves performance.

Effect of continuous propofol administration on memory

Using the method described above we (4) have studied working memory in a different group of volunteers with propofol infusions. In this study we compared infusion dose, plasma propofol concentration, WLR and an auditory evoked response method. When we compared psychological performance using the WLR test with simultaneous measurement of auditory evoked potential (AEP) there was a significant correlation ($p <$ 0.005). *However, there was no significant correlation between infusion dose and psychological performance or between infusion dose and plasma concentration. These data show that over the dose range of propofol required to produce the complete range of cognitive impairment from just sedated to unconscious the processed electroencephalogram (EEG) is a better measure of cognitive perform- ance than various measures of dose, including plasma concentration.*

Of considerable interest was the response to painful stimulation. The electrical stimulation test was designed to cause arousal and would have been unpleasant in non-sedated subjects. It did in fact produce arousal, i.e. subjects opened their eyes and looked around, but this either could not be remembered subsequently or if it was the experience was not recalled as painful.

Effects of different methods of sedation on memory

Investigators have questioned whether drugs either affect memory directly or whether the 'amnesic' effects may reflect impairments in attention, arousal or mood rather than memory processes. Veselis *et al.* (5) have demonstrated unequal amnesic effects of midazolam, propofol, thiopentone and fentanyl. For example, propofol shows a high likelihood of exceeding the criterion of memory impairment well before it meets criteria of sedation; in contrast, fentanyl exceeds the sedation criteria and shows a low probability for amnesia for the same concentration range. Propofol has equivalent amnesic effects to those of midazolam at equal sedation. Whilst these results suggest that memory and sedation are distinct processes which can be affected by drugs independently, the results should be interpreted with caution. A recent editorial suggests that combinations of powerful analgesics and sedative doses of anaes- thetics may result in a conscious patient during surgery with neither implicit or explicit memory of intraoperative events and it was proposed that this might be acceptable for routine surgery (2). As mentioned earlier, this was precisely the proposal of Artusio more than 40 years ago.

Subconscious perception with implicit memory

So far we have concentrated largely on the effects of anaesthetics on various aspects of sensation and *explicit memory* but we have also alluded to the rather contradictory evidence about anaesthetic effects on *implicit memory*. We defined explicit memory as the conscious effort needed to recall every detail of a particular event in the exact sequence that the event developed. *Implicit memory* is inferred when there is a change in behaviour as a result of a previous stimulus but the person has no recognition or recall of that stimulus. Implicit memory is revealed when previous experiences facilitate performance on tasks that do not require conscious or intentional recollection of these experiences. There is considerable interest in the possibility of *implicit memory* formation during general anaesthesia because this may have either advantageous or deleterious postoperative effects. The possibility of subconscious perception with implicit memory of intraoperative events is still a very controversial subject and will be outlined below.

We have shown that a gradual increase in anaesthetic concentration leads first to a progressive reduction in working memory then loss of consciousness. Implicit memory of intra-anaesthetic events may remain after loss of consciousness and, as a consequence, postoperative behaviour may be modified by the administration of auditory information (priming) during anaesthesia.

The evidence of explicit recall during anaesthesia can be detected postoperatively with tests of free recall. When explicit memory is lost, indirect tests of memory must be used to demonstrate evidence of implicit memory and learning. In such tests the subject is not required to retrieve information about the learning episode, rather implicit memory for the events is inferred from altered performance. Examples of such indirect memory tests include Category Generation, Free Association, Stem Completion and Forced Choice Recognition. There is considerable conflict about the possibility of implicit memory of intraoperative events. Some years ago Ghoneim and Block (see 1) listed 14 papers showing implicit memory during anaesthesia, whereas Merikle and Rondi (see 1) concluded that 'there is not a single consistent finding indicating that adequately anaesthetized patients do in fact remember events during anaesthesia'.

More recently, Merikle and Daneman (6) carried out a meta-analysis on 44 studies of memory for unconsciously perceived events by anaesthetized patients. They showed that positive suggestions had no effect on postoperative recovery but also showed that specific information can be registered as implicit memories as long as postoperative testing was not delayed longer than 36 h. *However, they suggested that unconsciously perceived information may have a longer lasting impact if the material is personally relevant and meaningful.*

Salience of the stimulus

In this regard the *salience of the stimulus* may be important. In the previously mentioned study of Newton *et al.* (see 1) shock words were learnt at higher (but subanaesthetic) doses of isoflurane than neutral words. Using incremental doses of isoflurane (0.1, 0.2 and 0.4 MAC), Newton *et al.* demonstrated that the absence of a response to a command generated no recall, whereas response to a command was not necessarily remembered. They were also able to demonstrate the effects of attention; subjects' memory for a list of neutral words was lost at 0.2 MAC, yet memory of a shock word was present at this concentration.

In many studies a neutral auditory stimulus is presented in the face of the far more salient (and frightening) stimulus of surgery. Andrade (personal communication) has recently shown that memory for events during anaesthesia is more likely during surgery than when anaesthetics are given for experimental studies in volunteers not scheduled for surgery. Cork *et al.* (see 1) have demonstrated the absence of explicit or implicit memory of words presented during sufentanil and N_2O/oxygen anaesthesia, yet nine of 25 patients reported vague dreamlike recollections of intraoperative events.

The studies investigating this subject utilize a wide variety of indirect memory tests making comparison of results difficult. The most appropriate type of test to detect evidence of implicit memory has yet to be determined. The timing of the postoperative testing may also influence the results and as mentioned above, Merikle and Daneman (6) in their meta-analysis found that up to 36 h was the most appropriate time.

Interaction between the effect of surgery and depth of anaesthesia on intraoperative memory – the Robinson Crusoe experiment

We have described the effect of gradually increasing anaesthetic concentration on working memory. It would seem intuitively obvious that the results generated by research into memory and learning during general anaesthesia would be influenced by anaesthetic depth, yet in the absence, until recently, of any generally accepted monitor of depth of anaesthesia, it was impossible to determine whether the stimuli were presented to the patients at equivalent depths of anaesthesia. There is now convincing evidence that unconscious processing of auditory information and implicit memory of intraoperative events occurs in patients in whom the early cortical potentials of the mid-latency auditory evoked potential (MLAEP) are preserved during general anaesthesia (see below for more detailed discussion of the MLAEP). Schwender *et al.* (see 1) studied patients undergoing cardiac surgery, anaesthetized with high-dose fentanyl and either flunitrazepam, isoflurane or propofol. During the operation the story of Robinson Crusoe was played to the patients and postoperatively they were asked to say what they associated with the word 'Friday'. Any association with the Robinson Crusoe story was regarded as evidence of implicit memory. Those with light anaesthesia, as demonstrated by the MLAEP, associated 'Friday' with some aspects of the Robinson Crusoe story, whereas those with deep anaesthesia did not.

This is a very important experiment which shows that the latencies of the MLAEP are related to the step-wise depression of consciousness, cognition and memory seen with *surgery* and *general anaesthesia*. A very short N_b latency in the AEP is associated with wakefulness and conscious awareness with explicit recall. As the latency increases, there is loss of explicit memory of contemporary events, followed by loss of consciousness and eventually loss of implicit memory as the MLAEP wave disappears.

That there is an interaction between surgical stimulation and depth of anaesthesia is also supported by the findings of Bethune *et al.* (7) who exposed 20 patients, receiving either propofol or methohexitone infusions, to a taped message during surgery and again during the postoperative recovery period. The tape was also played to another 20 patients in the postoperative period only. Only those patients who were exposed to the tape during the intraoperative period showed evidence of implicit recall, suggesting that suppression of auditory awareness is a function of both the pharmacological degree of sedation and the degree of surgical stimulation. In none of our studies in volunteers have we been able to demonstrate implicit memories of events during light anaesthesia (2) *even when they were still conscious*. It seems that there is a need for some other factor and recent research suggests that this may be fear conditioning.

Total intravenous anaesthesia and awareness

As shorter acting intravenous (IV) anaesthetic agents have become more readily available, there has been an increase in the enthusiasm for using these agents both for induction and for maintenance of anaesthesia. IV agents may be given by bolus or infusion. The loss of consciousness following bolus induction of anaesthesia is dependent upon the rate of injection, the arm brain circulation time, the initial volume of distribution of the agent and the susceptibility of the brain to the effects of the drugs. Infusion regimens for induction of anaesthesia produce rising curves of blood anaesthetic concentrations which are analogous to inhalation induction. The trough of anaesthetic concentration of the bolus must not be allowed to fall below the threshold for recovery of consciousness and the infusion is arranged to prevent this.

'MAC' leads to anaesthetic overdose

It cannot be overemphasized that general anaesthetics *abolish consciousness before they abolish movement in response to a painful stimulus*. The amount of volatile anaesthetic required to achieve the latter is known as the MAC and has previously been used as a measure of anaesthetic potency to compare different inhalation agents. The MAC is defined as the minimum alveolar concentration required to abolish movement in response to a surgical stimulus in 50% of patients. It is clearly related only to inhalation anaesthesia. As our thinking about general anaesthesia has evolved, a lower dose, that required to abolish cognition, the MAC^{awake} and MAC^{asleep}, is gaining increasing relevance. In fact, it is now being realized that the notion of MAC, the concentration to prevent movement, has held up thinking about the actual concentration of anaesthetic needed, i.e. that required to abolish consciousness. Consequently we have probably been overdosing patients with general anaesthetics for 30 years. To relate this concept to IV anaesthetics the blood concentrations of IV agents have been measured at these levels of anaesthesia, EC_{50}^{awake} and EC_{50}^{asleep}. These values are illustrated in Table 6.1, which shows data collected from a variety of sources. The recurring theme is that the abolition of consciousness occurs at approximately 50% of the anaesthetic required to ablate movement in response to a painful stimulus.

There are certain pitfalls which must be avoided when devising guidelines for administration of IV anaesthesia:

♦ Ensure that quoted values for MAC^{asleep} are measured and not calculated as there is often a considerable difference between predicted and measured concentrations.
♦ Another confusing factor, especially for $MAC^{awake/asleep}$, is exactly what end-points are used to judge the loss of consciousness and what intensity of stimulus was applied (8).
♦ The values for $MAC^{awake/asleep}$ are based on 50th centile probability curves; should we be using the EC_{95} to provide a greater margin of safety?
♦ The values are also condition dependent, e.g. opioids reduce anaesthetic agent requirements. Propofol requirement in the presence of alfentanil 250 ng/ml are reduced by 50% ; N_2O 67% in oxygen reduced the EC_{50} of propofol by 25–30% (9).
♦ Clinical signs are poor markers of anaesthetic depth; however, they should not be entirely ignored.

Table 6.1 A general anaesthetic dose equivalent to MAC compared to concentration required to abolish consciousness

	MAC^{awake} (%)	MAC (%)	MAC^{awake}/MAC
Halothane	0.4	0.74	55%
Isoflurane	0.5	1.28	39%
Desflurane	2.5	5.0	50%
Sevoflurane	0.7	1.7	41%
	Equivalent dose (µg/ml)		
Propofol	3.4–4.3	8.1–12.2	40%

The constantly changing drug concentrations during incremental IV drug dosage may result in periods of light anaesthesia followed by periods of excessive neurophysiological suppression. This has stimulated the design of often-complex infusion regimens in order to overcome these problems.

Target-controlled infusion systems – a computer-aided guess

This approach (e.g. 'Diprifusor'; Zeneca Pharma) has been designed to ease the administration of propofol for maintenance of anaesthesia. Astonishingly the system is based on a model that predicts plasma propofol levels according to the patients' weight! Such a system works in clinical practice only by overdosing the patient, which is the basis of all general anaesthetic delivery systems. The system adjusts the infusion flow rate including giving rapid increments or pausing when higher or lower levels of anaesthesia are required. However, such systems should be used carefully. *Estimated plasma concentrations are not a direct representation of the required propofol concentration in the brain.* For this reason several spurious entities have been described, such as 'the analog effect-site concentration' which has been incorporated into the latest generation of 'Diprifusor'. However, most anaesthetists are also quite unsure about the required functional end-point. Is it to prevent movement, to avoid unconsciousness or to prevent explicit memory? We (8) have argued for the latter.

To gain most from the use of expensive short-acting anaesthetic agents we should use as little drug as possible both to save on drug costs and to limit adverse effects such as prolonged recovery. Computer simulations can be used to estimate plasma propofol levels to achieve anaesthesia for surgery. The minimum blood propofol concentration to achieve loss of consciousness in 50% of patients is 3.4 µg/ml, whereas concentrations in excess of 10–15 µg/ml are needed to suppress responses to surgical stimuli in 95% of patients. The addition of alfentanil causes a reduction in the propofol concentration to achieve these end-points. Thus a plasma level of alfentanil of 350 µg/ml will reduce the propofol level to 2 µg/ml for 95% failure to move. Below this level unconsciousness cannot be assured. However, the therapeutic window is very large, the upper limit is still poorly defined but may be more than 20 µg/ml (10). This huge range brings into question the clinical relevance of estimated intraoperative blood concentration and expensive devices designed to predict these concentrations.

Comparison of manual with target-controlled concentrations

Russell *et al.* (11) have compared manual with target-controlled infusion (TCI) of propofol, and found that all anaesthetists quickly became familiar and confident with both techniques, with most expressing a preference for the TCI scheme. However, using TCI, significantly more propofol was used for induction, laryngeal mask insertion (201 against 160 mg) and during maintenance of anaesthesia (13.2 against 8.2 mg/kg/h). Using TCI was associated with a significant reduction in movement in response to surgical stimulation, suggesting that a deeper plane of anaesthesia was reached than that required to achieve loss of consciousness.

Incidence of awareness with different anaesthetic techniques

There are critics of TIVA who claim an increased risk of awareness. The overall incidence of awareness in all general anaesthetic techniques is 0–2 per 1000 with both IV and inhalation techniques being comparable (1) Experience in the use of IV techniques is clearly important. Sandin and Nordstrom (12) describe five cases in a series of 2500. Two were secondary to a failure to deliver the planned dose of anaesthesia, whilst three related to a greater than expected requirement for propofol. All cases were associated with cardiovascular changes and could have been avoided. In a similar study Nordstrom *et al.* (13) cite two cases who complained of awareness following TIVA for dental surgery. Again N_2O was not used and insufficient propofol was administered despite tachycardia and hypertension. One patient complained in the immediate postoperative period. The second recalled a bad dream on the first postoperative day and had explicit recall at 8 days. Dreaming associated with anaesthesia is common and when interviewing patients with a potential history of awareness, records must be clear about what the patient actually remembers. It is all too easy for them to confabulate, confusing dreams in the recovery room with knowledge gained elsewhere of the goings on in an operating theatre.

It is our view that the administration of a general anaesthetic with whatever computerized delivery system is little better than a guess if no measurement is made of end organ effect, i.e. depth of anaesthesia. We have discussed the different possible clinical end-points and we now outline the methods that may be used to measure the effects of general anaesthetics on the brain.

Methods for measuring depth of anaesthesia

The majority of methods for measuring depth of anaesthesia have been listed in Table 6.2 (see 1).

Depth of anaesthesia is the state of the brain which is the balance of depressant effects of anaesthetics and the stimulating effects of surgery. Clinical signs were the mainstay in the days before neuromuscular blockade. Later, blood pressure (P), heart rate (R), sweating (S) and tears

Table 6.2   Methods for measuring depth of anaesthesia

1. Clinical signs
2. Deductions based on anaesthetic dose
3. Oesophageal contractility
4. Frontalis EMG
5. Sinus arrhythmia
6. EEG
   - (i)   Power spectrum
   - (ii) BIS
   - (iii) AEP

(T) (PRST) were the principle signs used in assessing light anaesthesia in paralysed patients. However, Russell (see 1) showed that the PRST index correlated poorly with the presence of conscious awareness in apparently anaesthetized patients during surgery. Most of us use our own clinical experience to guess the general anaesthetic requirements.

Of all the methods for measuring depth of anaesthesia the majority of interest focuses on the EEG. Oesophageal contractility has been discarded. Frontalis electromyogram (EMG) and sinus arrythmia have not been fully evaluated. EEG power spectrum and AEP continue to be examined. The power spectrum has not proved to be entirely reliable, part of the problem being the different end-points chosen. Because of the traditional concept of MAC many workers, particularly in North America, focus on a limb movement as a clinical end-point, either spontaneous movement or a movement in response to noxious stimulus. Because we now know that such movement is determined at subcortical levels it is unlikely that the EEG, which reflects cortical activity, would give an accurate reflection of subcortical activity during light anaesthesia. Cortical function is more susceptible to the effects of anaesthetics than subcortical and movement in response to pain obviously occurs in unconscious patients.

Power spectrum

Rampil (14) has recently reviewed the subject of EEG signal processing during anaesthesia. The difficulties encountered with power spectrum derivations in relation to depth of anaesthesia may be attributed to the assumption made regarding EEG properties for the purpose of such analysis, i.e. stationarity and linearity. The first assumes that the statistical properties of the signal are constant over time. This is overcome by splitting the signal into discrete epochs, so that the statistical properties are approximately constant over these periods. However, there is no justification for assuming linearity in physiological systems, particularly those in which the output depends on some function of the input.

Feedback is an important component of physiological systems and it is also one of the characteristics of chaotic time series. Indices derived from the power spectrum have not proved to be reliable predictors either of sedation or of movement.

Bispectral analysis

Bispectral analysis is a method of signal processing which accommodates quadratic interactions between wave components making up the EEG trace by quantifying phase coupling (15). It was initially used to study phenomena such as ocean waves. Recently, with the availability of inexpensive high-speed computing it has been possible to obtain an on-line measure which may be useful to monitor anaesthesia. The bispectrum depends upon phase coupling and on the amplitude of relevant waves. This is normalized to eliminate wave amplitude learning bicoherence, a pure measure of phase coupling. Sigl and Chamoun (see 1) have devised a bispectral index (BIS) which uses 'a set of features that include EEG bispectrum, real triple products and bicoherence, as well as time domain features such as the level of burst suppression'. The location of the electrodes on the forehead suggests that there may also be a frontalis EMG contribution. We illustrate some typical patterns of BIS in awake, sleeping and anaesthetized subjects in Figure 6.4.

Predicting movement

Vernon *et al.* (16) suggest that the BIS is a good predictor of movement under anaesthesia although not independent of the anaesthetic regimen employed. Of course, as argued above, prediction of movement may be of much less interest and relevance as the ability to predict consciousness during anaesthesia. Furthermore, there are limitations about the assumptions made in calculating the concentration of propofol needed to produce a particular effect.

A measure of cognitive function

Liu *et al.* (17) used BIS, 95% spectral edge frequency (SEF), median frequency (MF), and δ, θ, α and β power bands during midazolam sedation. They used a five-point scale of Observer Assessment of Alertness/Sedation (OAA/S) from no response to wide awake. The BIS gave the best correlation with OAA/S but the 95% SEF showed similar changes. This study is of interest because it addresses a cognitive scale of arousal rather than subcortical responses.

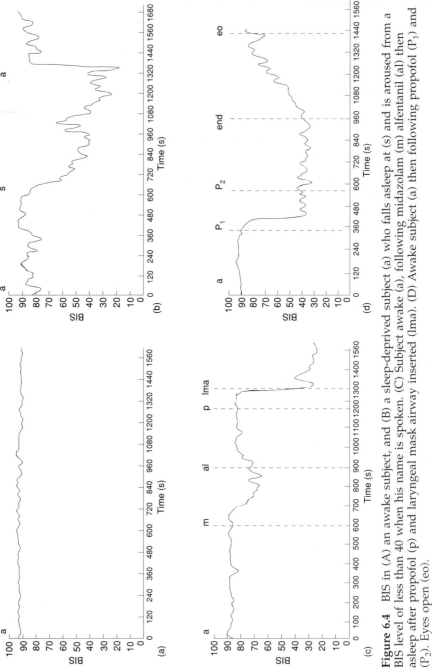

Figure 6.4 BIS in (A) an awake subject, and (B) a sleep-deprived subject (a) who falls asleep at (s) and is aroused from a BIS level of less than 40 when his name is spoken. (C) Subject awake (a), following midazolam (m) alfentanil (al) then asleep after propofol (p) and laryngeal mask airway inserted (lma). (D) Awake subject (a) then following propofol (P$_1$) and (P$_2$). Eyes open (eo).

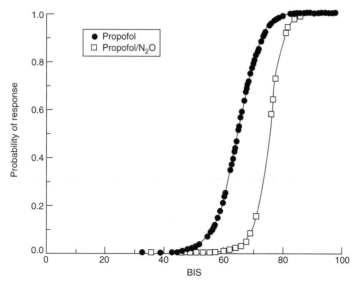

Figure 6.5   Probability curve of response to command at different BIS values using either propofol or propofol with N_2O. Note how N_2O reduces the probability of response at a given BIS. From Kearse *et al*. (18). Reproduced by permission of the publisher, Lippincott, Williams & Wilkins.

More recently, Kearse *et al*. (18) showed that the BIS accurately predicted response to verbal commands during sedation and hypnosis with propofol. The relationship between BIS and likelihood of response is shown in Figure 6.5.

Auditory evoked potentials

The AEP is the response in the EEG to a sound stimulus and is extracted by computer averaging (1). There are two types of AEP, the transient and the steady state.

The transient auditory evoked potential

The transient AEP consists of a series of positive and negative waves that represent the processes of transduction, transmission and processing of auditory information from the cochlea to the brainstem, the primary auditory cortex and the frontal cortex. The waveform of the transient AEP can be divided into three parts, depending upon the latency following the time of the auditory stimulus: waves originating in the brainstem (1–10 ms), early cortical or middle latency waves (10–100 ms) and late cortical waves (over 100 ms), which include the event-related potential (P_{300}) (Figure 6.6).

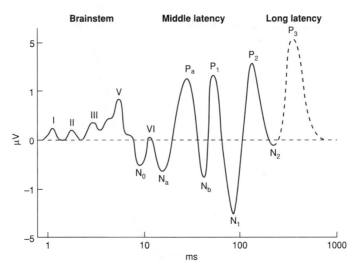

Figure 6.6   A diagrammatic representation of the auditory evoked response pattern indicating the different subdivisions and nomenclature. The MLAEP is also referred to as the early cortical response. The long latency waves include the P_3 or P_{300} wave.

The brainstem AEP is unsuitable as a monitor of the depth of anaesthesia because it is affected differently by different anaesthetics. There are few studies of anaesthetic action on the late cortical potentials. The P_{300} component of the evoked potential is reduced in a dose-dependent manner by N_2O, until reaching zero at 62% end-tidal N_2O, but its reappearance is delayed following awakening from anaesthesia.

The majority of studies of the AEP focus on the early cortical or middle latency waves. Both inhalational and IV anaesthetic agents result in progressive increases in latency, and reductions in amplitude of the P_a and N_b waves of the MLAEP, reversible upon cessation of the agent.

We showed that the changes in the amplitude and latencies of the waves within the MLAEP seen with increasing doses of anaesthetic agents can be reversed by surgical stimulation. This implies that the early cortical AEP or MLAEP is not merely a bioassay of the anaesthetic agent, but reflects the depth of anaesthesia, as a balance of the drug-induced cognitive depression and surgical stimulation. This implies that the early cortical AEP or MLAEP is not merely a bioassay of the anaesthetic agent, but reflects the depth of anaesthesia, as a balance of the drug-induced cognitive depression and surgical stimulation.

Several studies have addressed the changes in the MLAEP associated with loss of consciousness and memory during general anaesthesia. Bolus injection of thiopentone suppresses the MLAEP and as the patient begins to awaken, the latencies within the response return to the awake values.

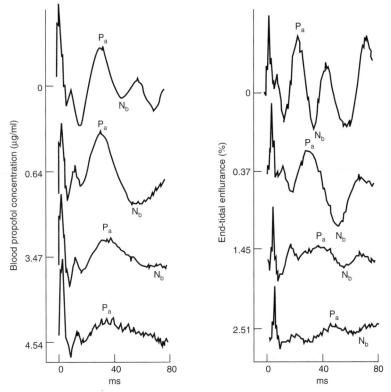

Figure 6.7   The effect of an increase either in propofol dose or enflurane dose on the morphology of the MLAEP. Note the reduction in amplitude and increase in latency in each case.

The transient method has been widely studied with a great variety of anaesthetics (1). Very extensive studies of the AEP have been reported by Schwender and co-workers (see 1). The pattern of the transient auditory evoked response is shown in Figure 6.7. The effect of general anaesthetics is to reduce wave amplitude, particularly of the middle latency (or early cortical waves) and to increase their latency. Davies *et al.* (19) studied the change in MLAEP during repeated transitions from consciousness to unconsciousness using propofol. With the first change from consciousness to unconsciousness (response to command) the latencies of N_a, P_b and N_b increased from 20, 32 and 43 to 23, 39 and 55 ms, respectively. During successive transitions from unconscious to conscious, the awake latencies were slightly higher than baseline awake values whereas anaesthetized latencies were the same as those during the first period of unconsciousness.

During anaesthesia for Caesarian section a prominent MLAEP is associated with intraoperative wakefulness, purposeful movements and postoperative recall of surgical manipulation. Using the isolated forearm technique we demonstrated during N_2O/oxygen anaesthesia, a threshold N_b latency of 44.5 ms was associated with the MLAEP containing three waves rather than the two waves seen with the longer latency. When the N_b latency decreased below this threshold four of their seven patients showed a positive response to command, indicating conscious awareness. However, when a volatile agent was added the responses were abolished and N_b latency increased to more than 44.5 ms. Similarly, at sub-MAC concentrations of isoflurane the ability to respond to command is associated with higher amplitudes and shorter latencies in the MLAEP.

Auditory evoked potentials and implicit memory during anaesthesia

As mentioned earlier in this chapter, there is now convincing evidence that unconscious processing of auditory information and implicit memory of intraoperative events occurs in patients in whom the early cortical potentials of the MLAEP are preserved during anaesthesia.

During anaesthesia, the story of Robinson Crusoe was played to the patients and postoperatively they were asked to say what they associated with the word 'Friday'. Any association with the Robinson Crusoe story was regarded as evidence of implicit memory. Of the patients who showed evidence of implicit memory, all exhibited an increase in P_a latency of less than 12 ms. None of the patients who demonstrated an increase in P_a latency of more than 12 ms showed evidence of implicit learning.

It therefore seems apparent that the latencies of the MLAEP are related to the step-wise depression of consciousness, cognition and memory seen with general anaesthesia. A short N_b latency is associated with wakefulness and conscious awareness with explicit recall. As the latency increases, amnesia occurs, followed by loss of consciousness and eventually loss of implicit memory.

Steady-state response auditory evoked potential

The steady-state response AEP has been less widely studied during anaesthesia. We have examined steady-state responses at different stimulating frequencies (4). With anaesthesia the largest amplitude response occurs at lower frequencies (below 20 Hz) and there is often a persistent, although greatly reduced, response at 40 Hz. There was a close correlation between cognitive function and the frequency of the maximum steady-state response.

As mentioned above, increasing anaesthetic depth is associated with an increase in latency of the waves within the middle latency part of the transient AEP. Therefore, it was suggested (Galambos, personal communication) that the stimulating frequency required to achieve phase locking of the P_a and P_b waves progressively decreases with increasing anaesthetic dose. This is the basis of the coherent frequency outlined below, and previously described by Munglani *et al.* (see 1) and Andrade *et al.* (4).

From our previous studies of the transient AEP, we predicted that as the anaesthetic concentration increased the maximum amplitude in the steady-state response would not be achieved at 40 Hz but at progressively lower frequencies. Thus, we varied the stimulating frequency from 6.5 to 50.5 Hz and in awake subjects we found maximum power near 40 Hz and with increasing sedation this fell to about 27 Hz at the point when consciousness was lost.

Steady-state 40 Hz auditory evoked potentials, working memory and anaesthesia

We have assessed cognitive function before and during the administration of the IV anaesthetic, propofol, using the WLR test (see above) (4).

Table 6.3 shows the median WLR score and mean infusion rate, plasma propofol concentration and maximum coherent frequency at each stage of the experiment. There was a significant decrease in WLR performance from awake to small propofol dose and from small dose to large dose ($P < 0.01$ for each comparison). Maximum coherent frequency varied likewise, decreasing significantly from 38 Hz awake to 30 Hz small dose and to 27 Hz for large dose (Figure 6.8).

The maximum coherent frequency plotted against WLR score for the propofol study and also, for comparison, for our previous study with isoflurane (see 1) is shown in Figure 6.9. The equations for these lines are $y = 25.6 + 0.74x$ for propofol and $y = 23.7 + 0.75x$ for isoflurane. The slightly different intercepts may be caused by changes in the method of calculating maximum coherent frequency in the propofol

Table 6.3 Median WLR score, mean propofol infusion rate, mean plasma concentration and mean maximum coherent frequency at each stage of the experiment

Measure	*Stage*				
	Awake	*Light sedation*	*Deep sedation*	*Light sedation (recovery)*	*Awake (recovery)*
WLR score	13	10.0	0.5	7.5	13
Maximum coherent frequency (Hz)	38	30	27	29	36
Infusion rate (mg/kg/h)	0	3.7	4.45	3.71	0
Plasma propofol concentration (μg/ml)	0	1.22	1.85	1.82	0.93

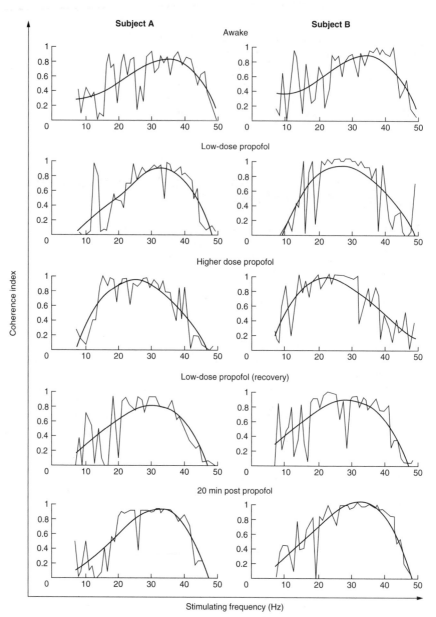

Figure 6.8 The coherence index (CI) obtained at different stimulating frequencies ranging from 8 to 50 Hz in two subjects given sedative doses of propofol. Note the shift of frequency to obtain maximum CI from about 40 Hz fully awake to about 23 Hz fully sedated.

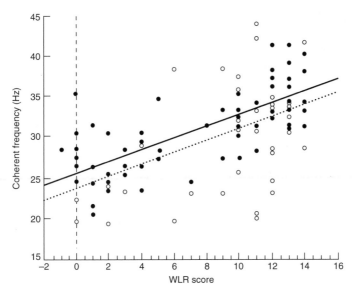

Figure 6.9 Comparison of the effects of propofol or isoflurane on WLR and coherence frequencies (see 1).

study. The very similar slopes of the two lines suggest that the coherent frequency predicts psychological function independently of the type of anaesthetic used. Overall, the change in WLR performance correlated with infusion dose, plasma concentration and maximum coherent frequency. It could be argued that these correlations are artifactually high because, when subjects are awake, there is no variation in infusion dose and only a small variation in WLR because performance is near its ceiling. We therefore repeated the correlational analyses for the propofol sedation stages only; there remained a correlation between WLR performance and maximum coherent frequency ($r = 0.47$, $P < 0.005$), and between WLR performance and plasma concentration ($r = -0.51$, $P < 0.05$).

Thus we have shown that the coherent frequency of the AEP correlates strongly with psychological performance at sedative doses of propofol and isoflurane. The relationship between maximum coherent frequency and WLR score is similar across subjects, despite large variations in the dose of propofol needed to bring about the required changes in psychological performance. During sedation, cognitive performance was predicted by coherent frequency, but not by propofol infusion rate. Coherent frequency thus measures fluctuations in depth of sedation and not just loss of awareness. These findings extend our earlier study with isoflurane, suggesting that coherent frequency measures depth of sedation regardless of the anaesthetic used.

Comparison of methods

Doi *et al.* (20) studied four EEG indexes [BIS, 95% SEF, MF and AEP index (AEPI)] in 10 patients during emergence from anaesthesia. They compared the signals with gradually decreasing calculated blood propofol concentrations, and evaluated the signal differences between preinduction and emergence from anaesthesia. Values of BIS, MF and SEF correlated with calculated blood concentrations of propofol during emergence from anaesthesia. The correlation was best with BIS, but was poor with MF and SEF at low calculated blood propofol concentrations. Although AEPI values did not correlate with calculated blood concentrations of propofol during emergence from anaesthesia, values after eye opening and before anaesthesia were well distinguished from those during emergence from anaesthesia. BIS correlated best with calculated blood concentrations of propofol. AEPI appeared to distinguish the awake from asleep state. This work confirms our belief that it is preferable to measure end organ response rather than deduce blood concentrations of drugs which have very indirect relationships with end organ.

Closed-loop feedback control of anaesthesia

Control theory distinguishes between open-loop control and closed-loop control. In open-loop control, the input to the system (e.g. drug dosage) is independent of the output (e.g. depth of anaesthesia), whereby in a closed-loop control systems the input at a given moment in time is a function of the previous output.

Closed-loop infusions of anaesthetic agents require an easily and rapidly measured end-point which has a low incidence of false-positive results. The model of the input/output relationship cannot be based purely on a mathematical model, since as discussed above there is great pharmacokinetic and pharmacodynamic variability. Measuring blood levels of anaesthetic agents are slow to perform and do not guarantee a lack of awareness. Consequently we have to turn to surrogate measures of anaesthetic depth to provide the controlling signal for the anaesthetic infusion rate. Ultimately, a closed-loop anaesthetic system may be envisaged, in which delivery of anaesthetic will be automatically controlled in order to achieve a programmed, predetermined depth of anaesthesia.

Awareness during anaesthesia – medico-legal aspects

Many patients have a fear of waking up from the anaesthetic while surgery is still in progress. This fear is fuelled by well-publicized cases of awareness under general anaesthesia reported in the news media. Although such situations are rare (between 0.2 and 0.01%) they are invariably the results of inadequate anaesthesia in patients with neuro-muscular blockade. If the complaint is deemed to be genuine, successful litigation results, as the patient has been subjected to a profound physical and psychological trauma. A patient in the UK was recently awarded £100 000 damages following awareness in theatre. However, all cases should be carefully investigated because fraudulent claims have been made. Recall of events in the recovery area may be mistakenly interpreted as intraoperative awareness. Recall of some painless intra-operative event is not rare, and it is easy for patients to fill in gaps and imagine more than they actually experienced, especially if considerable time elapsed between the anaesthetic and the taking of a full history of the event.

If a patient claims to have been aware when seemingly under general anaesthesia they should be treated sympathetically, as denial by medical staff of the authenticity of their experience may adversely influence the patients' subsequent psychological behaviour and fuel a need to proceed with legal action. If a patient complains of being aware, it is essential that the anaesthetist involved is notified without delay. The worst problems arise after long delays between the episode and notifying the anaesthetist. It is particularly unfortunate if the surgeon alone is informed and attempts to deal with the situation without informing the anaesthetist. If that anaesthetist is a trainee, he/she should inform a consultant. The anaesthetist must then visit the patient as soon as possible and make a detailed record of the patient's experience, including any memories of conversations that the patient may have heard in the operating theatre, as well as all specific instances of pain and discomfort, and try to determine whether the claim is genuine. If there is an obvious anaesthetic explanation the patient should be reassured that the anaesthetist believes them and an attempt should be made to explain the cause of the awareness, if it is known. The patient should be reassured that they can

Table 6.4 Check list following a complaint of awareness during general anaesthesia

---

1. Visit the patient as soon as possible, along with a witness
2. Take a full history and document the patient's exact memory of events
3. Attempt to confirm the validity of the account
4. Keep your own copy of the account
5. Give a full explanation to the patient
6. Offer the patient follow-up, including psychological support, and document that this has been offered
7. Reassure the patient that they can safely have further general anaesthetics, with minimal risk of a further episode of awareness
8. If the cause is not known, try to determine it
9. Notify your medical defence organization
10. Notify your hospital administration
11. Notify the patient's GP

---

safely have further anaesthetics, but it is often difficult to convince patients that such an episode will not be repeated. The patient should be offered psychological support and care must be taken in adequate follow up. In addition the anaesthetist must inform the hospital administration, his/her own medical defence organization and the patient's general practitioner (Table 6.4).

Post-traumatic stress disorder

Fortunately, not all patients suffer long-term sequelae. In the survey by Moerman *et al.* (see 1), eight of the 26 patients who reported conscious awareness had no sequelae. The remaining patients in her study reported sleep disturbances, nightmares, flashbacks and a preoccupation with death. In addition to a lasting fear of anaesthesia, a post-traumatic stress disorder may result, characterized by re-experience of the event, avoidance of stimuli associated with the event, numbing of general responsiveness and increased arousal. Although impossible to prove through controlled trials, anecdotal evidence suggests that early counselling may reduce the incidence of post-traumatic stress disorder following intraoperative awareness.

References

1. Bailey C, Jones JG. Patients memories of events during general anaesthesia. *Anaesthesia* 1997; **52**: 460–76.
2. Andrade J, Jones JG. Is amnesia for intraoperative events good enough? *Br J Anaesth* 1998; **80**: 575–6.
3. Tomlin PJ, Jones BC, Edwards R, Robin PE. Subjective and objective sensory responses to inhalation of nitrous oxide and methoxyflurane. *Br J Anaesth* 1973; **45**: 719–24.
4. Andrade J, Sapsford DJ, Jeevaratnum D, Pickworth AJ, Jones JG. The coherent frequency in the electroencephalogram as objective measure of cognitive function during propofol sedation. *Anaesth Analg* 1996; **83**: 1279–84.
5. Veselis RA, Reinsel RA, Feshchenko VA, Wronski M. The comparative amnesic effects of midazolam, propofol, thiopental, and fentanyl at equisedative concentrations. *Anaesthesiology* 1997; **87**: 749–64.
6. Merikle PM, Daneman M. Memory for unconsciously perceived events: evidence from anaesthetised patients. *Consciousness and Cognition* 1996; **5**: 525–41.
7. Bethune DW, Ghosh S, Gray B, *et al.* Learning during general anaesthesia: implicit recall after methohexitone or propofol infusion. *Br J Anaesth* 1992; **69**: 197–9.
8. Kazama T, Ikeda K, Morita K. Reduction by fentanyl of the Cp50 values of propofol and haemodynamic responses to various noxious stimuli. *Anaesthesiology* 1997; **87**: 213–27.
9. Davidson JAH, Macleod AD, Howie JC, Kenny GNC Effective concentration 50 for propofol with and without 67% nitrous oxide. *Acta Anaesthesiol Scand* 1993; **37**: 458–64.

10. Vuyk J, Mertens MJ, Olofsen E, Burm AG, Bovill JG. Propofol anaesthesia and rational opioid selection. *Anaesthesiology* 1997; **87**: 1549–62.
11. Russell D, Wilkes MP, Hunter JB, *et al.* Manual compared with target controlled infusion of propofol. *Br J Anaesth* 1995; **75**: 562–6.
12. Sandin R, Norstrom O. Awareness during total intravenous anaesthesia. *Br J Anaesth* 1993; **71**: 782–7.
13. Nordstrom O, Engstrom AM, Persson S, Sandin R. Incidence of awareness in total i.v. anaesthesia based on propofol, alfentanil and neuromuscular blockade. *Acta Anaesthesiol Scand* 1997; **41**: 978–84.
14. Rampil IJ. A primer for EEG signal processing in anaesthesia. *Anesthesiology* 1998; **89**: 980–1002.
15. Rosow C, Manberg PJ. Bispectral index monitoring. *Anesthesiol Clin North Am/Annu Anesthetic Pharmacol* 1998; **2**: 89–107.
16. Vernon JM, Lang E, Sebel PS, Manberg P. Prediction of movement using bispectral electroencephalographic analysis during propofol/alfentanil or isoflurane/alfentanil anesthesia. *Anesth Analg* 1995; **80**: 780–5.
17. Liu J, Singh H, White PF. Electroencephalogram bispectral analysis predicts the depth of midazolam induced sedation. *Anaesthesiology* 1996; **84**: 64–9.
18. Kearse LA, Rosow C, Zasiavsky A, *et al.* Bispectral analysis of the electroencephalogram predicts conscious processing of information during propofol sedation and hypnosis. *Anesthesiology* 1998; **88**: 25–34.
19. Davies FW, Mantzardis H, Kenny GNC, Fisher AC. Middle latency auditory evoked potentials during repeated transitions from consciousness to unconsciousness. *Anaesthesia* 1996; **51**: 107–13.
20. Doi M, Gajraj RJ, Mantzardis H, Kenny GNC. Relationship between calculated blood concentration of propofol and EEG variables. *Anaesthesia* 1997; **78**: 180–4.

7

Postoperative nausea, vomiting and recovery

J. M. Millar

- Impact of postoperative nausea and vomiting
- Causes of postoperative nausea and vomiting
- Physiology of postoperative nausea and vomiting
- Antiemetics
- Specific clinical problems

The 'big little problem' of postoperative nausea and vomiting (PONV) is increasingly recognized as more than a trivial inconvenience. Distressingly common, it has physiological, psychological and economic disadvantages for both the patient and the health care provider, and active efforts should be made to prevent or reduce it. The multiple factors and aetiology involved in PONV make it a continuing clinical challenge. However, severe PONV, like severe pain, is no longer acceptable in modern anaesthetic practice,

The impact of postoperative nausea and vomiting

Physiological and surgical effects

Postoperative vomiting and retching can result in a range of clinical complications which threaten both the success of the surgical procedure and the safety of the patients (Table 7.1). Nausea can delay eating and drinking, and result in dehydration and debility. For the patient persistent nausea is often more unpleasant and debilitating than a single vomit.

Recovery

All stages of recovery are delayed by persistent PONV. Scoring systems such as the Steward and Aldrete scores used to measure early recovery do not usually include PONV, although this may be an important determi-

Table 7.1 Clinical effects of postoperative vomiting and retching

- Oesophageal rupture
- Pulmonary aspiration of stomach contents
- Dehydration and electrolyte imbalance
- Raised intracranial and intraocular pressure
- Wound problems
    - bleeding and haematoma formation
    - increased pressure on suture lines
    - venous hypertension in skin flaps
    - wound dehiscence

nant of time spent in the recovery room. It has been associated with prolonged recovery room stays (1–3) and patients with PONV spent 30% longer in the recovery room after major gynaecological surgery (4). When different general anaesthetic techniques are compared, recovery is often similar in patients without PONV, but prolonged in those who suffer it.

Intermediate recovery is influenced by PONV. This is most significant in day case surgery, which is increasingly important in modern health care and currently accounts for 50% of elective surgery in the UK. PONV is the most important factor determining length of stay (5,6) and unplanned overnight admission after day case surgery. After day case oral surgery procedures lasting 3 h, propofol compared to isoflurane for maintenance (after propofol induction in both groups) significantly reduced PONV (8 versus 40%) and allowed more rapid discharge home (7). After laparoscopy, the use of desflurane was associated with delayed recovery and very high rates of overnight admission due to PONV, even when ondansetron was given prophylactically (5).

PONV delays patients' return to normal activities (8,9) and employment, as well as negatively influencing patient attitudes to day surgery.

Use of resources

PONV consumes resources – patient throughput is disrupted, nursing time is required to attend to patients and clean up afterwards, and extra drugs and intravenous (IV) fluids are required to control emesis and dehydration. Hospital bed stays and dependency are increased, and this may prevent other patients having their surgery. It is often difficult to ascribe an accurate financial cost to these resources, but it can adversely affect the care of all patients through a knock-on effect. The avoidance of PONV can mean more predictable and better use of resources.

Patient attitudes to postoperative nausea and vomiting

PONV is the postoperative side effect that patients dread most and it is often the yardstick by which they judge their anaesthetic. Patients ranked

PONV as the most undesirable outcome after anaesthesia (10). Orkin (11) found that in order to avoid PONV, 75% of individuals were willing to trade a variety of other unpleasant consequences, including dysphoria, increased pain and increased cost. In another study when patients were asked to score the PONV they had experienced, a single retrospective score correlated with the *worst* contemporaneous score recorded during their postoperative course (12). Patient satisfaction with their anaesthetic is always adversely affected by PONV.

The cost of postoperative nausea and vomiting

Cost-effectiveness can be overused to justify cheap health care. It is easy to add up the price of drugs used, but difficult to ascribe costs to the use of other resources – particularly the indirect costs such as reduced patient throughput or delay in return to work. The cost of an outcome may be different depending on the circumstances – if a bed is empty and a nurse is available, the cost of an unplanned stay is minimal. If the use of the bed means that another patient's operation is cancelled and an operating theatre and its staff stand idle, the human and financial cost is great. In addition, unpleasant side effects, patient satisfaction and quality are never included in cost calculations (13,14).

The drugs used in anaesthesia generally cost no more than 1% of the cost of the patient's hospital stay (15) and have the potential to save money if they significantly reduce PONV. Carroll *et al.* (16) found that patients with PONV incurred a additional cost of $14.95 in personnel, supplies and drugs, plus $7.12 in nursing time. Lost revenue was estimated at an average of $415 per patient with PONV if patient throughput was reduced. In operations and patient populations with low risk of PONV, the cost-effectiveness of a technique which reduces it may be more difficult to demonstrate.

Hitchcock and Rudkin (17) looked at the outcome in day surgery after anaesthesia with propofol induction followed by either propofol infusion or isoflurane or enflurane. Propofol infusion was associated with fewer postoperative complications, overnight admissions and post discharge consultations; overall costs were little different when these were taken into consideration.

The causes of postoperative nausea and vomiting

The multiple factors in PONV make investigating it, interpreting the results of clinical studies and treating it difficult. They can be divided into factors related to:

- The patient
- The surgery
- Perioperative drugs
- Other perioperative events

Table 7.2   Patient factors in PONV

◆ Individual susceptibility
◆ Females
◆ History of PONV
◆ History of motion sickness
◆ Age
◆ Anxiety?
◆ Obesity?
◆ Migraine

Patient factors (Table 7.2)

There is considerable variation in individual susceptibility to PONV. Women are 3 times more likely to suffer PONV under the same surgical circumstances. Although a relationship to the menstrual cycle has been found, there is lack of consensus as to the precise days. Clinically this is unhelpful, as surgery cannot usually be timed with accuracy; a better policy is treat women expectantly for PONV.

A history of PONV also increases the likelihood of further PONV by 3 times, as does a history of motion sickness. PONV is extremely common in young children and becomes less common with age.

Anxiety may be a factor, with increased catecholamine secretion or swallowed air suggested as causes. Obesity has also been blamed but this is not confirmed by other studies. Traditionally this has been ascribed to absorption of anaesthetic agent in fat and this may be less relevant with newer volatile agents with low blood gas solubility. The increased likelihood of gastro-oesophageal reflux in obese patients and of gastric inflation during mask ventilation has also been implicated.

Migraine occurring in the perioperative period is often unrecognized and can cause intractable emesis in susceptible patients. Anxiety, stress, fasting, hypoglycaemia and vasoactive drugs are perioperative trigger

Table 7.3   Disease-related factors in PONV

◆ Hiatus hernia and gastro-oesophageal reflux
◆ Delayed gastric emptying
    – shock
    – pregnancy
    – neuropathies, diabetes mellitus
◆ Intestinal obstruction
◆ Full stomach – food or blood
◆ Pain
◆ Infections
◆ Raised intracranial pressure
◆ Metabolic diseases

factors. Once identified, migraine responds well to the 5-hydroxy-tryptamine (5-HT₃) agonist sumatripin.

PONV may also be related to the patient's disease or preoperative condition (Table 7.3). The presence of food or, particularly, blood in the stomach is likely to cause postoperative vomiting.

Surgical factors

The relationship between PONV and certain surgical procedures (Table 7.4) is well recognized. A major offender is laparoscopy with incidences of up to 80% (5), so that it is frequently used in antiemetic studies. However, this may mean that the results are not necessarily transferable to other operations with different mechanisms of causing emesis.

What are the precipitating factors in procedures with high incidences of PONV? (Table 7.5):

- *Vagal stimulation.* Stretching of the peritoneum with insufflated gas is probably one of the mechanisms in laparoscopy. A gasless technique for laparoscopy, while not allowing as good a view or access, has been

---

Table 7.4   Surgical procedures with a high incidence of PONV

- Laparoscopy, especially for tubal sterilization and cholecystectomy
- Intra-abdominal operations
- Gynaecological procedures
- Breast surgery
- Strabismus correction
- Middle ear surgery
- Bat ear correction
- Dental procedures particularly wisdom teeth
- Tonsillectomy
- Acoustic neuroma

Table 7.5   Mechanisms involved in PONV in surgical procedures

---

- Vagal stimulation
    - stretching the peritoneum
    - oculocardiac reflex
    - cervical dilatation
- Spasm and ileus of hollow viscera
    - pain and spasm in tubal sterilization
    - ileus – overt or subclinical
- Vestibular stimulation
- Swallowed blood

---

shown to reduce PONV (18). Peritoneal stretching may cause vagal stimulation – bradycardia may also occur as the peritoneum is stretched. Other vagal influences on PONV are found in strabismus surgery (related to the oculocardiac reflex) and cervical dilatation in gynaecological procedures.

◆ *Spasm or ileus of hollow viscera*. The use of clips or rings for tubal sterilization causes more pain and nausea than diathermy cauterization, and this may be related to tubal spasm or ischaemia. Intra-abdominal operations and gynaecological operations may cause ileus, even if this is not clinically significant.

◆ *Vestibular stimulation*. This is responsible in surgery for acoustic neuroma, the middle ear and correction of bat ears.

◆ *Swallowed blood*. Oral surgery and tonsillectomy can result in considerable swallowed blood which is very emetic.

Duration of surgery may be important but probably due to the nature of the procedure rather than the time taken (19). Longer procedures are usually associated with more invasive surgery and with increased drug administration and postoperative pain.

Drug factors

Virtually every drug given in the course of an anaesthetic can trigger PONV and the cocktail of drugs given during the course of a routine anaesthetic can make determining the cause difficult. Few studies can be directly compared because of the different combinations of drugs, patients and procedures.

Premedication

Opioid premedication is associated with increased emesis. Benzodiazepine premedication is neutral or may reduce it if anxiety and catecholamine secretion are decreased (20).

Induction agents

Ketamine has the highest incidence of PONV of all the IV agents, perhaps because of its sympathomimetic effects, as α-adrenergic stimulation has been shown to cause emesis. Etomidate is the second most emetic induction agent. Thiopentone and methohexitone probably have a similar moderately high incidence. Benzodiazepines such as midazolam are neutral, neither causing or alleviating PONV.

Propofol is the anaesthetic agent with the lowest incidence of emesis and it is now generally considered to have antiemetic properties. One of the difficulties in studying its effects compared to other agents used in anaesthesia is that it may be used for both induction and maintenance and compared in studies where barbiturate and/or volatile techniques have been used. There are no studies of PONV where propofol has been compared to other induction agents alone without the confounding influences of volatile agents, nitrous oxide (N_2O) or opioids, but it has usually been found to reduce nausea compared to thiopentone (21,22) or methohexitone (23) in brief balanced anaesthetic techniques where the influence of the induction agent might be expected to be more important than the brief period of inhalation anaesthesia.

Volatile anaesthetic agents

Volatile agents are major culprits in PONV, particularly as operating time increases. Ether and chloroform were well recognized to be extremely emetic. Halothane, enflurane or isoflurane are great improvements, but there is no evidence that any one of them is significantly better than the others with regard to PONV.

Although desflurane and sevoflurane, newer agents with very low blood solubility, might be expected to reduce PONV or at least its duration, in practice this has not proved true. Desflurane seems to have a slightly higher incidence compared to isoflurane (24) or sevoflurane (25), which reduces the value of its fast wakeup. Sevoflurane and isoflurane compared for day case laparoscopy (26) resulted in similar PONV and time to discharge; overnight admission rates were 12.5 and 16%, respectively, due to prolonged PONV. In the 24 h following surgery only 17% of the sevoflurane group and 36% of the isoflurane group had no PONV. In a multicentre study, the incidence of PONV after sevoflurane was less that after isoflurane, but was still high – 35 versus 51% (27). A study in children showed no significant difference in PONV between halothane, sevoflurane and desflurane (28).

The conclusion is that all the volatile agents share the property of an equally high chance of causing postoperative emesis. Desflurane and sevoflurane have faster wake-up times but are expensive and may not improve recovery because of their emetic side effects.

Propofol versus volatile agents for maintenance

In general propofol used for maintenance has been found to significantly reduce emesis and improve well-being compared to maintenance with enflurane (29), isoflurane (30), desflurane (31) and sevoflurane (32,33), but not in every study (34,35). This may be explained by different patient groups and procedures, and by the use of long-acting opioids for postoperative analgesia.

Nitrous oxide

There is controversy about the emetic effects of N_2O, with many conflicting studies. Suggested mechanisms are its diffusion into the inner ear causing vestibular stimulation, diffusion in gut and/or central stimulation. Three separate meta-analyses have now concluded that it does increase emesis (36–38). However, the majority of studies considered in these meta-analyses compared thiopentone/volatile anaesthesia with or without N_2O. Tramer *et al.*'s meta-analysis of propofol infusion compared with anaesthesia of any kind with or without N_2O concluded that propofol was as good at reducing early and late vomiting as omitting N_2O but that propofol (but not omitting N_2O) also decreased early and probably late nausea (39). They also considered that the number and quality of the studies was a limitation to the validity of this conclusion.

Does adding N_2O to propofol anaesthesia increase PONV? A summary of the studies where propofol has been used to maintain anaesthesia with and without N_2O is given in Table 7.6 (40–51). The only significant increase in emesis with the use of N_2O was in children having mixed or strabismus surgery (40,41). However, two other studies in children having strabismus surgery failed to find any difference. In Reimer *et al.*'s (43) study of children having squint surgery, propofol with or without N_2O significantly reduced vomiting compared to thiopentone/halo-thane/N_2O in the immediate postoperative period, but not overall as vomiting increased in the first 24 h in all the groups. Squint surgery may be so emetic that it eventually overrides any antiemetic effect of propofol. (See discussion of strabismus surgery below.) A meta-analysis of propofol used for maintenance of anaesthesia found that this reduced PONV regardless of the presence or absence of N_2O or use of opiate (52).

The disadvantages of N_2O are difficult to show with any conviction. It may distend the gut, and has been considered to increase surgical difficulty and PONV in abdominal surgery, but this was not found to be true in laparoscopic cholecystectomy (53). No prospective study has demonstrated occupational health risks (54) or psychomotor impairment in theatre personnel (55).

There may be advantages from using N_2O in a propofol IV technique: it has analgesic properties, it reduces propofol requirements and cost, and the anaesthetic is generally smoother (56). The risk of awareness from omitting N_2O has been calculated from pooled data to be as high as 2% (37) and this may be a decisive factor in its continued use.

Opioids

Long-acting opioids, given by any route – oral, intramuscular (IM), IV, epidural or intradural – have a well-documented track record for making patients nauseated. They are probably responsible for the majority of emesis continuing beyond the first few postoperative hours and when patients relate that they were sick for a week after an anaesthetic, it is likely to have been due to the analgesia, not the anaesthetic. Patient-controlled analgesia (PCA) has been referred to as 'patient-controlled nausea'.

Day case patients, and children in particular, given morphine often only begin to feel sick after their discharge once they travel home in the car. A comparison of morphine and fentanyl in day case patients found no difference in early emesis but an increased incidence overall with morphine, the majority of which occurred after discharge (57). Morphine used for analgesia in day surgery has been associated with increased rates of overnight admission.

Table 7.6 Propofol anaesthesia with and without N_2O

Surgery[a]		Overall emesis (%)[b]		Significance[d]
		With N_2O[c]	Without N_2O[c]	
Crawford et al. (40)	mixed paed surgery	53	7	$P < 0.05$
Watcha et al. (41)	paed strabismus	60	23	$P < 0.05$
Klockgether et al. (42)	paed strabismus	27	40	NS
Reimer et al. (43)	paed strabismus	42	28	NS
Standl et al. (44)	paed strabismus	28	23	NS
Heath et al. (45)	gynae	12	16	NS
Aktar et al. (46)	gynae/urol, day	12	4	NS
Sukhani et al. (47)	gynae, lap, day	29	25	NS
Gunawardene et al. (49)	gynae, minor	3	0	NS
Gregory et al. (50)	gynae major	0	0	NS
Lindekaer et al. (48)	hernia, day	average scores only given		NS
Kalman et al. (51)	major abdo	emesis not given 'gastrointestinal symptoms'		NS

[a] Surgery: paed = paediatric; gynae = gynaecology; urol = urology; lap = laparoscopy; day = day cases; hernia = hernia repair; abdo = abdominal.
[b] Any patient with nausea and/or vomiting in first 24h.
[c] Propofol induction and maintenance with or without N_2O.
[d] $P > 0.05$ = NS = non-significant.

The long-lasting effects of morphine outlast any antiemetic effect of propofol used for anaesthesia. Marshall *et al.* (58) found that propofol maintenance reduced PONV after laparoscopy, but only in those patients who did not receive opioids. Women having breast surgery with morphine for postoperative analgesia (59) had a similar high incidence of PONV after propofol/propofol, propofol/isoflurane and thiopentone/isoflurane, all with air/oxygen. Other studies have found that the effect of propofol is short lived when morphine is required for postoperative analgesia (30). However, propofol infusion has been shown to be longer lasting and more effective than ondansetron in reducing PONV after breast surgery with morphine analgesia (60).

Short-acting opioids, such as fentanyl or alfentanil, may not have as profound or as prolonged an effect. They do not generally significantly increase nausea or vomiting (22), and their analgesic effects may contribute to postoperative analgesia (61), although this has been disputed (62). The role of the ultra short-acting opioid, remifentanil, is unclear – a significant increase in emesis has not been reported (63–65). However, there is recent evidence (66) that acute tolerance to opioids may be induced which may explain anecdotal reports of increased amounts of postoperative morphine. This may increase emesis.

The use of non-steroidal anti-inflammatory drugs (NSAIDs) and/or local or regional analgesia reduces the need for morphine, particularly in short-stay surgery, and it should be avoided wherever alternative analgesia can be used. A satisfactory alternative for severe pain has yet to be found.

Other drugs

A variety of other drugs given in association with anaesthesia and surgery may contribute to PONV:

◆ Muscle relaxants and their reversal: muscle relaxants are probably neutral in their effects unless they cause hypotension, e.g. tubocurarine. However, glycopyrrolate/neostigmine has been found to increase PONV compared with no reversal (67), atropine/neostigmine mixtures (68) or edrophonium (69). These findings are disputed (70). They are probably unimportant overall compared to the other assaults of anaesthesia and surgery.
◆ Prostaglandins given to facilitate termination of pregnancy are potent emetics, as are oxytocin and especially ergometrine given for uterine contraction.
◆ Antibiotics.

Other perioperative factors in postoperative nausea and vomiting (Table 7.7)

As well as the drugs, there are other factors in the perioperative period. Prolonged fluid fasting and hypoglycaemia may contribute to PONV, and

Table 7.7   Perioperative factors and PONV

- Fasting and hypoglycaemia
- Hypoxia and hypercarbia
- Hypotension
- Gag reflex from suction or oral airways
- Air in the stomach from mask ventilation
- Movement on trolleys
- Turning
- Pain

giving IV fluids has been found to reduce it in some day case studies (71). Hypoxia, hypercarbia and hypotension all cause PONV, and hypotension in the course of epidural or spinal anaesthesia may induce PONV even in the absence of general anaesthesia. In patients susceptible to motion sickness, 30–60% associated PONV with active or passive movement – being moved around on a trolley, turned or early ambulation (20).

The physiology of postoperative nausea and vomiting

See Figure 7.1.

- The vomiting centre (VC) in the lateral reticular formation in the medulla close to the tractus solitarius initiates and coordinates emesis
- The chemoreceptor trigger zone (CRTZ) which lies in the area postrema outside the blood–brain barrier and acts as a sensing organ for toxins, chemicals and drugs via blood and cerebrospinal fluid (CSF); drugs do not act directly on the VC
- The nucleus of the tractus solitarius and the vagal nuclei which lie in close proximity to the CTZ and receive input from the pharynx and gastrointestinal (GI) tract via the vagus
- The vestibular portion of the VIIIth cranial nerve
- Higher centres for sight, taste and smell, as well as emotion

The main receptors involved in PONV are:

- Dopamine D_2, found in the area postrema
- Serotonin 5-HT_3, found in the area postrema, vagal nuclei, solitary tract and its nucleus, and GI tract, as well as elsewhere in the CNS
- Histamine H_1, found in the nuclei of the solitary tract and vagus, and the vestibular pathway
- Muscarinic cholinergic found in nuclei of the solitary tract and vagus, and the vestibular pathway

The role of opioid receptors found in the area postrema and brain stem is less clear. Encephalins have a complex role and may have an antiemetic effect.

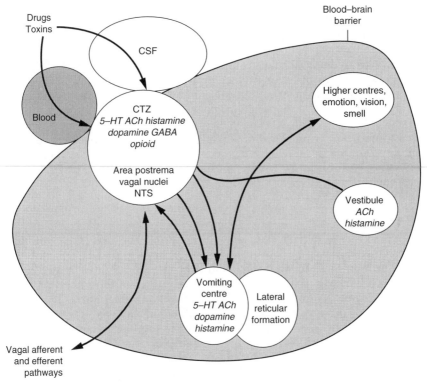

Figure 7.1 Physiology of PONV and transmitters. Reproduced with permission from Paxton LD. Physiology and control of nausea and vomiting. Reproduced by permission of Churchill Livingstone in: McCaughey W, Clarke R, Fee J, Wallace W, eds. *Anaesthetic pharmacology and physiology.* Edinburgh: Churchill Livingstone 1997.

Although it would be attractive to ascribe a single receptor to a particular trigger for PONV so that an appropriate antiemetic could be used, in practice there is considerable overlap in the triggers and receptors found in each of these afferent pathways to the VC. Morphine and opioids occupy a special place in this respect. They are capable of triggering nausea and vomiting not only via their direct effects on the CTZ, but also via a vestibular effect akin to motion sickness and a vagal effect from the GI stasis they produce.

Antiemetics

Classes of antiemetics and commonly used drugs in each group:

- ◆ Antidopaminergic D_2: droperidol, metoclopramide, chlorpromazine, prochlorperazine
- ◆ Antiserotonin 5-HT_3: ondansetron, granisetron, tropisetron

♦ Antihistamine H_1: cyclizine, promethazine, dimenhydrinate, chlorpromazine, prochlorperazine
♦ Anticholinergic: atropine, hyoscine

These drugs may not have a pure effect at a single receptor – there is some overlap. For instance, metoclopramide has a weak anti-5-HT_3 effect, promethazine has a weak anti-D_2 effect, cyclizine has weak anticholinergic effects, and prochlorperazine has both anti-H_1 and anti-D_2 actions. The use of these drugs in different clinical situations will be considered. The clinical use of some of them is limited by their sedative or psychomimetic side effects, and chlorpromazine, hyoscine, promethazine and dimenhydrinate are no longer first-line drugs for the treatment of PONV.

Droperidol

Droperidol, a potent D_2 antagonist, is popular because of its low cost, undoubted efficacy and presumed low incidence of side effects when used in low dose. This means 0.5–0.65 mg for an adult or 20 µg/kg for children; in doses greater than this there is little additional antiemetic effect (72) but a higher incidence of sedation and dysphoria. The use of low dose of droperidol has become popular in day case surgery and is considered to be 'cost-effective' compared to more expensive drugs such as ondansetron (73,74). However, there is increasing evidence of previously unrecognized side effects. Twenty-three percent of patients given 1.25 mg droperidol reported anxiety or restlessness (75). After a neurolept technique with thiopentone and droperidol 20 µg/kg, early recovery was prolonged, 37% of patients reported memory impairment and 53% had 'locked in feelings' compared to a propofol technique with no droperidol (76). These are not isolated reports – it seems these effects are more common than acknowledged even after low-dose droperidol. Foster *et al.* (77) followed up women given placebo, or droperidol 0.5 or 1 mg with a propofol/fentanyl/isoflurane anaesthetic. Nausea and vomiting was not reduced by droperidol, and akathisia, i.e. restlessness, was reported by 23% in the 0.5 mg group and 38% of the 1 mg group compared to 5% in the placebo group. In half the patients this restlessness was described as 'unpleasant'. Anxiety was only reported by women who received droperidol.

Patient distress after droperidol may therefore go unrecognized in day case patients. Interestingly when droperidol was used in PCA with morphine, sedation but no dysphoria or restlessness was reported, perhaps because of the euphoria and sedation produced by morphine (78).

Studies confirming the effectiveness of low-dose droperidol have used a thiopentone/volatile anaesthetic technique. With propofol/isoflurane anaesthesia, it did not reduce PONV after laparoscopy (79) or minor gynaecological procedures (77). Droperidol 75 µg/kg added to a propofol anaesthetic did not reduce vomiting after strabismus surgery (41). Droperidol does not appear to add any extra antiemesis with propofol and has even been reported to increase PONV used with it (80). It should not be given prophylactically with a propofol technique.

Because of its unpleasant side effects, droperidol should be restricted to a rescue antiemetic rather than given as routine prophylaxis, particularly in day cases.

Metoclopramide

Metoclopramide is a less reliable first-line treatment for PONV (81), although its gastrokinetic effects may be useful. It was no more effective than placebo for laparoscopy-induced PONV (72,79). Added to patient-controlled morphine analgesia, it reduced the severity but not the incidence of PONV (82).

Ondansetron

The 5-HT$_3$ antagonists, principally ondansetron, have become popular despite their high cost because of their efficacy and perceived lack of side effects, although this may not be entirely true. Tramer et al.'s (83) meta-analysis of the efficacy and side effects of ondansetron reported a 3% raised liver enzymes and 3% headache. They also concluded that ondansetron may be more effective at reducing vomiting than nausea. Many studies have not compared 5-HT$_3$ antagonists to established antiemetics, making the results difficult to interpret.

Despite this pessimistic view, there is good evidence that ondansetron is effective against PONV related to middle ear surgery and tonsillectomy (84), although no better than perphenazine. After laparoscopy it was as effective as droperidol in reducing nausea but better at reducing vomiting (85). It is effective in children perhaps due to its effects on vomiting which is common and easier to measure than nausea in the paediatric setting where it is as or more effective than droperidol (86).

When added to propofol/desflurane technique with a high incidence of PONV, ondansetron reduced emesis and improved recovery times (5), but the overall results were very much better after a propofol technique without ondansetron. Propofol anaesthesia has also been shown to be more effective and longer lasting than ondansetron 4 mg in reducing nausea for the first 6–12 h and vomiting for the first 24 h after breast surgery where morphine was used for analgesia (60).

There is some controversy as to the appropriate dosage and timing of its administration. Current recommendations seem to favour giving 8 mg IV towards the end of surgery (87) and 16 mg orally (83). It has been calculated that ondansetron is cost-effective when the risk of PONV is greater than 33% (88).

Antihistamines

Cyclizine, an underrated antiemetic, is less used than it should be because of its reputation for sedation. It is very effective against opioid-induced

PONV with few side effects (89) and was as successful as droperidol in controlling emesis with PCA after loading dose of 50 mg IV plus 2 mg cyclizine added to each 1 mg morphine in the syringe pump (90). Two studies have compared cyclizine with ondansetron in day case laparoscopy; it was ineffective in one (91) but as effective as ondansetron with significantly less rescue antiemetic needed in the second (92).

Propofol and antiemesis

In McCollum *et al.*'s classic study (93) which sought to establish whether propofol had antiemetic effects, it was compared to methohexitone after morphine or pethidine premedication. The incidence of PONV was greatly reduced for the 6 h postoperative period of the study in the propofol group. However, there was a tendency for PONV to increase by 6 h in both groups, although significantly less so in the propofol group. This suggests that any antiemetic effect of propofol is related to its serum level and that eventually this reduces below the effective level, leaving the longer acting effects of opioids. Gan *et al.* (94) looked at the serum concentration of propofol (given by target-controlled infusion) needed to treat established PONV. Ninety-three percent of patients were successfully treated without increased sedation and the mean calculated serum level for an antiemetic response was 343 ng/ml. This may be achieved with a 10 mg bolus followed by 0.6 mg/kg/h.

The use of subhypnotic doses of propofol has given conflicting results, probably because of confounding factors of the serum level and the aetiology of the emesis. Patients given a single dose of propofol 0.5 mg/ kg at the end of middle ear surgery with a non-propofol anaesthetic had no retching and vomiting for 6 h compared to 46% in controls, but the incidence of nausea was not reduced (95). After major gynaecological surgery with morphine PCA, propofol 0.1 mg/kg/h failed to reduce PONV (96), as did 30 mg/h (3 ml/h) after major orthopaedic surgery with intrathecal morphine (97). A higher infusion rate, 1 mg/kg/h, was effective after thyroidectomy (98) but not after gynaecological laparoscopy (99); 1 mg/kg/h was also an effective dose in chemotherapy patients with emesis refractory to 5-HT$_3$ antagonists (100).

Propofol may be more effective in controlling PONV in women – used for maintenance compared with isoflurane it significantly reduced PONV after thyroid surgery, but only in women (101).

The mode of antiemetic action of propofol is controversial. Any antiemetic effect from the lipid emulsion solvent has been excluded (102). Borgeat has suggested that surgery associated with vagal stimulation is less amenable to antiemesis with propofol and that its antiemetic effects are due to its subcortical effects (103). Its effects on reducing emesis refractory to 5-HT$_3$ antagonists suggests that its effects are additive to these and not mediated via serotonin antagonism. In a study looking at the effects of adding placebo, droperidol, metoclopramide and ondansetron to a propofol/isoflurane anaesthetic for laparoscopy (79), only ondansetron reduced PONV; droperidol and metoclopramide, both anti-D$_2$ antagonists, were no more effective than placebo. No study has shown any additional improvement in PONV when droperidol is added to propofol. Does this suggest that propofol's effects are mediated via dopamine antagonism? This has been contradicted by the failure of prolactin levels to increase during infusion of propofol as they do with anti-D_2 antagonists (104). The mechanism of the antiemetic effect of propofol remains unexplained.

Miscellaneous antiemetic interventions

There is a range of alternative treatments which have been found to reduce PONV.

♦ Ephedrine 0.5 mg/kg was found to be as effective an antiemetic as droperidol 40 µg/kg in reducing PONV for 24 h after laparoscopy, with significantly less sedation (105) but was not effective after paediatric inguinal hernioplasty. However, it is cheap, does not make patients sleepy and deserves further investigation.
♦ Dexamethasone is increasingly recognized as a useful antiemetic drug in a wide range of clinical situations. It has been reported to be effective after major gynaecological (106), thyroid (107), middle ear (108), laparoscopic (109), adenotonsillectomy (110) and oral surgery (111), as well as with epidural morphine (112) and chemotherapy (113). The antiemetic effects of dexamethasone appear to be additive in combination with 5-HT$_3$ antagonists (108,114). Droperidol, metoclopramide or granisetron with or without dexamethasone 8 mg given to patients having major gynaecological surgery (115,116) resulted in significantly less PONV in the granisetron group; dexamethasone only significantly reduced PONV when added to granisetron.
♦ Ginger root 0.5–1 g was variably effective after laparoscopic surgery (117,118).
♦ Nabilone, a cannabinoid, has not been adequately investigated for PONV and may have adverse effects on mood and sedation.
♦ Acupuncture/pressure. Acupuncture influences encephalin concentrations and stimulation of the P6 point has been shown to have an antiemetic effect. Electro-acupuncture (119) reduced vomiting after laparoscopy and acupressure with wrist bands reduced nausea and vomiting after Caesarean section. It needs to be administered to awake patients which may explain its lack of effect given during anaesthesia for tonsillectomy and strabismus repair in children. Side effects have not been reported.
♦ IV fluids may reduce nausea and vomiting if hypotension or hypoglycaemia are prevented; reduction in thirst may prevent vomiting early postoperative oral fluids. However, after propofol anaesthesia only modest benefits can be demonstrated (71,120). The effects of reducing preoperative fluid fasting have not been compared with IV fluids.

Many of these alternative approaches to emesis lack adequate evidence and merit further investigation.

Neurokinin 1 antagonists

A promising group of drugs, these block the output from the vomiting centre rather than the receptors which affect the input to the centre. This means that they are effective against PONV from any cause. They appear to have no important side effects but have so far only been tested in animals and are not yet clinically available.

Specific clinical problems

Laparoscopy (Table 7.8)

A propofol total IV anaesthetic (TIVA) with or without N_2O (47,121) is more effective than a volatile anaesthetic technique in reducing the very high incidence of PONV after laparoscopy (122–124), even when ondansetron and/or droperidol are used with the volatile technique (25,51). Droperidol does not appear to reduce PONV any further with a propofol technique, but ondansetron may have additive effects (79) and may be the most logical rescue antiemetic for established PONV after propofol.

Table 7.8   Reduction of PONV after laparoscopy

◆ Propofol induction and maintenance ± N_2O
◆ Reduce peritoneal stretching
  – limit gaseous distension
  – expulsion of a much gas as possible at end of surgery
◆ Avoid morphine if possible
  – short-acting opioids
  – non-steroidal analgesics
  – local anaesthetic into skin and peritoneum
◆ Ondansetron as rescue antiemetic
◆ Dexamethasone??

The combination of dexamethasone with a 5-HT$_3$ antagonist may be synergistic and seems to be particularly effective in gynaecological laparoscopy (126). Limiting abdominal gaseous distension and reducing the residual gas at the end of the procedure are simple measures that may also help (127). Avoiding morphine if possible by using NSAIDs, and wound and intraperitoneal local anaesthetic is also sensible (128,129).

Strabismus surgery

Vomiting after paediatric strabismus surgery is very common, about 60%, and it persists for some time – up to 24–48 h postoperatively. These procedures are commonly done as day cases and vomiting often becomes worse after discharge. Droperidol 75 µg/kg has been the main drug used to treat it and this is effective (130), although it may be no more effective than 20 µg/kg and droperidol 75 µg/kg was associated with restlessness in 65% of children (131). TIVA with propofol may improve vomiting (132) and recovery (42) but this is not confirmed by a meta-analysis of antiemesis after strabismus surgery (130); the incidence of oculocardiac reflex is increased with propofol (130). There is no evidence that $5-HT_3$ antagonists are effective. The prevention of vomiting in children having squint surgery remains a problem.

Middle ear surgery

Another clinical problem is the reduction of PONV after middle ear surgery. D_2 antagonists are less effective in vestibular-related vomiting. $5-HT_3$ antagonists are effective (133), especially in combination with dexamethasone (108). However, it has been suggested that $5-HT_3$ antagonists are only effective in patients with no history of motion sickness (134) and when given at the end of surgery (87). Propofol anaesthesia reduces PONV and improves recovery(135,136) but may be insufficient alone (137). H_1 antagonists would seem the logical drugs to use (138). Transdermal hyoscine is effective (139) but not completely and has side effects. There are no randomized controlled studies of cyclizine or prochlorperazine in middle ear surgery, although both are frequently used for it and in the treatment of Menière's disease. Avoiding morphine would seem prudent because of its vestibular effects. Middle ear surgery is another incompletely solved problem area in PONV.

Patient-controlled analgesia

Although PONV is similar with PCA compared to IM morphine, clinically it reduces the effectiveness of PCA as many patients do not use it effectively due to nausea (140). Mixing an antiemetic in with the morphine solution is an attractive idea. Droperidol is the most common addition and is effective using an initial bolus of 0.5–1 mg followed by 3–10 mg per 50–60 mg morphine (141). Drowsiness limits the usefulness of this technique and fewer patients receiving droperidol described their analgesia as excellent (142), although overt dysphoria has not been reported. Gan et al. (143) compared bolus droperidol 1.25 mg at the end of surgery, droperidol 10 mg per 60 mg morphine in PCA, or both together. Droperidol bolus or mixed in morphine PCA were equally effective and the combination of both increased sedation with no further reduction of PONV.

Ondansetron was effective given as a 4 mg bolus at the end of surgery plus 8 mg per 60 mg morphine (144). Given as single doses at the end of surgery, ondansetron 4 mg was as effective as droperidol 2.5 mg; the combination of both was significantly better than each alone and was 90% effective in preventing PONV in women after abdominal surgery (145). After breast surgery with postoperative morphine analgesia, propofol anaesthesia was better at controlling PONV than ondansetron (60).

Cyclizine as a 50 mg bolus plus 100 mg per 50 mg morphine PCA solution was as effective as droperidol with no more sedation, but other side effects were not measured (90). More studies into cyclizine and PCA are needed.

A combination of ondansetron and droperidol may be the most effective for controlling PONV with PCA, but with expense and side effects. The value of mixing antiemetic in the PCA solution is not confirmed and common sense would suggest using the lowest dose of droperidol or reserving it for rescue antiemesis. Propofol anaesthesia may be effective for 12–24 h and warrants further investigation, and cyclizine should also be considered.

Prophylactic versus rescue antiemetic

Should prophylactic or rescue antiemesis be used? Both propofol and ondansetron are expensive but they may have benefits in improving speed and quality of recovery. However, in procedures and patients with low risk of PONV, significant differences compared to less expensive techniques may be difficult to demonstrate (146). The greater the baseline risk the greater the benefit from using prophylactic antiemesis, so it should therefore be targeted to:

◆ Women
◆ Patients with a history of PONV and/or motion sickness
◆ Procedures associated with a high risk of PONV
◆ Morphine used for postoperative analgesia

Two or more of these factors should be an indication for prophylactic antiemesis, ideally TIVA with or without an appropriate antiemetic for the surgical procedure. Otherwise rescue antiemetics are sufficient and cost-effective.

And finally. . .

◆ No anaesthetic or antiemetic has been shown to be 100% effective in all situations – some individuals defy the best efforts, but their PONV can usually be reduced if not completely abolished
◆ Any intervention which is worthy of introduction into routine clinical practice should reduce the incidence of PONV by at least 50%
◆ As there are multiple factors and mechanisms involved in PONV, it may be necessary to use a multimodal technique with different approaches and classes of antiemetic drugs in order to control PONV

Recommended reading

Hirsch J. Impact of postoperative nausea and vomiting in the surgical setting. *Anaesthesia* 1994; **49** (suppl): 30–1.

Watcha MF, White PF. Postoperative nausea and vomiting. Its etiology, treatment and prevention. *Anesthesiology* 1992; **77**: 162–84.

Palazzo MGA, Strunin L. Anaesthesia and emesis. I: etiology. *Can Anaesth Soc J* 1984; **31**: 178–87.

Palazzo MGA, Strunin L. Anaesthesia and emesis II: prevention and treatment. *Can Anaesth Soc J* 1984; **31**: 407–5.

Paxton LD. Physiology and control of nausea and vomiting. In: McCaughey W, Clarke R, Fee J, Wallace W, eds. *Anaesthetic pharmacology and physiology.* Edinburgh: Churchill Livingstone 1997.

References

1. Metter SE, Kitz DS, Young ML, *et al.* Nausea and vomiting after outpatient laparoscopy: incidence, impact on recovery room stay and cost. *Anesth Analg* 1987; **66**: S116.

2. Siler JN, Horrow JC, Rosenberg H. Propofol reduces prolonged outpatient PACU stay. *Anesthesiol Rev* 1994; **21**: 129–32.

3. Marais M, Maher M, Wetchler B, *et al.* Reduced demands on recovery room resources with propofol (Diprivan) compared with thiopental-isoflurane. *Anesthesiol Rev* 1989; **16**: 29–40.

4. Morris RW, Ernst E, Greaves DJ, *et al.* An audit of the incidence and costs associated with post-operative nausea and vomiting (PONV) following major gynaecological surgery in an outpatient population. *Br J Anaesth* 1993; **70** (suppl 1): A2.

5. Eriksson H, Korttila K. Recovery profile after desflurane with or without ondansetron compared with propofol in patients undergoing outpatient gynecological laparoscopy. *Anesth Analg* 1996; **82**: 533–8.

6. Green G, Jonsson L. Nausea: the most important factor determining length of stay after ambulatory anaesthesia. A comparative study of isoflurane and/or propofol techniques. *Acta Anaesthesiol Scand* 1993; **37**: 742–6.

7. Valanne J. Recovery and discharge of patients after long propofol infusion vs isoflurane anaesthesia for ambulatory surgery. *Acta Anaesthesiol Scand* 1992; **36**: 530–3.

8. Carroll NV, Meiderhoff P, Cox FM, Hirsch JD. Postoperative nausea and vomiting after discharge from outpatient surgery centers. *Anesth Analg* 1995; **80**: 903–9.

9. Sung Y-F, Reiss N, Tillette T. The differential cost of anesthesia and recovery with propofol–nitrous oxide anesthesia versus thiopental sodium–isoflurane–nitrous oxide anesthesia. *J Clin Anesth* 1991; **3**: 391–4.

10. Macario A, Weinger M, Carney S, Kim A. Which clinical anesthesia outcomes are important to avoid? The perspective of patients. *Anesth Analg* 1999; **89**: 652–8.

11. Orkin F. What do patients want? Preferences for immediate postoperative recovery. *Anesth Analg* 1992; **74**: S225.

12. McIndoe AK, Warwick P, O'Connor M. A comparison of retrospective versus contemporaneous nausea scores with patient-controlled analgesia. *Anaesthesia* 1996; **51**: 333–7.

13. Cade L, Morley PT, Ross AW. Is propofol cost-effective for day surgery patients? *Anesth Int Care* 1991; **19**: 201–4.
14. Rosenberg MK, Bridge P, Brown M. Cost comparison: a desflurane versus a propofol-based general anaesthetic technique. *Anesth Analg* 1994; **79**: 852–5.
15. Churnside RJ, Glendinning GA, Thwaites RMA, Watts NWR. Resource use in operative surgery: UK general anaesthesia costs in perspective. *Br J Med Econ* 1996; **10**: 83–98.
16. Carroll NV, Miederhoff PA, Cox FM, Hirsch JD. Costs incurred by outpatient surgical centers in managing postoperative nausea and vomiting. *J Clin Anesth* 1994; **6**: 364–9.
17. Hitchcock M, Rudkin G. The real cost of total intravenous anaesthesia: cost versus price. *Ambulatory Surg.* 1995; **3**: 43–8.
18. Koivusalo A-M, Kellokumpu K, Lindgren L. Gasless laparoscopic cholecystectomy: a comparison of postoperative recovery with conventional technique. *Br J Anaesth* 1996; **77**: 576–80.
19. Larson S, Lundberg D. A prospective survey of postoperative nausea and vomiting with special regard to incidence and relations to patient characteristics, anaesthetic routines and surgical procedures. *Acta Anaesthesiol Scand* 1995; **39**: 539–45.
20. Kamath B, Curran J, Hawkey C, *et al.* Anaesthesia, movement and emesis. *Br J Anaesth* 1990; **64**: 728–30.
21. Sampson IH, Plosker H, Cohen M, Kaplan JA. Comparison of propofol and thiamylal for induction and maintenance of anaesthesia for outpatient surgery. *Br J Anaesth* 1988; **61**: 707–11.
22. Millar JM, Jewkes CF. Recovery and morbidity after daycase anaesthesia. A comparison of propofol with thiopentone–enflurane with and without alfentanil. *Anaesthesia* 1988; **43**: 738–43.
23. Grant IS, Mackenzie N. Recovery following propofol ('Diprivan') anaesthesia – a review of three different anaesthetic techniques. *Postgrad Med J* 1985; **61** (suppl): 133–7.
24. Jakobsson J, Rane K, Ryberg G. Anaesthesia during laparoscopic gynaecologcal surgery: a comparison between desflurane and isoflurane. *Eur J Anaesthesiol* 1997; **14**: 148–52.
25. Song D, White PF. Comparison of sevoflurane and desflurane to propofol for maintenance of outpatient anesthesia. *Anesth Analg* 1997; **84**: S24.
26. Eriksson H, Haasio J, Korttila K. Recovery from sevoflurane and isoflurane anaesthesia after outpatient gynaecological laparoscopy. *Acta Anaesthesiol Scand* 1995; **39**: 377–80.
27. Philip BK, Kallar SK, Bogetz MS, *et al.* A multicenter comparison of maintenance and recovery with sevoflurane or isoflurane for adult ambulatory anesthesia. The Sevoflurane Multicenter Ambulatory Group. *Anesth Analg* 1996; **83**: 314–9.
28. Welborn LG, Hannallah RS, Norden JM, *et al.* Comparison of emergence and recovery characteristics of sevoflurane, desflurane, and halothane in pediatric ambulatory patients. *Anesth Analg* 1996; **83**: 917–20.
29. Raftery S, Sherry E. Total intravenous anaesthesia with propofol and alfentanil protects against postoperative nausea and vomiting. *Can J Anaesth* 1992; **39**: 37–40.
30. Phillips AS, Mirakhur RK, Glen JB, Hunter SC. Total intravenous anaesthesia with propofol or inhalational anaesthesia with isoflurane for major abdominal surgery. *Anaesthesia* 1996; **51**: 1055–9.

31. Rapp S, Conhan T, Pavlin D, *et al.* Comparison of desflurane with propofol on outpatients undergoing orthopedic surgery. *Anesth Analg* 1992; **75**: 572–9.

32. Fredman B, Nathanson M, Smith I, *et al.* Sevoflurane for outpatient anesthesia: a comparison with propofol. *Anesth Analg* 1995; **81**: 823–8.

33. Smith I, Terhoeve PA, Hennart D, *et al.* A multicentre comparison of the costs of anaesthesia with sevoflurane or propofol. *Br J Anaesth* 1999; **83**: 564–70.

34. Nelskyla K, Eriksson H, Soikkeli A, Korttila K. Recovery and outcome after propofol and isoflurane anesthesia in patients undergoing laparoscopic hysterectomy. *Acta Anaesthesiol Scand* 1997; **41**: 360–3.

35. Jellish W, Lien C, Fontenot H, Hall R. The comparative effects of sevoflurane versus propofol in the induction and maintenance of anesthesia in adult patients. *Anesth Analg* 1996; **82**: 479–85.

36. Hartung J. Twenty-four of twenty-seven studies show a greater incidence of emesis associated with nitrous oxide than with alternative anesthetics. *Anesth Analg* 1996; **83**: 114–6.

37. Tramer M, Moore A, McQuay H. Omitting nitrous oxide in general anaesthesia: meta-analysis of intraoperative awareness and postoperative emesis in randomized controlled trials. *Br J Anaesth* 1996; **76**: 186–93.

38. Divatia JVD, Vaidya JS, Badwe RA, Hawalder RW. Omission of nitrous oxide during anesthesia reduces the incidence of postoperative nausea and vomiting. *Anesthesiology* 1996; **85**: 1055–62.

39. Tramer M, Moore A, McQuay H. Meta-analytic comparison of prophylactic antiemetic efficacy for postoperative nausea and vomiting: propofol anaesthesia vs omitting nitrous oxide vs total i.v. anaesthesia with propofol. *Br J Anaesth* 1997; **79**: 256–9.

40. Crawford MW, Lerman J, Sloan MH, *et al.* Recovery characteristics of propofol anaesthesia with and without nitrous oxide: a comparison with halothane/nitrous oxide anaesthesia in children. *Paediatr Anaesth* 1998; **8**: 49–54.

41. Watcha MF, Simeon RM, White PF, Stevens JL. Effect of propofol on the incidence of postoperative vomiting after strabismus surgery in pediatric outpatients. *Anesthesiol* 1991; **75**: 204–9.

42. Klockgether-Radke A, Junge M, Braun U, Muhlendyck H. Influence of propofol on postoperative vomiting in children undergoing strabismus surgery. *Anaesthesist* 1995; **44**: 755–60.

43. Reimer EJ, Montgomery CJ, Bevan JC, *et al.* Propofol anaesthesia reduces early postoperative emesis after paediatric strabismus surgery. *Can J Anaesth* 1993; **40**: 927–33.

44. Standl T, Wilhelm S, von Knobelsdorff G, Schulte am Esh J. Propofol reduces emesis after sufentanil supplemented anaesthesia in paediatric squint surgery. *Acta Anesthesiol Scand* 1996; **40**: 729–33.

45. Heath KJ, Sadler P, Winn JH, McFadzean WA. Nitrous oxide reduces the cost of intravenous anaesthesia. *Eur J Anaesthesiol* 1996; **13**: 369–72.

46. Akhtar TM, Kerr WJ, Kenny GNC. Effect of nitrous oxide on post-operative nausea and vomiting during propofol anaesthesia for short surgical operations. *Eur J Anaesthesiol* 1993; **10**: 337–41.

47. Sukhani R, Lurie J, Jabamoni R. Propofol for ambulatory gynecologic laparoscopy: does omission of nitrous oxide alter postoperative sequelae and recovery? *Anesth Analg* 1994; **78**: 831–5.

48. Lindekaer AL, Skielboe M, Guldager H, Jensen EW. The influence of nitrous oxide on propofol dosage and recovery after total intravenous anaesthesia for day-case surgery. *Anaesthesia* 1995; **50**: 397–9.

49. Gunawardene RD, White DC. Propofol and emesis. *Anaesthesia* 1988; **43** (suppl): 65–7.
50. Gregory MA, Gin T, Yau G, *et al.* Propofol infusion for Caesarian section. *Can J Anaesth* 1990; **37**: 514–20.
51. Kalman S, Jensen A, Ekberg K, Entrei C. Early and late recovery after major abdominal surgery. Comparison between propofol anesthesia with and without nitrous oxide and isoflurane anaesthesia. *Acta Anaesthesiol Scand* 1993; **37**: 730–6.
52. Sneyd JR, Carr A, Byrom WD, Bilski AJT. A meta-analysis of nausea and vomiting following maintenance of anaesthesia with propofol or inhalational agents. *Eur J Anaesthesiol* 1998; **15**: 433–45.
53. Taylor E, Feinstein R, White PF, Soper N. Anesthesia for laparoscopic cholecystectomy. Is nitrous oxide contraindicated? *Anesthesiology* 1992; **76**: 541–3.
54. Halsey M. *Occupational exposure to inhalation anaesthetics.* Abingdon, UK: The Medicine Group (Education) Ltd for Zeneca Pharma 1996.
55. Stollery B, Broadbent D, Lee W, *et al.* Mood and cognitive functions in anaesthetists working in actively scavenged operating theatres. *Br J Anaesth* 1988; **61**: 446–55.
56. De Grood PM, Harbers JB, van Egmond J, Crul JF. Anaesthesia for laparoscopy. A comparison of five techniques including propofol, etomidate, thiopentone and isoflurane. *Anaesthesia* 1987; **42**: 815–23.
57. Claxton AR, McGuire G, Chung F, Cruise C. Evaluation of morphine versus fentanyl for postoperative analgesia after ambulatory surgical procedures. *Anesth Analg* 1997; **84**: 509–14.
58. Marshall CA, Jones RM, Bajorek PK, Cashman JN. Recovery characteristics using isoflurane or propofol for maintenance of anaesthesia: a double blind controlled trial. *Anaesthesia* 1992; **47**: 461–6.
59. Oddby-Muhrbeck E, Jakobsson J, Andersson L, Askergren J. Postoperative nausea and vomiting. A comparison between intravenous and inhalation anaesthesia in breast surgery. *Acta Anaesthesiol Scand* 1994; **38**: 52–6.
60. Gan TJ, Ginsberg B, Grant AP, Glass PSA. Double-blind, randomized comparison of ondansetron and intraoperative propofol to prevent postoperative nausea and vomiting. *Anesthesiology* 1996; **85**: 1036–42.
61. Jakobsson J, Davidson S, Andreen M, Westgreen M. Opioid supplementation to propofol anaesthesia for outpatient abortion: a comparison between fentanyl and alfentanil. *Acta Anaesthesiol Scand* 1991; **35**: 767–70.
62. Sukhani R, Vazquez J, Pappas AL, *et al.* Recovery after propofol with and without intraoperative fentanyl in patients undergoing for ambulatory gynecologic laparoscopy. *Anesth Analg* 1996; **83**: 975–81.
63. Rowbotham DJ, Peacock JE, Jones RM, *et al.* Comparison of remifentanil in combination with isoflurane or propofol for short-stay surgical procedures. *Br J Anaesth* 1998; **80**: 752–5.
64. Philip BK, Scuderi PE, Chung F, *et al.* Remifentanil compared with alfentanil for ambulatory surgery using total intravenous anesthesia. *Anesth Analg* 1997; **84**: 515–21.
65. Davis PJ, Lerman J, Suresh S, *et al.* A randomized multicenter study of remifentanil compared with alfentanil, isoflurane, or propofol in anesthetized pediatric patients undergoing elective strabismus surgery. *Anesth Analg* 1997; **84**: 982–9.
66. Vinik HR, Kissin I. Rapid development of tolerance to analgesia during remifentanil infusion in humans. *Anesth Analg* 1998; **86**: 1307–11.

67. Ding Y, Fredman B, White P. Use of mivacurium during laparoscopic surgery: effect of reversal drugs on postoperative recovery. *Anesth Analg* 1995; **80**: 450–4.
68. Salmenpera M, Kuoppamaki R, Salmenpera A. Do anticholinergic agents affect the occurrence of postoperative nausea. *Acta Anaesthesiol Scand* 1992; **36**: 445–8.
69. Watcha MF, Safavi FZ, McCulloch DA, *et al*. Effect of antagonism of mivacurium-induced neuromuscular block on postoperative emesis in children. *Anesth Analg* 1995; **80**: 713–7.
70. Huang C, Wang M, Susetio L, *et al*. Comparison of the combined effects of atropine and neostigmine with atropine and edrophonium on the occurrence of postoperative nausea and vomiting. *Ma Tsui Hsueh Tsa Chi* 1993; **31**: 113–6.
71. Elhakim M, el Sebiae S, Kaschef N, Essawi GH. Intravenous fluid and postoperative nausea and vomiting after day-case termination of pregnancy. *Acta Anaesthesiol Scand* 1998; **42**: 216–9.
72. Pandit SK, Kothary SP, Pandit UA, *et al*. Dose–response study of droperidol and metoclopramide as antiemetics for outpatient anesthesia. *Anesth Analg* 1989; **68**: 798–802.
73. Fortney JT, Gan TJ, Graczyk S, *et al*. A comparison of the efficacy, safety, and patient satisfaction of ondansetron versus droperidol as antiemetics for elective outpatient surgical procedures. *Anesth Analg* 1998; **86**: 731–8.
74. Tang J, Watcha MF, White PF. A comparison of costs and efficacy of ondansetron and droperidol as prophylactic antiemetic therapy for elective outpatient gynecologic procedures. *Anesth Analg* 1996; **83**: 304–13.
75. Melnick B, Sawyer R, Karembelkar D, *et al*. Delayed side effects of droperidol after ambulatory general anaesthesia. *Anesth Analg* 1989; **69**: 748–51.
76. Linnemann MUS, Guldager H, Nielsen J, *et al*. Psychomimetic reactions after neurolept and propofol anaesthesia. *Acta Anaesthesiol Scand* 1993; **37**: 29–32.
77. Foster PN, Stickle BR, Laurence AS. Akathisia following low-dose droperidol for antiemesis in day-case patients. *Anaesthesia* 1996; **51**: 491–4.
78. Roberts CJ, Millar JM, Goat VA. The antiemetic effectiveness of droperidol during morphine patient-controlled analgesia. *Anaesthesia* 1995; **50**: 559–62.
79. Paxton LD, McKay AC, Mirakhur RK. Prevention of nausea and vomiting after day case gynaecological laparoscopy. A comparison of ondansetron, droperidol, metoclopramide and placebo. *Anaesthesia* 1995; **50**: 403–6.
80. Wagner BJK, Berman SL, Devitt PA, O'Hara DA. Retrospective analysis of postoperative nausea and vomiting to determine antiemetic activity of droperidol added to propofol: a possible drug interaction. *Pharmocotherapy* 1994; **14**: 586–91.
81. Diemunsch P, Conseiller C, Clyti N, *et al*. Ondansetron compared with metoclopramide in the treatment of established postoperative nausea and vomiting. *Br J Anaesth* 1997; **79**: 322–6.
82. Walder AD, Aitkenhead AR. Antiemetic efficacy of metoclopramide when included in a patient-controlled analgesia infusion. *Anaesthesia* 1994; **49**: 804–6.
83. Tramer MR, Reynolds JM, Moore A, McQuay HJ. Efficacy, dose-response, and safety of ondansetron in prevention of postoperative nausea and vomiting. *Anesthesiology* 1997; **87**: 1277–89.
84. Splinter WM, Rhine EJ. Prophylaxis for vomiting by children after tonsillectomy. *Br J Anaesth* 1998; **80**: 155–8.

85. Koivuranta Mk, Laara E, Ryhsnen PT. Antiemetic efficacy of prophylactic ondansetron in laparoscopic cholecystectomy. *Anaesthesia* 1996; **51**: 52–5.
86. Davis PJ, McGowan FX Jr, Landsman I, *et al.* Effect of antiemetic therapy on recovery and hospital discharge time: a double-blind assessment of ondansetron, droperidol, and placebo in pediatric patients undergoing ambulatory surgery. *Anesthesiology* 1995; **83**: 956–60.
87. Sun R, Klein KW, White PW. The effect of timing of ondansetron administration on outpatients undergoing otolaryngologic surgery. *Anesth Analg* 1997; **84**: 331–6.
88. Watcha MF, Smith I. Cost-effectiveness analysis of antiemetic therapy for ambulatory surgery. *J Clin Anesth* 1994; **6**: 370–7.
89. Dundee JW, Loan WB, Morrison JD. A comparison of the efficacy of cyclizine and perphenazine in reducing the emetic effects of morphine and pethidine. *Br J Clin Pharmacol* 1975; **2**: 81–5.
90. Walder AD, Aitkenhead AR. A comparison of droperidol and cyclizine in the prevention of postoperative nausea and vomiting with patient-controlled analgesia. *Anaesthesia* 1995; **50**: 654–6.
91. Watts SA. A randomized double-blinded comparison of metoclopramide, ondansetron and cyclizine in day case laparoscopy. *Anaesth Int Care* 1996; **24**: 546–51.
92. Cholwill JM, Wright W, Hobbs GJ, Curran J. Comparison of ondansetron and cyclizine for prevention of nausea and vomiting after day-case gynaecological laparoscopy. *Br J Anaesth* 1999; **83**: 611–4.
93. McCollum J, Milligan K, Dundee J. The antiemetic effect of propofol. *Anaesthesia* 1988; **43**: 239–40.
94. Gan TJ, Glass PS, Howell ST, *et al.* Determination of plasma concentrations of propofol associated with 50% reduction in postoperative nausea. *Anesthesiology* 1997; **87**: 779–84.
95. Honkavaara P, Saarnivaara S. Comparison of subhypnotic doses of thiopentone vs propofol on the incidence of postoperative nausea and vomiting following middle ear surgery. *Acta Anaesthesiol Scand* 1998; **42**: 211–5.
96. Montgomery JE, Sutherland CJ, Kestin IG, Sneyd JR. Infusions of subhypnotic doses of propofol for the prevention of postoperative nausea and vomiting. *Anaesthesia* 1996; **51**: 554–7.
97. Grattidge P. Nausea and vomiting after major arthroplasty including morphine: a randomised trial of subhypnotic propofol infusion as prophylaxis. *Acta Anaesthesiol Scand* 1998; **42**: 124–7.
98. Ewalenko P, Janny S, Dejonckheere M, *et al.* Antiemetic effect of subhypnotic doses of propofol after thyroidectomy. *Br J Anaesth* 1996; **77**: 463–7.
99. Scuderi PE, D'Angelo R, Harris L, *et al.* Small-dose propofol by continuous infusion does not prevent postoperative vomiting in females undergoing outpatient laparoscopy. *Anesth Analg* 1997; **84**: 71–5.
100. Borgeat A, Wilder-Smith OHG, Rifat K, *et al.* Adjuvant propofol is effective in preventing refractory chemotherapy associated nausea and vomiting. *Anesthesiology* 1992; **77**: A208.
101. Sonner JM, Hynson JM, Clark O, Katz JA. Nausea and vomiting following thyroid and parathyroid surgery. *J Clin Anesth* 1997; **9**: 398–402.
102. Ostman PL, Faure E, Glosten B, *et al.* Is the antiemetic effect of the emulsion formulation of propofol due to the lipid emulsion? *Anesth Analg* 1990; **71**: 536–40.
103. Borgeat A, Wilder-Smith O, Saiah M, Rifat K. Subhypnotic doses of propofol possess direct antiemetic properties. *Anesth Analg* 1992; **74**: 539–41.

104. Borgeat A. Subhypnotic doses of propofol do not possess antidopaminergic properties. *Anesth Analg* 1997; **84**: 196–8.
105. Rothenberg DM, Parnass SM, Litwack K, *et al.* Efficacy of ephedrine in the prevention of postoperative nausea and vomiting. *Anesth Analg* 1991; **72**: 58–61.
106. Liu K, Hsu CC, Chia YY. Effect of dexamethasone on postoperative emesis and pain. *Br J Anaesth* 1998; **80**: 85–6.
107. Wang JJ, Ho ST, Lee SC, *et al.* The prophylactic effect of dexamethasone on postoperative nausea and vomiting in women undergoing thyroidectomy: a comparison of droperidol with saline. *Anesth Analg* 1999; **89**: 200–3.
108. Fujii Y, Toyooka H, Tanaka H. Prophylactic antiemetic therapy with a combination of granisetron and dexamethasone in patients undergoing middle ear surgery. *Br J Anaesth* 1998; **81**: 754–6.
109. Rothenberg DM, McCarthy RJ, Peng CC, Normoyle DA. Nausea and vomiting after dexamethasone versus droperidol following outpatient laparoscopy with a propofol based general anaesthetic. *Acta Anaesthesiol Scand* 1998; **42**: 637–42.
110. Pappas AL, Sukhani R, Hotaling AJ, *et al.* The effect of preoperative dexamethasone on the immediate and delayed postoperative morbidity in children undergoing adenotonsillectomy. *Anesth Analg* 1998; **87**: 57–61.
111. Baxendale BR, Vater M, Lavery KM. Dexamethasone reduces pain and swelling following extraction of third molar teeth. *Anaesthesia* 1993; **48**: 961–4.
112. Wang JJ, Ho ST, Liu YH, *et al.* Dexamethasone reduces epidural morphine-related nausea and vomiting. *Anesth Analg* 1999; **89**: 117–20.
113. Goedhals L, Heron JF, Kleisbauer JP, *et al.* Control of delayed nausea and vomiting with granisetron plus dexamethasone or dexamethasone alone in patients receiving highly emetogenic chemotherapy: a double-blind, placebo controlled, comparative study. *Ann Oncol* 1998; **9**: 661–6.
114. Lopez Olaondo L, Carrascosa F, Pueyo FJ, *et al.* Combination of ondansetron and dexamethasone in the prophylaxis of postoperative nausea and vomiting. *Br J Anaesth* 1996; **76**: 835–40.
115. Fujii Y, Tanaka H, Toyooka H. The effects of dexamethasone on antiemetics in female patients undergoing gynecologic surgery. *Anesth Analg* 1997; **85**: 913–7.
116. McKenzie R, Roliey TJ, Tantisera B, Hamilton DL. Effect of propofol for induction and ondansetron with or without dexamethasone for the prevention of nausea and vomiting after major gynecologic surgery. *J Clin Anesth* 1997; **9**: 15–20.
117. Phillips S, Rugger R, Hutchinson SE. Zingiber officinale (Ginger) – an antiemetic for day case surgery. *Anaesthesia* 1993; **48**: 715–7.
118. Arfeen Z, Owen H, Plummer H, *et al.* A double blind randomized controlled trial of ginger for the prevention of postoperative nausea and vomiting. *Anaesth Int Care* 1995; **23**: 449–52.
119. Ho RT, Jawan B, Fung ST, *et al.* Electro-acupuncture and postoperative emesis. *Anaesthesia* 1989; **45**: 327–9.
120. Yogendran S, Asokumar B, Cheng DCH, Chung F. A prospective randomized double-blinded study of the effect of intravenous fluid therapy on adverse outcomes in outpatient surgery. *Anesth Analg* 1995; **80**: 682–6.
121. Sengupta P, Plantevin OM. Nitrous oxide and day case laparoscopy: effects on nausea, vomiting and return to normal activity. *Br J Anaesth* 1988; **60**: 570–3.

122. Van Hemelrijck J, Smith I, White PF. Use of desflurane for outpatient anesthesia. A comparison with propofol and nitrous oxide. *Anesthesiology* 1991; **75**: 197–203.
123. Ding Y, Fredman B, White PF. Recovery following outpatient anesthesia: use of enflurane versus propofol. *J Clin Anesth* 1993; **5**: 447–50.
124. Randel G, Levy L, Kothary S, Pandit S. Propofol versus thiamylal–enflurane anesthesia for outpatient laparoscopy. *J Clin Anesth* 1992; **4**: 185–9.
125. Raeder JC, Mjaland O, Aasbo V, *et al.* Desflurane versus propofol maintenance for outpatient laparoscopic cholecystectomy. *Acta Anaesthesiol Scand* 1998; **42**: 106–10.
126. Fujii Y, Tanaka H, Toyooka H. Granisetron–dexamethasone combination reduces postoperative nausea and vomiting. *Can J Anaesth* 1995; **42**: 387–90.
127. Lindgren L, Koivusalo A-M, Kellokumpu I. Conventional pneumoperitoneum compared with abdominal wall lift for laparoscopic cholecystectomy. *Br J Anaesth* 1995; **75**: 567–72.
128. Wheatley SA, Millar JM, Jadad AR. Reduction of pain after laparoscopic sterilization with local bupivacaine: a randomised, parallel, double-blind trial. *Br J Obstet Gynaecol* 1994; **101**: 443–6.
129. Loughney AD, Sarma V, Ryall EA. Intraperitoneal bupivacaine for the relief of pain following day case laparoscopy. *Br J Obstet Gynaecol* 1994; **101**: 449–51.
130. Tramer M, Moore A, McQuay H. Prevention of vomiting after paediatric strabismus surgery: a systematic review using the numbers-needed-to-treat method. *Br J Anaesth* 1995; **75**: 556–61.
131. Brown RE, James DJ, Weaver RG, *et al.* Low-dose droperidol versus standard-dose droperidol for prevention of postoperative vomiting after paediatric strabismus surgery. *J Clin Anesth* 1991; **3**: 306–9.
132. Weir PM, Munro HM, Reynolds PI, *et al.* Propofol infusion and the incidence of emesis in pediatric outpatient strabismus surgery. *Anesth Analg* 1993; **76**: 760–4.
133. Fujii Y, Toyooka H, Tanaka H. Granisetron reduces the incidence of nausea and vomiting after middle ear surgery. *Br J Anaesth* 1997; **79**: 539– 42.
134. Honkavaara P. Effect of nausea and vomiting after middle ear surgery during general anaesthesia. *Br J Anaesth* 1996; **76**: 316–8.
135. Jellish WS, Leonetti JP, Murdoch JR, Fowles S. Propofol-based anesthesia as compared with standard anesthetic techniques for middle ear surgery. *J Clin Anesth* 1995; **7**: 292–6.
136. Woodward WM, Barker I, John RE, Peacock JE. Propofol infusion vs thiopentone anaesthesia for prominent ear correction in children. *Paediatr Anaesth* 1997; **7**: 379–83.
137. Habre W, Sims C. Propofol anaesthesia and vomiting after myringoplasty in children. *Anaesthesia* 1997; **52**: 544–6.
138. Takeda N, Morita M, Hasegawa S, *et al.* Neuropharmacology of motion sickness and emesis. A review. *Acta Oto Laryngol Suppl* 1992; **501**: 10–15.
139. Honkavaara P. Effect of transdermal hyoscine on nausea and vomiting during and after middle ear surgery under local anaesthesia. *Br J Anaesth* 1996; **76**: 49–53.
140. Taylor NM, Hall GM, Salmon P. Patients' experiences of patient-controlled analgesia. *Anaesthesia* 1996; **51**: 525–8.
141. Roberts F, Dixon J, Lewis G, *et al.* Induction and maintenance of propofol anaesthesia. A manual infusion scheme. *Anaesthesia* 1988; **43** (suppl): 14–7.

142. Russell D, Duncan LA, Frame WT, *et al.* Patient controlled analgesia with morphine and droperidol following caesarean section under spinal anaesthesia. *Acta Anaesthesiol Scand* 1996; **40**: 600–5.
143. Gan TJ, Alexander R, Fennelly M, Rubin AP. Comparison of different methods of administering droperidol in patient-controlled analgesia in the prevention of postoperative nausea and vomiting. *Anesth Analg* 1995; **80**: 81–5.
144. Wrench IJ, Ward JE, Walder AD, Hobbs GJ. The prevention of postoperative nausea and vomiting using a combination of ondansetron and droperidol. *Anaesthesia* 1996; **51**: 776–8.
145. Pueyo FJ, Carrascosa F, Lopez L, *et al.* Combination of ondansetron and droperidol in the prophylaxis of postoperative nausea and vomiting. *Anesth Analg* 1996; **83**: 117–22.
146. Gupta A, Kullander M, Ekberg K, Lennmarken C. Assessment of recovery following day-case arthroscopy. A comparison between propofol and isoflurane-based anaesthesia. *Anaesthesia* 1995; **50**: 937–42.

PART 3

TYPES OF ANAESTHESIA

8

Day case surgery

W. L. Rowe

- The need for high quality care in day case surgery
- Patient selection
- Patient assessment
- Choice of drugs
- Cost–benefit analysis

Introduction

Most surgical units are now, or soon will be, performing at least 50% of their elective surgery on a day case basis. Day surgery has the potential for achieving significant cost savings, increased patient satisfaction and lower infection rates when compared to in-patient treatment. The development of less invasive surgical procedures associated with less postoperative morbidity, in conjunction with newer anaesthetic and analgesic drugs, has increased the number of patients who could be treated as day cases. The economic pressure to control heath care expenditure in many countries has provided further stimulus to the expansion of day surgery. It is vital, however, that these patients, who are scheduled to return home within hours of surgery, receive optimum standards of care from initial diagnosis until full recovery from the effects of anaesthesia and surgery. The quality of anaesthetic care delivered to these patients can have a major impact on the success or failure of day case surgery. Consumer groups have pointed out major deficiencies in the delivery of care in some units and have been highly critical of this type of service with good justification. Intravenous (IV) anaesthesia, conducted competently, offers patients high quality anaesthesia with rapid and relatively uncomplicated recovery to 'street fitness'. This chapter outlines the processes surrounding good quality day case anaesthesia and the use of IV agents in particular.

Selection of patients and operations for day surgery

Selecting the right patients for day surgery is vital. Key reasons for a selection process are the need to reduce the risks of patients developing serious complications at home or during the journey home. Large follow-up surveys have shown day case surgery to be an extremely safe practice with very low incidences of mortality and major complications. As experience has grown over recent years, more centres are extending the range of procedures done as day cases, and are selecting less fit and more elderly patients for day surgery.

Selection of operations

Suitable operations need to have:

- A low incidence of severe pain requiring complex forms of pain control
- A low risk of major haemorrhage or other major complications requiring intervention such as laparotomy

Long duration of surgery has traditionally been seen as a barrier to day case surgery. However, using appropriate total IV anaesthetic (TIVA) techniques, and attention to details such as IV fluids and body warming devices, it is still possible to achieve rapid recovery from anaesthesia without major complications even after more than 2 h of body surface surgery, e.g. bilateral varicose vein surgery. Intelligent use of operating sessions can help by scheduling more extensive procedures early in the day in order to give these patients longer to recover before they have to go home. Some units discharge patients having more extensive procedures to a 'patient hotel' situated on or near a major hospital campus for an overnight stay before going home. Most patients prefer to be in familiar surroundings and provided that adequate information about what to expect and how to get help is provided, then day surgery is a popular alternative to the traditional overnight stay in hospital for many operations. Examples where traditional attitudes are changing include laparoscopic cholecystectomy, tonsillectomy and some types of trans-urethral prostatectomy.

Patient assessment for day surgery

The aim of patient selection is to identify patients who may need urgent medical or nursing care following anaesthesia. All patients should be assessed as individual cases and the planned procedure is an important factor in determining suitability for day surgery. Trained nurses using detailed guidelines can assess most cases effectively, although borderline or unusual cases must be referred to an experienced anaesthetist before final decisions are made. If more difficult cases are accepted then they must be scheduled when experienced anaesthetic and surgical staff are available.

Age

Age should not be a barrier to day surgery provided the patient is otherwise reasonably fit and there is a competent carer at home. Indeed some elderly patients benefit from a rapid return to familiar surroundings.

Body mass index

Caution needs to be exercised in patients with a body mass index (BMI) > 30 as these patients are more likely to have problems such as difficult airway management, hiatus hernia, hypoxaemia and delayed recovery from anaesthesia. However, experience has shown that it is perfectly reasonable to offer day case surgery to obese patients provided that experienced personnel and facilities for overnight admission are available if required. Pre-operative preparation should include acid aspiration prophylaxis with H_2 antagonists or proton-pump inhibitors. Most units set an upper limit for BMI although there is no clear evidence as to what this limit should be. Several leading day surgery units in the UK have set a limit of 34 for BMI.

ASA level of fitness

Current attitudes to ASA fitness levels in day surgery patients have also changed, as anaesthetic techniques have improved and surveys have shown little effect of ASA grade on morbidity following day case surgery. Many units will now accept patients with severe systemic illness, with some functional impairment (ASA 3) provided the illness is stable.

Chronic medical conditions

Patients with hypertension, diabetes, asthma, other chronic pulmonary diseases and patients taking oral steroid therapy can be suitable for day surgery but need careful individual assessment with appropriate investigation. For a comprehensive review of selection, investigation and preparation of patients for day surgery the relevant chapters in Millar *et al.*, *Practical Anaesthesia for Day Surgery*, are highly recommended (see Further reading).

The challenge of day case anaesthesia

The unpremedicated, anxious patient, undergoing a short but potentially painful surgical procedure, presents the anaesthetist with a difficult challenge. That is to provide high quality anaesthesia for a relatively short period of time, following which the patient is expected to recover full consciousness, without severe pain and nausea, so that he or she can be mobile enough to negotiate the journey home.

Early return to full function is highly desirable to enable patients or their carers to return to work or childcare. Much of the economic benefit of day surgery would be lost if these patients required long periods of recovery at home needing care from relatives, general practitioners or community nurses. It is vital, therefore, that appropriate drugs and techniques are used for the procedure, experienced anaesthetic and surgical staff are involved, and that appropriate analgesia is prescribed for the patient to take at home for an adequate period of time.

Selection of drugs: anaesthetic drugs

Propofol

Induction and maintenance of anaesthesia with propofol offers many advantages for the day surgery patient, so much so that for many it has become the day case anaesthetic of choice (see Figures 8.1–8.3):

- Rapid induction with few airway complications
- Rapid titration of anaesthetic delivery according to response and varying surgical stimulus
- Rapid recovery from anaesthesia to street fitness without residual effects
- Low incidence of nausea and vomiting
- High patient acceptability

The commonest reason for unplanned admission following day surgery is uncontrolled postoperative nausea and vomiting (PONV). IV anaesthesia with propofol is associated with a lower incidence of PONV than any of the currently available volatile agents. Even though the newer volatile agents (desflurane and sevoflurane) are associated with comparable recovery times to propofol, the quality of recovery following propofol makes it very popular with patients and anaesthetists. Propofol can been used as a sole anaesthetic agent when given by repeated intermittent boluses, constant infusion regimes or, more recently, by computer-assisted target-controlled infusion (TCI).

Pain on injection may be experienced with propofol, but can easily be prevented by the concomitant injection of 20–40 mg lignocaine during induction. Alternatively lignocaine 20–40 mg can be mixed in the propofol syringe immediately before use. Using a large vein whenever possible helps to reduce the incidence of pain and is an advantage during IV anaesthesia by enabling rapid entry of IV drugs into the central circulation.

Other IV anaesthetics

Thiopentone

The elimination half-life of thiopentone is long (11.5 h) and although recovery from anaesthesia is due to redistribution, which is relatively

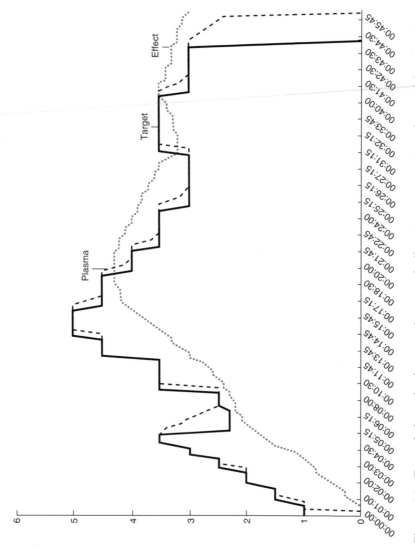

Figure 8.1 Expanded graph of target, plasma and effect-site concentration of propofol against time (see Figure 8.2).

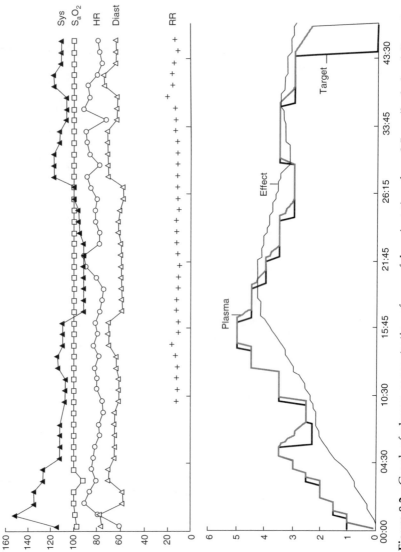

Figure 8.2 Graph of plasma concentration of propofol against time for a 2.5 mg/kg bolus followed by 10 mg/kg/h constant infusion (data from Stanpump computer simulation).

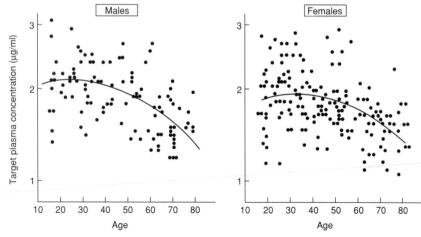

Figure 8.3   Effect of age on target plasma concentration of propofol required to induce anaesthesia in unpremedicated subjects. From Dundee JW, Wyant GM, eds. *Intravenous anaesthesia*, 2nd edn. London: Churchill Livingstone 1988: 174.

rapid, patients have impaired psychomotor function for several hours following administration. Clinical studies have showed that compared with propofol, thiopentone anaesthesia is followed by a period of hyperalgesia for up to 4 h. The slow clearance of the drug also makes accumulation likely to occur with repeated boluses or an infusion. These features make it unsuitable for use as the sole anaesthetic in day case patients.

Methohexitone

Methohexitone has a shorter elimination half-life (4 h) than thiopentone and has been used for IV anaesthesia by infusion. Accumulation may occur with prolonged use and excitatory effects are common, especially in patients who have not been premedicated.

Etomidate

Etomidate has a rapid elimination half-life (75 min), but is difficult to use as a sole anaesthetic agent due to difficulties assessing the depth of anaesthesia. It is associated with an unacceptably high incidence of PONV, which also makes its use unsuitable for day surgery.

Summary

Observations on common IV anaesthetic drugs are summarized in Table 8.1.

Table 8.1   Observations on common IV anaesthetic drugs for use in day case surgery

Drug	Half-life	Comments
Propofol	$t_{1/2\alpha}$: 2.5 min	Rapid recovery to street fitness
	$t_{1/2\beta}$: 35–45 min	Good laryngeal relaxation for airway insertion
	elimination: 200–300 min	Antiemetic properties
		Good patient acceptability
Thiopentone	11.5 h	Prolonged hang-over effect even after short administration
		Hyperalgesia for up to 4 h
		Unsuitable for infusion
Methohexitone	4 h	High incidence of excitatory effects in unpremedicated patients
Etomidate	1.25 h	High incidence of PONV
		Suppression of hypopituitary–adrenal axis

Selection of drugs: analgesic drugs

Opioid drugs

Short-acting opioid drugs are preferred in patients who are to become ambulant soon after surgery. Longer-acting drugs such as morphine and pethidine are associated with postural hypotension, sedation and nausea. The commonest opioid drugs used in day case anaesthesia in the UK are fentanyl, alfentanil and remifentanil.

Fentanyl

A slightly longer duration of action than alfentanil and a long elimination half-life make fentanyl unsuitable for use by infusion. It can be used very effectively though, by single or intermittent bolus injection in combination with a propofol infusion. Small (25–50 µg) boluses may be given intermittently to maintain a respiratory rate between 10 and 14 breaths per minute. Further boluses can be given in anticipation of stimulating parts of the procedure.

Alfentanil

Alfentanil has a shorter elimination half-life compared to fentanyl and can be used by infusion or intermittent bolus. Its pharmacokinetic profile is similar to propofol for short procedures, so it can be used in the same syringe in concentrations up to 1.25 mg per 500 mg propofol. For longer procedures a separate infusion is advisable due to the effect of the context sensitive half-life, where half-life increases with increasing duration of infusion.

Remifentanil

Remifentanil has the shortest duration of action of all currently available opioid drugs. It is metabolized by cholinesterases, so its elimination is predictable and unaffected by changes in hepatic function or blood flow. It is a very potent opioid agonist and is best given by infusion so that dose can be titrated to effect. For short cases, and in particular when patients will be required to breathe spontaneously, a dilute solution (e.g. 20 µg/ml) should be used to avoid low infusion rates. At low infusion rates titration to effect on respiratory rate is more difficult to control. Also inaccuracies in what is actually delivered to the patient due to syringe pump design become more significant at low infusion rates. There is a significant degree of inter-patient variability with remifentanil, so the dose required for adequate analgesia, while still allowing the patient to breathe spontaneously, may vary from 0.02 to 0.2 µg/kg/min.

Postoperative analgesia

When short-acting drugs are used intra-operatively it is vital that adequate postoperative analgesia is provided before the short-acting drugs wear off. It is common practice to use a variety of postoperative drugs in order to avoid giving long-acting opioid drugs. Local anaesthetic drugs are often used in this context, used by local infiltration, specific nerve blockade or topical administration. In addition non-steroidal anti-inflammatory drugs (NSAIDs), especially diclofenac and ketorolac, are commonly used in combination with oral codeine and paracetamol formulations. NSAIDs are often prescribed preoperatively or can be given IV or rectally during the operation. The use of combinations of different types of analgesic drugs, sometimes called 'balanced analgesia', is often successful in eliminating the need for long-acting opioid drugs altogether.

Tramadol is sometimes used for analgesia in day case patients. It has weak opioid activity, and also blocks the re-uptake of noradrenaline and 5-hydroxytryptamine in the central nervous system. It has a potency similar to that of pethidine, but is associated with a high (30–35%) incidence of nausea and vomiting.

Some patients undergoing more painful day case procedures (e.g. laparoscopic sterilization) may need more analgesia. It may still be possible to avoid the use of long-acting drugs by giving small boluses of fentanyl in the recovery unit until pain is controlled and oral or rectal drugs become effective. Alternatively, if equipment and staff are available it may be possible to continue the opioid infusion used in theatre into the recovery period, or use a patient-controlled analgesia (PCA) device containing alfentanil or remifentanil.

Summary

- Avoid long-acting opioid drugs where possible
- Use dilute infusions in theatre for easier titration to effect
- Ensure adequate postoperative analgesia before short-acting drugs wear off
- Use 'balanced' techniques for postoperative analgesia
- Consider continued infusions or PCA devices using short-acting opioids for more painful procedures where equipment and supervision are available

Economic aspects of TIVA in day case surgery

Propofol anaesthesia has often been regarded as an 'expensive' form of anaesthesia compared with low-flow volatile anaesthesia. In fact, for a 65 kg patient at 6 mg/kg/h maintenance infusion rate the anaesthetic is costing 12.6 pence/min at current prices. For 2% isoflurane using a fresh gas flow of 2 l/min the cost is 8.0 pence/min – a difference of 4.6 pence/min. These are hardly large sums of money, and appear totally irrelevant when compared to surgical costs, staff costs and the day surgery unit's overhead costs (heating, lighting, stationary, laundry services, etc). Also, for cases lasting 20 min or less most anaesthetists using volatile agents will not reduce fresh gas flows enough to make significant savings.

All volatile agents are associated with more PONV than propofol and this is the commonest cause of overnight admission following day surgery. These unplanned admissions can be expensive for the admitting unit, especially during winter months when emergency medical admissions can limit the number of beds available for elective surgery. Cost-benefit analysis, where all direct and indirect costs are considered, suggests that a small increase in the cost of the anaesthetic agent would be more than compensated for by a four-fold reduction in PONV, fewer unplanned admissions, faster recovery time in the first stage recovery unit and earlier discharge home. In some health care systems an earlier return to work has also been shown to be an extra cost-benefit associated with the use of propofol anaesthesia. Enlund in Sweden showed that even after a very short day case procedure, patients went back to work one day earlier following propofol anaesthesia compared with thiopentone anaesthesia and this more than compensated for the increased cost of anaesthesia.

The economic benefits associated with propofol anaesthesia can be summarized as:

- Faster throughput in the operating department
- Earlier discharge home
- Lower incidence of PONV
- Fewer unplanned admissions for PONV and delayed recovery
- Earlier return to work following day surgery

Further reading

Books

Cahill H, Jackson I. *Day surgery principles and nursing practice*. London: Ballière Tindall 1997.

Millar JM, Rudkin GE, Hitchcock M. *Practical anaesthesia and analgesia for day surgery*. Oxford: Bios 1997.

Wetchler BV, ed. *Anesthesia for ambulatory surgery*. Philadelphia, PA: JB Lippincott 1990.

Dundee JW, Wyant GM. *Intravenous anaesthesia*. Edinburgh: Churchill Livingstone 1988.

Articles

Coates D. 'Diprifusor' for general and day-case surgery. *Anaesthesia* 1998; **53** (suppl 1): 46–8.

Carroll PH, Ogg TW. Total intravenous anaesthesia in day case surgery. *Ambulatory Surg* 1995; **3**: 165–70.

Carroll PH, Ogg TW. Recovery after day surgery with intravenous agents. *Ambulatory Surg* 1996; **4**: 19–23.

Enlund M, Kobosko P, Rhodin A. A cost–benefit evaluation of using propofol and alfentanil for a short gynecological procedure. *Acta Anaesthesiol Scand* 1996; **40**: 416–20.

Hitchcock M, Rudkin GE. The real cost of total intravenous anaesthesia: cost versus price. *Ambulatory Surg* 1995; **3**: 43–8.

Raftery S, Sherry E. Total intravenous anaesthesia with propofol and alfentanil protects against nausea and vomiting. *Can J Anaesth* 1992; **39**: 37–40.

Rowe WL. Economics in anaesthesia. *Anaesthesia* 1998; **53**: 782–8.

Watcha MF, White PF. Economics of anesthetic practice. *Anesthesiology* 1997; **86**: 1170–96.

White PF, Smith I. Impact of newer drugs and techniques on the quality of ambulatory anesthesia. *J Clin Anesth* 1993; **5** (suppl 1): 3–13.

White PF, Smith I. Ambulatory anesthesia: past, present, and future. *Int Anesthesiol Clin* 1994; **32**: 1–16.

Websites

Intravenous infusion computer simulation software available on the internet at:
http://pkpd.icon.palo-alto.med.va.gov/

Stanpump: original text-based program for infusing 19 different drugs
            source code available

Stelpump: excellent graphical version of Stanpump
            allows two simultaneous infusions

9

Cardiac surgery

J. D. Kneeshaw and R. Mills

- Total intravenous anesthesia (TIVA) can be used for cardiac anaesthesia from induction to postoperative sedation
- TIVA is applicable to all cardiac surgical patients
- TIVA may facilitate extubation
- TIVA is economically viable
- Propofol-based TIVA produces acceptable haemodynamic stability
- Propofol-based TIVA is predictable even during hypothermic cardiopulmonary bypass
- Propofol-based TIVA may help to attenuate stress responses
- Propofol-based TIVA may exert a cerebral protective effect

Introduction

The aim of anaesthesia for cardiac surgery is to maintain cardiovascular stability, whilst ensuring an adequate depth of anaesthesia. Total intravenous anaesthesia (TIVA), as well as meeting the above criteria, solves the problem of loss of the lungs as a route of anaesthetic administration during cardiopulmonary bypass (CPB) by eliminating the need for volatile agents.

The physiological changes produced by CPB affect the pharmacokinetics and pharmacodymanics of the agents used in cardiac anaesthesia, and a brief discussion of CPB is therefore necessary later in this chapter.

Cardiac anaesthesia is in many ways the ideal arena for TIVA. Early techniques were based largely on high-dose IV opioid, usually morphine. Although these techniques reliably produced considerable cardiovascular stability, they were associated with the need for prolonged postoperative respiratory support and carried an unacceptable risk of awareness during surgery. Current techniques of TIVA for cardiac surgery are suitable for the induction and maintenance of anaesthesia, and can be continued for transfer to the postoperative ICU, and if required for postoperative sedation. The administration of hypnotic drugs by continuous infusion is also associated with a reduced risk of awareness.

Infusion rates can be adjusted rapidly to achieve the level of anaesthesia required at any stage of the perioperative period and the use of drugs without significant cumulative effects can facilitate earlier extubation of many patients; so called 'fast tracking'.

General considerations of patients with cardiac disease

Patients presenting for cardiac surgery may have congenital lesions, acquired valvular disease, coronary artery disease or lesions of the great vessels. In the developed world around 60–70% of cardiac surgical procedures involve patients with coronary artery disease and are designed to revascularize ischaemic myocardium. Many patients have impaired ventricular function, seen in the most extreme form in those patients with end-stage disease presenting for cardiac transplantation. Patients with cardiac disease are more vulnerable to the adverse haemodynamic effects of anaesthetic agents. They are less able to compensate for the effects of these agents because of their disease process and because of concomitant drug therapy such as β-blockade. Anaesthesia in these patients should be directed at maintaining haemodynamic stability and should promote a positive myocardial oxygen balance.

Co-existing systemic disease is common in patients presenting for cardiac surgery. Hypertension, peripheral vascular disease, cerebrovascular disease, diabetes, renal disease and pulmonary disease are frequently encountered as increasing numbers of high-risk and or elderly patients are being considered for surgical treatment. Intercurrent systemic disease may be encountered in any population of surgical patients, but the effect of systemic disease in cardiac surgery and anaesthesia is often magnified by the profound physiological changes associated with CPB.

Anaesthesia and cardiopulmonary bypass

CPB, the use of a pump and an oxygenator to take over the function of the heart and lungs during surgery, is one of the major factors which differentiates cardiac anaesthesia from anaesthesia for other surgical procedures. CPB produces profound changes in patient physiology, and in the distribution, metabolism and elimination of anaesthetic agents.

At the onset of CPB the patient's blood volume is mixed with the priming volume of the CPB circuit. In adult practice the prime is usually a crystalloid solution, but colloid or blood may be included in paediatric cases and for other specific reasons. The onset of CPB is associated with a decrease in mean arterial pressure secondary to vasodilation, haemodilution and the introduction of non-pulsatile flow. The overall effect is to produce a decrease in peripheral blood flow with relative preservation of the central circulation. Hepatic, renal, cerebral and skeletal perfusion have all been shown to be reduced during CPB.

A flow rate of 1.8–2.4 l/min/m^2 is maintained by the pump and the mean arterial blood pressure is determined by the systemic vascular resistance (SVR). Vasodilators or vasoconstrictors are used to manipulate the SVR to maintain the mean arterial pressure in the range 40–80 mmHg.

Frequently a heat exchanger in the CPB circuit is used to reduce the patient's body temperature to 28–32°C during CPB. This cooling reduces the patient's total metabolic rate and therefore oxygen consumption during CPB, providing some degree of protection from ischaemic damage. The distribution of drugs is changed by haemodilution, alterations in regional blood flow and by changes in protein binding. Drug elimination is reduced because of impaired hepatic metabolism and renal clearance, both resulting from decreased perfusion. Hypothermia also reduces metabolism and elimination of anaesthetic agents. Many drugs bind to components of the CPB circuit and there is sequestration of some drugs in relatively poorly perfused tissues such as the lungs. A few patients are cooled profoundly to 18°C or less if there is to be a limitation of CPB flow or a period of circulatory arrest to facilitate surgery. Patients are usually rewarmed before the discontinuation of CPB. Recently there has been an increasing trend toward the use of normothermic CPB in adult cardiac surgical practice.

When CPB is initiated there is generally a reduction in the plasma concentration of most anaesthetic agents resulting from haemodilution and drug sequestration. The plasma levels tend to increase subsequently during CPB because of reduced redistribution and clearance. Although plasma drug levels are often lower during CPB, free drug concentrations may remain relatively unchanged because a greater proportion of drug remains unbound to plasma proteins. All opioids exhibit a decrease in total plasma concentration at the start of CPB. This is particularly marked in the case of fentanyl, a drug that binds significantly to the CPB circuit, as well as being sequestered in the lungs during the period of low pulmonary blood flow. The decrease in drug concentration seen at onset of CPB is less significant for drugs that have a large volume of distribution. This is because the relative haemodilution caused by the addition of the priming volume of the CPB circuit is less significant than for drugs with a small volume of distribution. This is also true for drugs which equilibrate rapidly following haemodilution.

Anaesthetic regimes for operations involving CPB should take account of the influence of these factors on the pharmacokinetics of the anaesthetic agents to ensure safe, adequate and predictable anaesthesia.

Awareness during cardiac surgery, particularly during CPB, has been well documented. It occurs more commonly when predominantly opioid techniques were used to promote cardiovascular stability. Awareness is a potential hazard with any anaesthetic technique and may be more likely where there is difficulty in predicting the pharmacokinetics of anaesthetic agents during CPB. More stable levels of anaesthesia can be achieved by continuous drug infusions rather than repeated bolus doses of drugs. This form of administration is more appropriate for cardiac anaesthesia providing there is no significant accumulation of the agents used. Consciousness is usually lost below a brain temperature of 30°C and therefore the potential for awareness may be greater with the current trend towards normothermic CPB. Normothermia also implies less impairment of drug metabolism and elimination. In common with TIVA used for other types of surgical procedures, the route of administration must be secure to prevent inadequate anaesthesia. Anaesthetic agents are best administered via central venous catheters during cardiac surgery because venous access via peripheral cannulae cannot be confirmed easily.

Ventilation of the lungs is suspended during CPB and hence inhalation is not an available route of anaesthetic administration. It is possible to administer volatile agents during CPB by the provision of a vaporizer in the gas supply to the pump oxygenator. This mode of anaesthesia has the disadvantage that it is not under the direct control of the anaesthetist.

CPB is known to cause activation of the complement cascade. The complement system, consisting of over 20 plasma proteins, plays an important role in the body's defence to trauma, infection and immunological challenge. Complement activation leads to the release of histamine, cell lysis, contraction of smooth muscle, increased vascular permeability and activation of phagocytic cells. Exposure of blood to foreign surfaces such as the CPB circuit can trigger the cascade via the alternative pathway. This pathway can also be triggered by Hageman factor, XIIa, which is produced by activation of the coagulation cascade. Although on CPB, heparin inhibits activation of the coagulation cascade, sufficient factor XIIa is produced to promote complement activation. Activation of the complement system leads to direct membrane injury, neutrophil activation, enhanced phagocytosis and release of lysosomal enzymes. Cytotoxic materials thus released can produce tissue damage, particularly in the pulmonary vascular bed. It is thought that complement activation plays an important role in the genesis of 'post perfusion syndrome'. This is an important cause of morbidity in cardiac surgical patients. There may be one or more of the following: pulmonary and renal dysfunction, postoperative bleeding, fever, increased interstitial fluid, leukocytosis and haemolysis. Propofol, which has free radical scavenging properties, may limit some of the adverse effects associated with CPB.

It has been suggested that lipid-based drugs like propofol can, in high doses, interfere with the membrane function of the oxygenator during CPB through physical obstruction. This could adversely affect gas exchange in the device. In clinical practice this is not a problem, although if boluses of propofol are used on CPB, lipid globules can be seen to collect on the membrane. These are rapidly reabsorbed over a few minutes.

Cerebral perfusion is often decreased during CPB and hypothermia is still commonly used to provide some degree of cerebral, as well as myocardial, protection during surgery. It may also be helpful if the anaesthetic agents used cause a reduction in cerebral metabolic rate and hence some extra protection from relative ischaemia. High-dose thio-pentone (25–30 mg/kg) is considered to be the most effective drug in providing pharmacological cerebral protection from ischaemia. However, the prolonged postoperative effects of such a regime make it unsuitable for the routine management of cardiac surgical patients. Propofol is known to decrease cerebral metabolic rate and itself may confer some advantage in this respect.

Drugs used for total intravenous anaesthesia in cardiac surgery

General considerations

The ideal agent for cardiac anaesthesia should cause minimal myocardial depression, should not promote arrhythmias, and should have predict-able effects upon the peripheral and pulmonary vascular resistances. This must hold true at doses high enough to avoid awareness.

Drug administration by infusion is preferable to bolus techniques because infusions avoid large swings in plasma drug concentrations that may be associated with cardiovascular instability. Infusion also eliminates trough concentrations of agents associated with a high risk of awareness.

Agents should not have cumulative effects. This implies that drugs with short plasma half-lives are preferred. Agents should not be metabolized to active products and obviously should have no nephro-toxic or hepatotoxic effects.

Nitrous oxide (N_2O) has a depressant effect upon the myocardium which is particularly marked in the right ventricle. The depressant effect is often offset by the sympathetic stimulation associated with surgery, but in association with high-dose opioids and β-blockade this depressant effect may be clinically significant. In patients with pulmonary hyper-tension, N_2O may cause a marked increase in pulmonary artery pressure. N_2O will cause any air bubbles entering the circulation to increase in size. This increases the risk of systemic embolization during cannulation of the heart, during CPB and after a period of CPB. Systemic air embolism is a contributory cause of the many minor cognitive changes and neuro-psychiatric abnormalities that some patients experience after cardiac surgery. These considerations, in addition to the risk of vitamin B_{12} oxidation with prolonged exposure, have led to N_2O being discarded by most cardiac anaesthetists.

Hypnotic agents

Propofol

Propofol is increasingly becoming the agent of choice for cardiac anaesthesia. It fulfils many, but not all, of the properties of the ideal agent for cardiac TIVA. It is suitable for the induction and maintenance of anaesthesia, and for postoperative sedation. Propofol administered by infusion is not cumulative, it is rapidly metabolized and does not produce active metabolites.

The ideal anaesthetic agent for cardiac anaesthesia should not produce any haemodynamic disturbance. Propofol is, however, known to produce hypotension caused by a reduction in SVR, combined with some degree of myocardial depression. This hypotensive effect is clearly seen when anaesthesia is induced with a bolus sleep dose of propofol. However, the administration of propofol by infusion is associated with much less hypotension than administration by bolus injection and co-induction of anaesthesia by propofol infusion combined with a suitable opioid will usually produce cardiovascular stability. If hypotension does occur during propofol administration, it can and should be treated rapidly with IV fluid and if necessary a small dose of vasopressor. Many studies have now demonstrated that propofol infusion, at a rate 3–4 mg/kg/h in combination with moderate dose fentanyl (10–20 µg/kg), is not associated with significant haemodynamic disturbance in patients undergoing either myocardial revascularization or valvular cardiac surgery. It should be noted, however, that most studies have examined the effects of propofol anaesthesia in patients with good left ventricular function.

Greater caution should be taken with patients who have documented ventricular impairment. One animal study demonstrated a dose-dependent reduction in isolated left ventricular myocyte shortening velocity following exposure to propofol at anaesthetic concentrations (2–4 µg/ml). In the same study increasing concentrations of propofol produced a dose-dependent decrease in the responsiveness of myocytes to β-adrenergic stimulation. The effects of propofol on myocyte preparations subjected to conditions equivalent to hypothermic, hyperkaelemic cardioplegic arrest (HHCA) were also investigated. Propofol caused a dose-dependent reduction in indices of myocyte contractile function after simulated HHCA, but did not consistently produce a further decline in myocyte β-adrenergic responsiveness in addition to that produced by HHCA alone. Another *in vitro* study demonstrated a negative effect of propofol on the contractile function of isolated papillary muscle and of myocardial strips. This effect was quantitatively less than the effect of either thiopentone or ketamine on isolated human atrial muscle. *In vivo* work on the haemodynamic effects of propofol on left ventricular contractility have produced contradictory results which may reflect the different conditions under which the studies were performed.

The precise molecular basis for the negative inotropic effect of propofol is unclear. It has been postulated that propofol may have selective effects on sarcolemmal calcium flux, which alters myocyte contractile function. Despite the limitations of studies using isolated mechanically unloaded preparations, it seems likely that propofol does have some negative inotropic effect. Caution is therefore sensible when propofol is used in patients with significant ventricular dysfunction. Despite this caveat, propofol is successfully being used for anaesthesia in patients with poor ventricular function and in those with end-stage heart failure undergoing heart transplantation. In summary, the adverse effects of propofol are probably less significant than equipotent doses of other hypnotic agents.

On initiating CPB using TIVA with propofol there is an initial fall in the plasma drug concentration. This is predominantly due to haemodilution but there is also some binding of propofol to the CPB circuit. As CPB proceeds the plasma propofol concentration returns to, or even exceeds, the pre-CPB concentration, possibly due to decreased hepatic clearance. Despite these changes the free propofol concentration appears to vary very little, and infusions of 3–4 mg/kg/h maintain adequate anaesthesia during cold and warm CPB.

The lipid nature of propofol does not adversely affect gas exchange during CPB nor does it cause problems if haemofiltration is used to remove excess volume on CPB.

CPB produces a profound stress response with release of plasma catecholamines. High-dose opioid techniques do not effectively suppress this response. A study comparing patients receiving either propofol infusion or morphine and diazepam increments during CPB, showed that the increases in plasma cortisol, adrenaline and noradrenaline concentrations were significantly reduced in the propofol group. The stress response produced by surgery results in substrate mobilization, catabolism with a negative nitrogen balance and retention of salt and water. The magnitude of this response is generally related to the severity of operative trauma. There are theoretical advantages to obtunding this process, but as yet there are no known studies in cardiac patients demonstrating improved outcome attributable to attenuation of the stress response.

Postoperative bleeding can be a major cause of morbidity in cardiac surgery. A contributory factor in this problem is relative thrombocytopaenia caused by platelet loss in the CPB circuit. Lipid emulsions such as propofol can be taken up by platelets and might potentially interfere with their function. In clinical practice this does not appear to be a problem and an increased bleeding tendency has not been demonstrated in cardiac surgical patients anaesthetized with propofol.

Benzodiazepines

Benzodiazepines have for many years been popular induction agents in cardiac anaesthesia. They have also been recommended as supplements to anaesthesia at times of increased risk of awareness, in particular during CPB. There is, however, an increasing feeling amongst some cardiac anaesthetists that the benzodiazepines are amnesic rather than anaesthetic drugs when used in this way. Benzodiazepines are generally administered as boluses since most of the drugs of this type are cumulative if administered by continuous infusion. Delayed recovery may result from the cumulative effects of benzodiazepines, especially in the elderly, since both diazepam and midazolam are metabolized to active products. Additionally, a small but unpredictable subset of patients (approximately 6%) appear to metabolize midazolam extremely slowly. Benzodiazepines are used in conjunction with opioids to induce anaesthesia to combine cardiovascular stability with adequate hypnosis. However, midazolam in combination with high-dose opioid may produce significant hypotension secondary to myocardial depression.

There seems little place in modern cardiac anaesthetic practice for the use of boluses of drugs to maintain anaesthesia with the inherent risk of haemodynamic instability and fluctuating levels of anaesthesia when there are agents available that are safe and effective when administered by continuous infusion.

The benzodiazepines all exhibit a decrease in total drug concentration on CPB, but the effect on free drug levels is unclear. This group of drugs is largely protein bound and therefore changes in protein binding and acid base balance are likely to have significant effects upon free drug levels.

The elimination of benzodiazepines is prolonged following CPB.

Barbiturates

Both thiopentone and methohexitone have been used successfully by infusion for cardiac anaesthesia. Thiopentone, being extremely fat soluble, is particularly prone to accumulation after large doses or infusions, resulting in delayed recovery.

Thiopentone may produce a decrease in cardiac output and blood pressure, with a compensatory reflex tachycardia, although the tachycardia may not be seen in β-blocked patients presenting for coronary artery surgery. The haemodynamic profile of thiopentone does not preclude its careful use for the induction of anaesthesia in cardiac patients and some would argue that the haemodynamic effects of bolus sleep doses of thiopentone and propofol are clinically indistinguishable. If it is used for the maintenance of cardiac anaesthesia the plasma thiopentone concentration falls during CPB because of significant binding to the CPB circuit. However, an increase in the proportion of unbound drug maintains a relatively stable free thiopentone concentration. Although both infusions and incremental boluses have been used for maintenance anaesthesia during cardiac surgery, in either case marked cumulative effects of the drug are inevitable.

Thiopentone still retains an important role in cardiac anaesthesia in the area of prophylaxis against ischaemic cerebral damage associated with low-flow CPB or induced circulatory arrest (see above).

Methohexitone has a similar haemodynamic profile to thiopentone in equipotent doses. The elimination half-life of methohexitone is far shorter, approximately 3–4 h, and delayed recovery is less likely. Like propofol and thiopentone, plasma methohexitone concentration is reduced on CPB but free drug concentrations remain relatively constant. If combined with moderate doses of opioid, anaesthesia can be induced by infusing methohexitone at a rate of 6–8 mg/kg/h. Anaesthesia can then be maintained by an infusion of 3–4 mg/kg/h before, during and after CPB.

In adult cardiac surgery a methohexitone/fentanyl anaesthetic technique has been shown to compare favourably with a propofol/fentanyl technique. No differences in haemodynamic variables or times to extubation were demonstrated and indeed less vasoconstrictor was required to maintain an adequate perfusion pressure on CPB.

Etomidate

Etomidate infusions have been used for induction, maintenance and postoperative sedation for cardiac surgery. Although haemodynamic stability is good, the associated adrenal suppression may be undesirable and in certain circumstances etomidate infusions have been associated with an increased incidence of sepsis. This effect may be evident even after a single induction dose. Despite this, in a few centres, etomidate is still a popular agent particularly in patients with impaired ventricular function.

Ketamine

Ketamine has been used both for induction and maintenance of anaesthesia for cardiac surgery. It has a relatively short distribution half-life and an elimination half-life of 3–4 h making it suitable for use as an infusion. Ketamine does cause a degree of direct myocardial depression, but clinically this effect is hidden by a centrally mediated sympathetic response. If it is used as a sole agent this effect of ketamine may produce an unacceptable increase in myocardial oxygen consumption. This may lead to myocardial ischaemia in patients with critical coronary artery lesions. Co-induction of anaesthesia with a benzodiazepine should reduce the risk of ischaemic episodes and is said to produce relative haemodynamic stability. Further, the addition of a benzodiazepine tends to decrease the incidence of emergence delirium characteristic of ketamine.

Opioids

From as early as the 1960s high-dose opioid anaesthesia was advocated for its cardiovascular stability. The technique was introduced by Lowenstein, who used high-dose morphine in patients with poor ventricular function undergoing valve surgery. Morphine, fentanyl, alfentanil, sufentanil and now remifentanil have all been used in cardiac anaesthesia, occasionally as sole agents but more frequently in combination with one of the hypnotic agents discussed above.

Fentanyl

Anaesthesia using high-dose fentanyl (60–100 µg/kg) was first suggested by Stanley in the 1970s. In this technique a single large dose of fentanyl was used to both induce and maintain anaesthesia. The technique was widely used and met the criterion of producing haemodynamic stability.

This technique, which is still in favour in some centres, presents two major problems. First, the large dose of opioid leads to postoperative respiratory depression resulting in the need for a prolonged period of postoperative positive pressure ventilation. Secondly, despite producing a high initial plasma fentanyl concentration at the onset of CPB, the plasma fentanyl concentration falls leading to a significant risk of awareness. The reduction in the plasma concentration of fentanyl at this time is caused by binding of drug to components of the CPB circuit, haemodilution by the prime volume of the CPB circuit and sequestration of drug in the lungs.

It is likely that this high-dose fentanyl anaesthetic technique, when employed without hypnotic supplementation, led to cardiac anaesthesia gaining its once deserved reputation for producing an unacceptably high incidence of awareness during surgery. The incidence of awareness during unsupplemented fentanyl anaesthesia can be reduced by adding an infusion of fentanyl at a rate of 0.5–0.75 µg/kg/min after the initial bolus. The addition of this infusion will usually maintain a plasma fentanyl level greater than 20 ng/ml. Despite this, many patients still exhibit tachycardia and hypertension at the time of sternotomy. Plasma fentanyl concentrations in excess of this do not appear to produce any further haemodynamic protection, or indeed hypnotic effect, but they are associated with a prolongation of the period during which postoperative ventilatory support is required.

The administration of a large dose of fentanyl (above 50 µg/kg) at the induction of anaesthesia is often associated with the development of muscle rigidity which may make ventilation of the lungs difficult until neuromuscular blockade is established.

The difficulties with the unsupplemented fentanyl technique led to the use of fentanyl as part of a balanced anaesthetic in which anaesthesia is induced with an IV bolus of fentanyl (10–30 µg/kg) combined with a hypnotic agent such as propofol or midazolam. Incremental doses of fentanyl are often added at the time of sternotomy.

The decrease in concentration at the start of CPB is less when fentanyl is being infused rather than being administered by bolus injection. Following CPB the elimination half-life of fentanyl is prolonged and the release of drug sequestered in the lungs may increase the plasma fentanyl concentration.

Alfentanil

Unlike fentanyl, alfentanil does not appear to bind to the plastic of the CPB circuit. Although total plasma concentration is reduced on CPB, the free alfentanil concentration remains relatively constant. The clearance of alfentanil, unlike that of fentanyl, is not reduced on CPB.

The elimination half-life of alfentanil is shorter than that of fentanyl and therefore it is appropriate that alfentanil is used as a continuous infusion. Alfentanil has been proposed as a suitable sole agent for cardiac anaesthesia. Despite the use of very high doses, producing plasma levels of over 2000 ng/ml, the haemodynamic stability demonstrated by the technique has been shown to be inferior to that produced by fentanyl anaesthesia. The technique also tends to result in prolonged respiratory depression. As the anticipated benefit of earlier extubation following high-dose alfentanil anaesthesia has not been realized, there seems little reason to advocate its use in preference to fentanyl.

Sufentanil

Sufentanil is a more recent addition to the available opioid drugs suitable for cardiac anaesthesia. It appears to produce better haemodynamic control during periods of intense stimulation than fentanyl, but more severe hypotension has been reported during induction.

The elimination half-life of sufentanil is about 2.5 h and is therefore shorter than that of fentanyl. Sufentanil is therefore best administered by infusion for maintenance of anaesthesia following an induction bolus dose. This regimen will produce adequate plasma levels, but because there is a direct relationship between sufentanil clearance and hepatic temperature during hypothermic CPB, there may be some accumulation.

Sufentanil does not bind to the CPB circuit, but the total plasma concentration is reduced by approximately 30–55% at the start of CPB. The concentration remains relatively stable during hypothermic CPB and then increases with rewarming. This is probably caused by release of the large amount of sufentanil, sequestered in tissues during the period of hypothermia. The changes in free sufentanil concentration during CPB have not been completely defined. About 90% of the drug is protein bound, and the free component may vary considerably with temperature and pH without obvious changes in the total plasma concentration.

Published work has shown a dose of 10 µg/kg of sufentanil to shorten the time to extubation in comparison with fentanyl (95 µg/kg) but the mean time to extubation in this study was greater than 10 h after surgery. This is rather longer than is desirable in modern cardiac anaesthetic practice.

Remifentanil

Remifentanil is a relatively new opioid with a potency comparable to that of fentanyl. It is a selective µ opioid agonist, and is structurally similar to both fentanyl and alfentanil. Remifentanil, however, differs from the more established opioids in that it is broken down by esterases in the blood and tissues. These enzymes are different from the plasma cholinesterases responsible for the degradation of suxamethonium and are unaffected by anticholinesterase drugs. Remifentanil metabolism occurs in all tissues and therefore the elimination half-life is very short, of the order of 10 min.

The dose can be rapidly adjusted to suit the requirements of individual patients and this allows smooth control of haemodynamic variables. Because the clearance of remifentanil is rapid and its metabolism is not prolonged even after long periods of administration, large doses can be given without the risk of delayed recovery.

The rate of recovery from remifentanil is so rapid that great attention must be paid to ensuring that there is no interruption to the drug delivery system, which might cause a decrease in plasma concentration with consequent awareness occurring within a few minutes.

Remifentanil, despite its analgesic potency, is unsuitable for use without the concomitant administration of a hypnotic drug. Offset of the action of remifentanil is so rapid that 5–10 min after termination of an infusion there will be no residual opioid effect. Adequate postoperative analgesia must therefore be established prior to discontinuation of remifentanil. This is particularly important in the context of cardiac surgery where a sudden loss of analgesia may produce extreme haemodynamic instability. Sudden termination of the effect of remifentanil at the end of surgery without the prior establishment of some other means of analgesia may increase myocardial work and oxygen consumption in the early postoperative period.

A study comparing a group of patients receiving a fentanyl/volatile anaesthetic with a remifentanil/propofol infusion group demonstrated earlier extubation in the remifentanil TIVA group. This suggests that remifentanil, with its rapid clearance, may confer an advantage in patients for whom early extubation is a goal after cardiac surgery. Further work is required to document a real advantage for the use of remifentanil in cardiac anaesthesia.

Neuromuscular blocking agents

Theoretically muscle relaxants used in cardiac anaesthesia should produce minimal haemodynamic disturbance and provide smooth intubating conditions. Traditionally a single large dose of neuromuscular blocking agent is given at induction. This reduces the time to onset and ensures profound muscle relaxation at the time of laryngoscopy and tracheal intubation. A rapid onset of neuromuscular blockade also helps to overcome difficulty with positive pressure ventilation sometimes encountered if a large dose of opioid has caused muscle rigidity.

Duration of effect is not a primary concern in the majority of cardiac procedures which are several hours long. Predictable termination or reversal of these agents is more important in briefer operations, particularly with an increasing trend towards less invasive cardiac surgery in which the duration of the procedure is less predictable.

Pancuronium

Despite the arrival of newer drugs, pancuronium remains the most popular neuromuscular blocker for many cardiac anaesthetists. It is cheap and its relatively long duration of action obviates the need for incremental boluses. Pancuronium causes minimal histamine release and is not associated with hypotension. It has an indirect sympathomimetic effect, mediated by the inhibition of noradrenaline re-uptake. This helps to maintain systemic blood pressure and may produce tachycardia in non-β-blocked patients. These effects would appear unsuitable in patients with ischaemic heart disease, but in practice these effects offset the vagotonic effects of high-dose opioids.

Vecuronium

Vecuronium has the reputation of being the muscle relaxant associated with the greatest cardiovascular stability even at high doses. Its use can sometimes precipitate bradycardia in heavily β-blocked patients given large doses of opioid. The duration of action of vecuronium has been shown to be prolonged during hypothermic CPB.

Other muscle relaxants

Intubating doses of atracurium when used for cardiac anaesthesia may cause a significant reduction in blood pressure secondary to histamine release. Administration by continuous infusion is preferable if atracurium is to be used. It should be noted that the degradation of atracurium is temperature dependent and occurs more slowly during hypothermic CPB. Atracurium has an important place in the management of cardiac surgical patients with impaired renal function.

Mivacurium has failed to make any serious impact in cardiac anaesthesia. Like atracurium, intubating doses may cause substantial histamine release. Doses of 2 mg/kg have been documented to produce transient, but significant, decreases in mean arterial blood pressure, cardiac index and SVR. This may be accompanied by generalized erythema and bronchospasm. The magnitude of the histamine release associated with mivacurium is inversely related to the rate of injection.

The newer agents pipecuronium, rocuronium and cisatracuruim have not yet been shown to confer any advantages over the currently used relaxants, and are not widely used in cardiac anaesthesia.

Transfer to the ICU and postoperative sedation

When TIVA has been used during cardiac surgery the patient can be transferred to the ICU without interruption of the existing anaesthetic drug regime. This avoids abrupt changes in the level of sedation, which may result in haemodynamic disturbance.

Postoperative sedation with continuous IV infusions produces a more controllable level of sedation than bolus administration and is much preferred by nursing staff. Propofol combined with a suitable opioid infusion is ideal for sedation and its rapid recovery characteristics allow for predictable awakening either for extubation or for neurological assessment.

The continuation of infusions established in the operating theatre for postoperative sedation avoids unnecessary wastage of drugs, and reduces medical and nursing staff workload. This presents an economic advantage.

At the end of the procedure the infusion rate can be reduced to 1–2 mg/kg/h to maintain sedation for transfer to, and for the initial phase of postoperative management in, the cardiac recovery area or intensive care unit. It also eliminates abrupt changes in the level of anaesthesia or sedation and hence avoids sudden haemodynamic disturbances associated with rapid awakening or circulatory depression associated with over sedation. Recovery of consciousness following the discontinuation of propofol infusion is predictable and rapid. This allows easy weaning from mechanical ventilation and extubation. Propofol anaesthesia and sedation are particularly useful in patients for whom early extubation is planned.

Propofol TIVA techniques are ideal for promoting early extubation providing that patients are adequately warm and are haemodynamically stable. Although early extubation may not automatically lead to an earlier ICU discharge, it does alter the nursing dependency of patients, which can lead to financial and staffing benefits. A frequent criticism of the use of propofol for TIVA and for postoperative sedation is that such a regime is expensive. However, a British study of drug and nursing costs incurred by cardiac surgical patients compared a propofol/fentanyl group with a midazolam/fentanyl group. Although the drug cost per patient was slightly greater in the propofol group, the overall patient cost, which included staffing levels, was in fact lower in the propofol group. This was because patients were ready to be extubated earlier, nursing dependency was reduced and discharge from ICU occurred earlier. These results supported those of an earlier study conducted in Spain. There is still debate about the benefits or otherwise of early extubation following cardiac surgery. Arguments for or against early extubation are outside the scope of this chapter except to note that TIVA is suitable whether the patients are extubated 20 min or 20 h after surgery.

Almost all patients recovering from cardiac surgery will require IV continuous opioid analgesia. A few centres employ epidural analgesia for postoperative pain relief. This has not gained wide acceptance, largely due to the perceived risk of epidural haematoma formation in the presence of heparinization.

Propofol is, without doubt, the most popular agent for postoperative sedation of cardiac surgical patients. This is true even where a non-TIVA technique has been used in theatre. The injudicious use of boluses of propofol is likely to reduce systemic blood pressure and, if required, sedation should be deepened by adjustment of the infusion rate. Neuromuscular blockade is seldom required during sedation with propofol in the postoperative period. Intermittent positive pressure is usually well tolerated because of the depressant effect of propofol on the laryngeal reflexes.

Regrettably, some cardiac surgical patients will need to return to the operating theatre for re-exploration of the chest for postoperative bleeding or for cardiac tamponade. In this circumstance the infusion rates of the agents are easily adjusted to produce adequate anaesthesia for transfer and re-operation.

Anaesthesia for innovative cardiac surgical procedures

Minimally invasive surgery

Minimally invasive cardiac surgery is an area of recent development which presents new challenges to the anaesthetist. In common with their colleagues in other surgical specialities, cardiac surgeons are keen to undertake increasingly major procedures through smaller and smaller holes. This may range from not using CPB for coronary artery CPB surgery with median sternotomy to operating through a limited anterior thoracotomy or even through endoscopic ports in the thoracic wall.

The surgical aim is to reduce the size of incisions and to reduce surgical trauma. The almost universal implication for the anaesthetist is that these procedures take rather longer than traditional surgery and that the time taken is unpredictable. TIVA with its controllability and predictability of recovery is appropriate especially when the duration of the procedure is unpredictable.

With the development of newer instrumentation, especially in the field of beating heart coronary artery CPB, minimally invasive cardiac surgery is almost certainly here to stay. Smaller wounds do appear to decrease the requirement for postoperative analgesia, particularly if local anaesthetics are used either in paravertebral or intercostal blocks, or directly injected into wounds and drain sites.

At our institution, where direct coronary artery anastamosis without CPB is becoming more common, propofol infusion is used for induction of anaesthesia with a single initial bolus of fentanyl and muscle relaxant and a propofol infusion is continued for the maintenance of anaesthesia. At the end of surgery, providing that body temperature has been adequately maintained by a heated water mattress and lower body forced air warming, the propofol infusion is discontinued and residual neuromuscular relaxation is reversed. The patient is extubated in theatre or shortly after transfer to the recovery ward.

Trans myocardial laser revascularization

Trans myocardial laser revascularization (TMR) is an experimental treatment for patients suffering from angina caused by coronary artery disease which is unsuitable for treatment by conventional means. It involves the use of a CO_2 laser to create channels from the left ventricular cavity into ischaemic myocardium. It is claimed that these channels persist as sinusoids supplying blood directly to the myocardium and it is further claimed that symptomatic relief of angina is achieved in many patients. It is as yet unclear if this symptomatic improvement is due to improved myocardial blood supply. It has been suggested that the relief of symptoms may be caused by thermal denervation of the heart or by the placebo effect.

The procedure is conducted through a left thoracotomy and takes about 1 h to perform. Many of the patients involved have undergone previous coronary artery surgery and most have impaired left ventricular function. In our experience TIVA combined with continuous thoracic epidural analgesia works well in these patients. The anaesthetic technique which has been developed avoids haemodynamic instability during surgery, even in those patients with extremely poor ventricular function, and allows immediate postoperative awakening and extubation.

Although TMR is being combined with conventional cardiac surgery in some centres, its routine use cannot be condoned until there is substantial published evidence of its efficacy.

Anaesthesia for non-surgical procedures

The cardiac anaesthetist is frequently required to anaesthetize patients for diagnostic or therapeutic procedures in the catheter laboratory. The majority of adult procedures are now performed under local anaesthesia, but children and a few adults will require general anaesthesia.

TIVA is an appropriate technique for short cases such as DC cardioversion, left or right heart catheters, and for longer procedures such as balloon valvuloplasty or the implantation of pacemakers and internal cardioversion devices. If necessary, the depth of anaesthesia can be rapidly adjusted during periods of increased stimulation, such as the ablation of abnormal cardiac conduction pathways in patients undergoing electrophysiological procedures.

Infusion anaesthetic techniques are particularly useful where the duration of the procedure is unpredictable and rapid recovery is desirable. This is often the case because of the lack of adequate postoperative recovery facilities in the non-surgical areas of many hospitals.

TIVA produces no anaesthetic atmospheric pollution – a great benefit in X-ray departments and catheter laboratories where gas scavenging facilities are rarely provided.

Further reading

Bacon R, Chandrasekan V, Haigh A, *et al*. Early extubation after open-heart surgery with total intravenous anaesthetic technique. *Lancet* 1994; **345**: 133–4.

Bell J, Sartain J, Wilkinson GAL, Sherry KM. Propofol and fentanyl anaesthesia for patients with low cardiac output state undergoing cardiac surgery: comparison with high dose fentanyl anaesthesia. *Br J Anaesth* 1994; **73**: 162–6.

Bethune DW, Ghosh S, Gray B, *et al*. A comparative study with methohexitone and propofol as supplement to a fentanyl technique: assessment of implicit recall. In: Prys-Roberts C, ed. *Focus on infusion*. London: Current Medical Literature 1991: 42–3.

Carrasco G, Molina R, Costa J, *et al*. Propofol vs midazolam in short-, medium-, and long-term sedation of critically ill patients. A cost benefit analysis. *Chest* 1993; **103**: 557–64.

Gedney JA, Ghosh S. Pharmacokinetics of analgesics, sedatives, and anaesthetic agents during cardiopulmonary bypass. *Br J Anaesth* 1995; **75**: 344–51.

Hall RI, Murphy JT, Landymore R, *et al*. Myocardial metabolic and haemodynamic changes during propofol anesthesia for cardiac surgery in patients with reduced ventricular function. *Anesth Analg* 1993; **77**: 680–9.

Hebbar L, Dorman BH, Roy RC, Spinale FG. The direct effects of propofol on myocyte contractile function after hypothermic cardioplegic arrest. *Anesth Analg* 1996; **83**: 949–57.

Ng A, Tan SSW, Lee Chew SL. Effect of propofol infusion on the endocrine response to cardiac surgery. *Anaesth Int Care* 1995; **23**: 543–7.

Sherry KM, McNamara J, Brown JS, Drummond M. An economic evaluation of propofol/fentanyl on recovery in the ICU following cardiac surgery. *Anaesthesia* 1996; **51**: 312–7.

Appendix

An example TIVA regime for adult cardiac anaesthesia

Premedication	morphine	0.2–0.3 mg/kg
	hyoscine	5 µg/kg
Pre-induction (inserting of monitoring lines, etc.)	midazolam or propofol	1–3mg 10–15 mg
Induction	fentanyl	12–15 µg/kg
	propofol infusion	10 mg/kg/h for 5 min
	pancuronium	0.1–0.15 mg/kg
Maintenance	propofol infusion	3–5 mg/kg/h
	fentanyl	3–4 µg/kg at sternotomy
Blood pressure control (to lower BP)	sodium nitroprusside or glyceryl trinitrate	infusion infusion
Blood pressure control (to raise BP)	metaraminol or phenylephrine	0.25–0.5 mg aliquot 0.25–0.5 mg aliquot
Postoperative	propofol infusion	1.5–3 mg/kg/h for sedation
	morphine infusion (± droperidol)	20–50 µg/kg/h

NB. This is one of several TIVA regimes in current use at our institution. It is used for all types of cardiac surgery including transplantation. It should be noted, however, that the above doses of propofol are effective only with adequate premedication and with the opioid doses quoted above. Patients in whom premedication is omitted or who receive lower doses of fentanyl will require greater infusion rates of propofol to achieve cardiovascular stability and to avoid the risk of awareness. Also patients undergoing coronary artery surgery who do not receive β-adrenergic blocking drugs on the day of surgery may require more propofol and/or fentanyl than above to maintain cardiovascular stability.

10

Thoracic surgery

R. Feneck

- Benefits of TIVA in thoracic surgery
- Pathophysiology in thoracic surgery
- Maintenance of blood gas homeostasis
- Surgical conditions
- One lung ventilation
- Which TVA technique to use

Introduction

Total intravenous anaesthesia (TIVA) may be appropriate in many clinical situations, but in thoracic surgery there may be specific benefits to TIVA which may make it not just an acceptable alternative but clearly the technique of choice. The main potential benefits of TIVA in thoracic surgery are as follows:

- Avoidance of the need for inhalational agents in circumstances where delivery of volatile anaesthetics through a conventional vaporizer into the breathing circuit is either difficult or impractical
- Avoidance of the adverse physiological effects of some volatile anaesthetics
- Use of IV agents with a good profile of early recovery from anaesthesia, thereby maximizing postoperative mobilization and physiotherapy

Before considering the relative merits of TIVA and non-TIVA techniques in thoracic surgery, we should first consider the important cardiopulmonary physiological considerations in patients undergoing thoracic surgery.

Airway reactivity

Although airway reactivity and the presence of bronchospasm is important in any surgical patient, their are two reasons why this problem may be more prevalent, and more common, in thoracic surgical patients.

Firstly, many of these patients have a long history of cigarette smoking, which is often associated with an increased incidence of chronic obstructive pulmonary disease, excess airway secretions and increased bronchial reactivity leading to bronchospasm. Many thoracic surgical patients will show a response to, and benefit from, bronchodilator drugs when given preoperatively.

Secondly, the epithelial lining of the airway may be considered to be a metabolically active structure, in some ways comparable to the vascular endothelium. Certainly the airway epithelium is able to produce and inactivate both bronchodilator and bronchconstrictor substances and inflammatory mediators including prostaglandins (1). Epithelial damage may result in the loss of enzymes that degrade bronchoconstrictor peptides (2) and may permit excitation of afferent nerve fibres resulting in reflex bronchoconstriction. Reflex bronchoconstriction is a frequent response to upper respiratory tract instrumentation in susceptible individuals, particularly if the depth of anaesthesia is inadequate. Thoracic surgery, whether through diagnostic instrumentation or mediastinal resection, involves an increase in external and internal physical contact with the epithelium which potentially promotes epithelial damage resulting in an increased incidence and severity of this problem.

The effects of the lateral decubitus position on gas exchange

The effects of gravity on the distribution of pulmonary ventilation and blood flow in the erect posture have been long identified (3). The gravitational effect is such that the lung can be considered as comprising three zones (Figure 10.1). In the upper zone (Zone 1), the perfusion pressure in the pulmonary artery is reduced by the gravitational effect such that little or no blood flow occurs at the apices of the lungs. The lung is thus relatively compliant, and therefore receives an amount of pulmonary ventilation which results in a significant mismatch of ventilation and perfusion. Alveolar pressure is greater than pulmonary artery (input) pressure, and as a result the area of lung ventilated is unable to take part in effective gas exchange and is described as ineffective, or 'dead space'. In the mid-zone, the pulmonary input pressure is greater than alveolar pressure, but alveolar pressure is greater than pulmonary venous (output) pressure, thereby still limiting pulmonary blood flow and resulting in ventilation/perfusion (V/Q) mismatch. As pulmonary artery pressure increases down Zone 2 and alveolar pressure remains relatively constant, V/Q mismatch decreases towards the bottom of Zone 2. In Zone 3, since both pulmonary input and output pressure exceed alveolar pressure, it is the pulmonary arterial–venous pressure difference that determines blood flow. Strictly speaking, at the very bottom of the lung, the pressure difference between the pulmonary artery and the pulmonary interstitial fluid becomes the determining driving pressure.

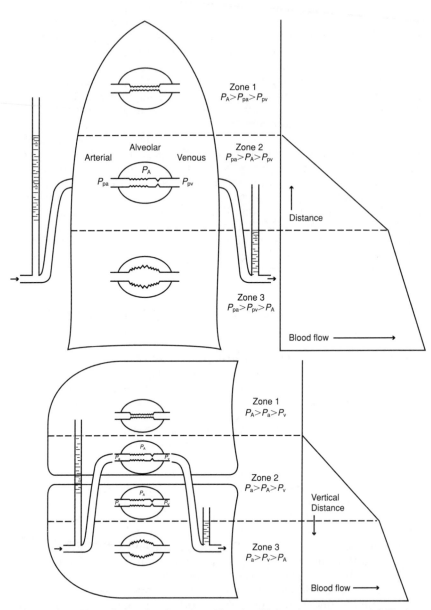

Figure 10.1 The relationship between alveolar (P_A) pulmonary arterial (P_{pa}) and pulmonary venous (P_{pv}) pressures in the upright and lateral decubitus positions.

The same situation applies in the lateral decubitus position, except that the vertical gradient is less than in the upright position and therefore the effects of gravity are less important. Nevertheless, the overall result is that, in the lateral position, the non-dependent (up) lung is again more compliant and preferentially ventilated, and the dependent (down) lung receives the greater part of pulmonary blood flow. This situation becomes exaggerated under anaesthesia, where the reduction in lung volume and weight of the mediastinum serves to make the dependent (down) lung that receives the majority of the blood flow less compliant and more prone to develop atalectatic areas (4). In the open-chested patient, the non-dependent lung becomes even more compliant since the effect of chest wall compliance is lost and further maldistribution of ventilation to the non-dependent lung may occur. Finally, with the cessation of ventilation to the non-dependent lung (i.e. during one-lung ventilation), all of the pulmonary ventilation is distributed to the dependent lung, but a variable amount of blood flow is distributed to the non-dependent lung. This is partly determined by the pulmonary hypoxic vasoconstrictor response, which results in pulmonary vasoconstriction in areas of lung that are atalectatic and therefore underventilated. Hypoxic-induced vasoconstriction therefore serves to minimize perfusion to unventilated areas and therefore to minimize V/Q mismatch. However, numerous factors may have an effect on the integrity of the hypoxic pulmonary vasoconstrictor response (HPV), including pulmonary arterial hypertension, mitral stenosis, volume overload, lung disease, thromboembolism, hypothermia and pulmonary vasoconstrictors. These will all serve to increase pulmonary artery pressure and act in opposition to pulmonary vasoconstriction thereby reducing HPV. Furthermore, any additional intrathoracic pressure in the dependent lung may have the effect of increasing the resistance of blood flow through the dependent lung and thereby effectively increasing the tendency to shunt blood through the non-dependent lung. Finally, drugs that have direct vasodilator effects may directly oppose the physiological vasoconstrictor response; these would includes nitrates, sodium nitroprusside, isoprenaline and of course volatile anaesthetics.

Cardiac disease

A consideration of those factors prevalent in patients presenting for thoracic surgery (males, elderly, history of smoking) immediately suggests that such patients would be at increased risk for developing ischaemic heart disease and thoracic surgery patients should be considered to be in a high-risk cardiac group. Studies in patients undergoing both endoscopic and open thoracic procedures have shown that thoracic surgery patients are at risk from perioperative myocardial ischemia and infarction (5–7). Furthermore, thoracic surgery is recognized as being associated with a large degree of surgical stress and risk factor determinations that estimate the degree of risk for patients with cardiac disease undergoing non-cardiac surgery clearly identify thoracic surgery as a source of increased risk (8).

Perioperative haemodynamic instability and myocardial oxygen imbalance may be a major cause of morbidity. The factors required to maintain myocardial oxygen balance are well described (9). However, these factors may be more difficult to control during thoracic surgery, when surgical stress may cause a significant increase in factors determining myocardial oxygen demand, or if cardiac decompensation and hypoxaemia during one-lung ventilation causes a significant reduction in myocardial oxygen supply.

The drug treatment of myocardial ischaemia may also interact adversely with thoracic surgery. Many patients with significant obstructive lung disease are intolerant of β-blockers and, conversely, non-selective β-blockade may have adverse effects on bronchomotor tone. Anti-anginal vasodilators, including nitrates, may have an impact on the integrity of the HPV response during surgery. None of these drugs should be withheld in thoracic surgery patients, but they may make the perioperative management of the patient with ischaemic heart disease undergoing thoracic surgery more difficult.

Endoscopic procedures including rigid bronchoscopy

Many of the most difficult surgical procedures are those which require the surgeon and anaesthetist to share the airway. Although the best example of this is in ENT surgery, thoracic surgery, which includes direct laryngoscopy and rigid bronchoscopy, is also an appropriate example of airway sharing. The most common such technique is rigid bronchoscopy and the anaesthetic techniques that are used in this setting are shown in Table 10.1.

Table 10.1   Anaesthetic techniques for rigid bronchoscopy

Awake
   topical analgesia to the larynx and trachea
General anaesthesia
   inhalational induction and maintenance, spontaneous ventilation with topical
     anaesthesia or neuromuscular blockade and controlled ventilation
   IV induction and inhalational maintenance, spontaneous ventilation with
     topical anaestheisa or neuromuscular blockade and controlled ventilation
   IV anaesthesia, muscle relaxation and IV anaesthesia by intermittent bolus or
     continuous infusion (TIVA)
Ventilation via
   'apneic oxygenation' using a high flow through fine bore catheter
   controlled ventilation using a conventional breathing circuit
   jet ventilation (Sanders injector) at low or high frequencies, either manually
     or using an automatic ventilator

In considering the relative merits of each anaesthetic technique it is best to consider the following criteria:

♦ Ventilation and maintenance of blood gas homeostasis
♦ Ease of delivery of anaesthesia
♦ Effects of anaesthesia on the circulation
♦ Surgical conditions
♦ Quality and speed of recovery

Maintenance of blood gas homeostasis

Examination of the tracheobronchial tree with a rigid bronchoscope results in considerable stimulation of the autonomic nervous system. The effect on the respiratory system is to produce copious salivation and coughing, and possibly bronchospasm. Salivation may be controlled by preoperative anticholinergic medication such as intramuscular atropine, but IV atropine given immediately before induction has negligible value as an anti-sialogue. The result of copious salivation may be airway obstruction and coughing. In the spontaneously breathing patient, the depth of anaesthesia needed to suppress the cough reflex needs to be considerable, and there may therefore be a significant reduction in ventilation resulting in inadequate gas exchange with consequent hypoxia and hypercapnia. Therefore techniques that rely on spontaneous ventilation during bronchoscopy are rarely used.

Any anaesthetic technique that relies on the use of an open breathing system will suffer from difficulties in scavenging exhaust gases. Whatever the method of induction of anaesthesia, it is hard to avoid an open breathing system during the bronchoscopic examination; it is virtually impossible to do so if bronchial biopsies need to be taken. This problem is more severe if the anaesthetic technique relies on the use of high concentrations of volatile anaesthetic agents.

The problem of tracheobronchial stimulation and coughing may be solved by use of neuromuscular blocking drugs. In practice, complete muscular relaxation is required at the start of the procedure and therefore a rapid onset short-acting neuromuscular relaxant is most appropriate. Despite the development of short-acting non-depolarizing relaxants, suxamethonium remains the relaxant most commonly used unless the bronchoscopy is prolonged or is immediately followed by another procedure. In this later case, which is not uncommon, a relatively short-acting non-depolarizing agent (e.g. vecuronium, atracurium or rocuronium) may be used.

After achieving full neuromuscular blockade, maintaining adequate blood gas homeostasis may be achieved by a number of mechanism. Briefly, these are as follows.

♦ *Permissive apnea during the procedure.* Following adequate preoxygenation and administration of 100% oxygen either during spontaneous or controlled ventilation, the bronchoscopy is undertaken without any form of ventilation. The rate of fall of oxygen saturation may vary, and is dependent on the initial percentage of oxygen saturation, the cardiac output and the metabolic state of the tissues determining the rate of oxygen consumption. In practice, the bronchoscopist usually has a few minutes in which to complete the procedure, which is frequently enough time to complete a simple visual examination but not enough time to take biopsies, etc. The level of oxygen saturation is easily monitored by a pulse oximeter. The rate of rise of CO_2 tension is less easy to measure. Expired gas analysis is not possible during apnea, and any attempt to aspirate gas out of the lungs will not collect a sample which is truly end-tidal and therefore will be an inconstant and variable reflection of arterial CO_2 tension. End-tidal CO_2 concentrations are notoriously unreliable in open breathing circuits and should not be used to estimate arterial CO_2 tension. Trancutaneous CO_2 tension monitoring is less accurate than transcutaneous pulse oximetry, and intermittent blood gas analysis is invasive and requires ready access to analysers. Other techniques of CO_2 tension monitoring have been described including transcorneal CO_2 monitoring, although in practice the anaesthetist usually relies on an estimated rate of rise of CO_2 tension of up to 6 mmHg/min of apnea in an adult patient, based on the patient's rate of CO_2 production. This is usually described as 200 ml/min in a 70 kg adult, but may in fact be considerably greater under conditions of acute surgical stress. With the technique described above, anaesthesia cannot be maintained by the inhalational route during the procedure. Inhalational anaesthesia established before the apneic period, or intermittent or continuous IV anaesthesia are the options available.

◆ *'Apneic' high-flow oxygenation.* The essentials of the technique are described above, but in addition a fine-bore catheter is placed through the patients vocal chords and oxygen is insufflated into the lungs, usually at a rate of 6–8 l/min. The effectiveness of the technique is partly related to the effectiveness of providing a transbronchial pressure at sufficiently high flow rates. Such a technique has been used experimentally in small animals to control both oxgenation and CO_2 elimination. However, to be effective in adult patients, a flow rate of 70 l/min would be required, which is both impractical and dangerous. In practice although this is an effective method of oxygenation for a number of minutes, CO_2 elimination should be assumed as being near zero and therefore CO_2 build up at a rate of 3–6 mmHg/min will occur.

◆ *Intermittent positive pressure ventilation (IPPV)* may be used and a number of ventilating side arms have been developed. However, unless a glass window or telescope and seal is used, gas will escape from the proximal end of the bronchoscope causing ventilation to be inadequate. The use of other devices, including biopsy brush and/or forceps, makes the technique very impractical and it is not widely used. However, anaesthesia could be maintained by either IV or inhalational agents.

♦ *Ventilation using the Sanders (venturi) jet injector.* This technique exploits the effect of gas accelerated through a fine nozzle. Under these conditions, the pressure of the gas escaping from the nozzle falls markedly, such that an area of negative pressure is created and gas is entrained into the jet stream. The amount of gas entrained (entrainment ratio) depends on a number of factors including the size of the nozzle and the flow rate of gas through the nozzle. One potential drawback of a jet ventilation technique is the limitations it imposes on the technique for anaesthesia. Gases must be delivered to the injector nozzle at a high pressure if the physical process of acceleration through a nozzle, reduction in pressure immediately distal to the nozzle and entrainment of ambient gas are to occur. Modern calibrated vaporizers are operational only at or near atmospheric pressure and certainly cannot be subjected to gases at or near pipeline pressures. The use of volatile anaesthetics with the jet injector is therefore only possible with highly specialized vaporizers designed and constructed for use with high gas pressures. Thus IV anaesthesia is not merely an alternative but the technique of choice in this setting.

Ease of delivery of anaesthesia

Given the problems of delivery of adequate ventilation referred to above, the delivery of volatile agents becomes cumbersome at best.

In contrast, IV anaesthesia can be easily provided in this setting, usually through a small cannula in a peripheral vein, although the exact nature of vascular access is decided by other considerations, including the general state of the patient and the nature of any other thoracic surgery. In short cases IV drugs including anaesthetics, analgesics and muscle relaxants may be given by intermittent bolus injection. In longer cases, or where a smoother conduct of anaesthesia is desirable, a continuous infusion of anaesthetic using a modern electronic syringe pump may be considered ideal. Specimen techniques for this procedure are shown in Table 10.2.

Effects of anaesthesia on the circulation

It has long been recognized that instrumentation of the upper respiratory tract may produce a marked autonomic response (10), including a hyperdynamic response as a result of sympathetic activation resulting in tachycardia, systemic and pulmonary hypertension. In addition, arrhythmias are not infrequent, particularly ventricular and supraventricular ectopic activity. However, occasionally the effects of parasympathetic activation are seen, e.g. a profound slowing of the heart rate possibly with the development of a junctional rhythm. This bradycardia may be associated with either hypertension or hypotension.

The haemodynamic response to laryngoscopy and intubation has been described as a more fundamental physiological response to a noxious

Table 10.2 Specimen techniques for TIVA and bronchoscopy. Patient premedicated with atropine only

---

Ultra-short case (1–2 min)
  Propofol induction (1.5–2.5 mg/kg); suxamethonium (1–1.5 mg/kg) for muscle relaxation.

Short case (2–5 mins)
  Propofol induction (1.5–2.5 mg/kg) plus repeated boluses of 20 mg every 1–2 min or as dictated clinically; **OR** zero order propofol infusion initially set at 35 ml/h (5 mg/kg/h) and adjusted clinically.
  Suxamethonium (1–1.5 mg/kg) plus repeat boluses of 25 mg as required (n.b. prior atropine) **OR** mivacurium (0.1–0.2 mg/kg).

Medium case (5–15 mins)
  Propofol induction (1.5–2.5 mg/kg) followed by continuous infusion; initially 6–8 mg/kg/h reducing to 3–5 mg/kg/h after 5 min.
  Plus alfentanil 0.5–1 mg at induction.
  Plus bolus of suxamethonium or mivacurium (see above) followed by repeat boluses of suxamethonium (see above) or vecuronium 1–2 mg.

Long case (>15 min)
  Propofol induction dose and continuous infusion as above.
  Plus alfentanil (1–2 mg) at induction **OR** remifentanil infusion (0.25–0.5 ug/kg/min).
  Plus vecuronium 0.12 mg/kg at induction; further doses of 1–2 mg as indicated clinically.

---

stimulus than, for example, limb withdrawal (11). Roizen *et al.* have described the minimum alveolar concentrations (MAC) of volatile anaesthetics required to prevent the responses to noxious stimuli (12). The MAC for prevention of haemodynamic responses to noxious stimuli can be seen to be substantially in excess of that required to prevent other more conventional responses, i.e. movement, lacrimation, etc. (Table 10.3). This has two practical consequences:

◆ If such a high concentration of volatile anaesthetic agent is used in the unstimulated patient, there would be a risk of significant haemodynamic depression
◆ If the depth of anaesthesia is insufficient, instrumentation of the upper respiratory tract would be associated with a substantial and potentially damaging hyperdynamic circulatory response

The difficulty in achieving a considerable depth of anaesthesia without haemodynamic depression may be easily recognizable as a feature of volatile anaesthesia. However, the problem of achieving haemodynamic stability may become evident with either volatile or IV anaesthetics. We found that IV anaesthesia to be unpredictable in preventing haemodynamic responses to rigid bronchoscopy, and success was in part

Table 10.3 Standard MAC values for halothane and enflurane compared with MAC values to prevent movement (MAC-EI) and pressor responses (MAC-BAR) to laryngoscopy and intubation

	Halothane	Enflurane
MAC_{50}	1.0 MAC ($0.74 \pm 0.03\%$)	1.0 MAC ($1.68 \pm 0.04\%$)
$MAC\ EI_{50}$	1.3 MAC	1.4 MAC
$MAC\text{-}BAR_{50}$	1.5 MAC	1.6 MAC
MAC_{95}	1.2 MAC	1.1 MAC
$MAC\text{-}EI_{95}$	1.7 MAC	1.9 MAC
$MAC\text{-}BAR_{95}$	2.1 MAC	2.6 MAC

These values have been age-adjusted.

dictated by the choice of IV anaesthetic and the use of opioid supplementation (13).

If anaesthesia is likely to be at all prolonged, a continuous infusion of IV anaesthetic is more appropriate both to ensure adequacy of anaesthesia and to promote haemodynamic stability throughout the procedure. This naturally favours the use of IV anaesthetics whose pharmacokinetic profile is such that they can easily be given by constant infusion (see later).

Surgical conditions

The surgical requirements for bronchoscopy are relatively straightforward, but they may nonetheless be relatively hard to achieve:

◆ Relaxation of the jaw and paralysis of the vocal chords
◆ A dry airway
◆ Absence of movement or coughing, either during positioning of the bronchoscope or alternatively during biopsies, brushings, etc.
◆ Good haemodynamic control to minimize bleeding from biopsy sites
◆ Rapid return to spontaneous ventilation, rapid return of the cough reflex and preferably rapid return to consciousness in order to maximize clearance of any blood or sputum in the tracheobronchial tree

Clearly IV induction of anaesthesia followed by muscular relaxation is the quickest and most effective way of achieving suitable conditions for insertion of the bronchoscope. The need for good conditions at this point cannot be overstated. The insertion of a rigid bronchoscope is not the easiest of tasks, and poor quality relaxation may play a part in any resulting trauma to the lips, gums and teeth. Similarly, bronchoscopic intubation through partially closed vocal cords may also be significantly traumatic.

The value of a dry airway also cannot be overstated, particularly in patients undergoing prolonged bronchoscopy. Copious salivation may on occasion render the bronchoscopic examination almost impossible.

The rapid onset of anaesthesia and muscle relaxation will ensure good conditions for a rapid examination, and where necessary these conditions can be easily continued for a more prolonged examination or for therapeutic procedures such as laser resection of endobronchial or tracheal lesions.

Quality and speed of recovery

Rapid recovery is desirable in many circumstances in thoracic surgery and rigid bronchoscopy is no exception. If a simple examination is all that is planned, the procedure may take only 5 min, ideally followed by a rapid and full return to consciousness. If biopsies have been taken, if an endobronchial lesion has been resected or if the pre-existing pathology is such that sputum production is copious, then an early return to consciousness is even more important, since this will allow the patient to cough effectively and clear any blood or secretions that may be present.

Mediastinoscopy, anterior mediastinotomy and median sternotomy

These procedures are performed to carry out examination of and biopsy from the anterior and superior mediastinum. They are difficult and not without complications, and are therefore best carried out under general anaesthesia.

The surgical technique consists of making a small incision at the suprasternal notch and carrying out blunt dissection of the pretracheal fascia into the mediastinum and then inserting the mediastinoscope under the manubrium sternum. When positioned behind the thoracic aorta but anterior to the trachea, the mediastinoscope may be used to gain access to the superior mediastinal lymph nodes, including the anterior and lateral para-tracheal, the para-mainstem and the anterior subcarinal lymph nodes. Left-sided lesions are more easily approached via a left anterior mediastinotomy via the second rib interspace. This approach gives useful access to centrally located and left-sided pathology, as well as the thymus and structures of the anterior mediastinum. The relative indications and contra-indications to these procedures vary between different authorities, but certainly they will be more hazardous in the presence of superior vena cava (SVC) obstruction, severe tracheal deviation and thoracic aortic aneurysm.

The clinical condition of the patient may be very variable. However, of major concern is the presence of SVC obstruction, particularly if there has been no development of collateral venous channels, compression or deviation of the airways including the trachea and main bronchii, and evidence of significant impairment of the cerebral circulation.

If the patient has SVC obstruction without collateral channel development, then the venous return to the right side of the heart will be poor via any vein which drains into the SVC. Thus IV access for anaesthetic drugs, muscle relaxants and fluids should be secured via a vein that drains into the inferior vena cava. A peripheral lower limb vein may be used, but it is probably easiest and most secure to cannulate a femoral vein using a seldinger wire technique. This will also allow easy placement of a wide bore cannula, which may be necessary for rapid transfusion should haemorrhage occur. However, it is preferable to use a separate cannula for TIVA since should haemorrhage occur this may require massive blood transfusion. Although many surgeons do not consider SVC obstruction to contra-indicate mediastinotomy or mediastinoscopy, there is no doubt that major haemorrhage is more likely in these patients.

Evaluation of the patients airway should also be undertaken before surgery. Chest X-ray, chest computed tomography (CT) and fibre optic bronchoscopy will reveal the extent and level of any tracheal deviation, and external compression of the trachea or main bronchii. This is an important consideration, since control of the airway is of vital importance and, where there is any doubt, many would consider an IV technique to be contra-indicated and anaesthesia should be both induced and maintained using volatile agents and during spontaneous ventilation.

Fibre optic evaluation of the airway has changed this somewhat, for it not only allows a detailed examination of the airway but also provides an indication of the patients respiratory reserve. Put bluntly, if the patient can tolerate a fibre optic examination then in all probability they can tolerate IPPV, which removes a major contra-indication to IV anaesthesia in this setting. Indeed, we and others have utilized TIVA techniques exclusively for endobronchial laser resection based on these criteria and with no adverse consequences (14,15). Nonetheless, if there is any doubt about the patients ability to tolerate IPPV, and particularly in cases of trauma, inhalational techniques should be considered.

The authors experience is to use a TIVA technique, supplementing a propofol induction and maintenance infusion with alfentanil (dose/weight) and atracurium (dose/weight). The patients lungs are ventilated with either oxygen and nitrous oxide (N_2O) or oxygen-enriched air as appropriate. The aim should be to awaken and extubate the patient at the end of the procedure.

The usual minimum monitoring standards should be observed, but it may be best to place the blood pressure cuff on the left arm and gain access to palpate the right radial artery in order to exclude mediastinoscopic compression of the major vessels during the procedure. Compression of the innominate, right subclavian or carotid arteries may occur theoretically. If an indwelling arterial cannula is placed it may be most suitably placed in the right wrist for the same reason.

Both cervical mediastinoscopy and anterior mediastinotomy are not without complications, and clearly haemorrhage is a major complication. Blood should be available particularly in the higher-risk cases. Catastrophic hemorrhage is rare, but emergency sternotomy or thoracotomy may be necessary to locate and stem the source. Consideration should be given to the fact that, in circumstances of massive haemorrhage, the delivery route for anaesthesia may be jeopardized. Certainly access for TIVA should be separate from a large bore transfusion cannula.

Venous air embolism is rare (less than 0.1%), particularly if the patient is being ventilated with IPPV rather than breathing spontaneously.

Resection of large masses in the anterior mediastinum

Large masses at or near the anterior medistinum are frequently associated with problems of compression, and symptoms and signs of compression most frequently affect the airway (trachea and main bronchii), the heart (right ventricle and pulmonary artery) and the SVC. In some patients, very large tumours will produce symptoms and signs of compression affecting all three.

Major airway compression may be caused by cystic hygroma, teratoma, thymoma, retrosternal thyroid tumour and lymphoma. Patients who have symptoms of airway compression are more likely to suffer from serious respiratory complications perioperatively, but a proportion of patients who are relatively asymptomatic will also suffer a stormy perioperative course. Anaesthesia in these patients must therefore be recognized as hazardous at all times and steps taken accordingly. Where intrathoracic airway obstruction is suspected a flow-volume loop, preferably in the erect and supine positions, may help to identify the level of obstruction.

A needle biopsy under local anaesthesia and CT guidance is commonly performed and initial radiotherapy, chemotherapy or both is carried out to produce shrinkage of the tumour, thereby reducing the effects of the compression. This latter point is important, since following treatment the tumour size and effects of compression may be profoundly reduced.

The detailed anaesthetic technique is less important than the guiding principles, which are as follows:

♦ Pre-operative evaluation of the state of the airway, including simple spirometry, flow-volume loop assessment, fibre optic bronchoscopy and other lung function tests as appropriate.
♦ Needle biopsy under local anaesthesia if possible.
♦ Chemotherapy or radiotherapy to shrink the tumour and reduce the immediate life-threatening aspects of the procedure.
♦ Induction of anaesthesia in whatever position the patient will tolerate best, preferably supine with mild head up tilt, but be prepared to move the patient quickly if respiratory obstruction should occur.
♦ A wide range of endotracheal tube sizes and lengths should be available as well as a rigid bronchoscope.
♦ The patient should be fully pre-oxygenated to allow for maximum time if problems in securing the airway do occur.
♦ An IV induction of anaesthesia is usually acceptable, but an inhalational induction or the use of helium/oxygen mixture may be necessary.

- Muscle relaxants should only be used after checking that the patient's lungs can be adequately ventilated artificially. Remember that adequate ventilation of the lungs should be rechecked after the endotracheal tube has been passed. It may be necessary to change the patients posture, and remove the endotracheal tube and start again if necessary.
- Airway management problems may become apparent in the post-extubation period. Removal of the tumour may not relieve the symptoms of obstruction, particularly if resection leads to partial collapse of the tracheal wall.

Compression of the pulmonary artery and right ventricle is rare because these structures lie underneath the aortic arch and tracheobronchial tree, and thus they are partially protected by them. However, in patients with evidence of severe tracheobronchial compression, compression of the pulmonary outflow tract may occur. Obstruction may be caused by lymphoma; obstruction caused by a cyst has also been described.

The consequences of pulmonary outflow tract compression are worsening right ventricular function, right ventricular dilatation, functional tricuspid regurgitation and raised central venous pressure, shift of the intraventricular septum leading to a reduced left ventricular end diastolic volume and reduced cardiac output. As pulmonary blood flow is reduced pulmonary gas exchange is worsened and hypoxia may ensue.

It may be important to vary the patients posture in order to reduce the effects of the obstruction and steps should be taken to ensure that this is possible quickly at any time during surgery. The anaesthetic technique should take into account both airway considerations, and the preservation of right ventricular filling and contractile function. In this regard, ketamine may be a useful agent for induction of anaesthesia and analgesia. Volume loading should also be available, although care must be taken not to overload the right ventricle particularly in the presence of poor contractile function.

Obstruction or compression of the SVC is a particularly sinister sign in patients with mediastinal pathology. Although the cause may be benign, lesions responsible for SVC obstruction are frequently malignant, and such causes include bronchial carcinoma and lymphoma. The SVC syndrome is characterized by obstruction to and therefore engorgement of veins that drain into the SVC, most obviously from the head and neck and upper limbs. The venous pressure in these veins may be markedly raised and flow from the veins to the right atrium will be sluggish at best. There may be an increased incidence of venous thrombosis as a result.

Dyspnea and cough are frequent, and orthopnea may be marked due to further postural venous engorgement. If the central venous is markedly raised, cerebral venous engorgement may occur leading to headache, cerebral oedema and irritation, and altered mental state. These problems are more likely to occur in patients in whom SVC obstruction develops rapidly. A slower onset is more likely to be met by the development of an adequate collateral circulation, characterized by prominent veins on the upper chest wall.

SVC obstruction may complicate the use of TIVA, since the IV route chosen becomes critically important. The veins of the head and neck and upper limbs drain into the SVC rendering these unavailable for use. Even if the obstruction is only partial, trauma to the SVC may result in surgical plication and loss or interruption of the anaesthetic. Veins that drain into the IVC must be chosen both for volume replacement and to deliver IV anaesthesia.

The main points of management are summarized below:

♦ Preoperative radiotherapy should be undertaken in all but the mildest of cases. Nonetheless, every attempt should be made to reduce upper airway and head and neck oedema, and the patients airway should be carefully evaluated since the haemorrhagic consequences of even the mildest trauma may be severe. The use of an anticholinergic drying agent is recommended.
♦ The patient may be at risk from postural exacerbation of the compression, similar to patients with tracheobronchial compression.
♦ Radial arterial monitoring and lower limb venous access is preferable in all but the mildest cases. Cannulation of central veins that drain into the SVC should be avoided.
♦ Induction of anaesthesia may be associated with a reduction in venous pressure and thus a substantial fall in cardiac output. Consider an agent that preserves venous tone such as ketamine. Vasopressors should be available.
♦ Blood should be cross-matched and in severe cases available in the operating theatre at the time of surgery.
♦ Great care should be taken during induction and emergence to avoid coughing, straining, etc., that may further increase venous pressure.

Median sternotomy

This is the usual route of access for cardiac surgery, but in addition resection of the thymus and retrosternal thyroid is usually undertaken via this route.

Thymectomy and myasthenia gravis

Myasthenia gravis was first described by Thomas Willis in 1672, although the electrophysiological diagnosis was described much later by Freidrich Jolly. The condition was named myasthenia gravis by Campbell in 1900.

It is a disease of neuromuscular transmission resulting in early fatigue. The exact signs and symptoms will depend on which groups of muscles are affected.

In normal tissues, acetylcholine is released from vesicles in the nerve terminal and combines with acetylcholine receptors at the postsynaptic receptor on the motor end plate. Acetylcholine is hydrolysed by cholinesterase and choline is taken up into the nerve terminal to aid further synthesis of acetylcholine. The receptors on the postsynaptic terminal are constantly being formed and sequestrated, and the lifespan of an acetylcholine receptor is normally about 7 days.

In myasthenia, the postsynaptic receptors are attacked by the immuno-globulin G autoantibody, thereby leading to the binding of autoantibody to the receptor, and consequently a substantial reduction in the number of functional receptors at the motor end plate and hence reduced neuro-muscular function. Not only is the number of receptors reduced but the average lifespan of a postsynaptic acetylcholine receptor is reduced to approximately 1 day.

The pathological processes involved in myasthenia indicate that there are three broad therapeutic strategies available.

First, to increase the amount of acetylcholine available in order to maximize occupancy of a reduced mass of receptors. This entails the use of anticholinesterases (neostigmine, pyridostigmine). Secondly, to modify the autoimmune process by pharmacological means, which entails the use of corticosteroids and, more rarely, azothiaprin. Thirdly, thymectomy to remove the source of the autoantibody.

Surgery is generally very effective in myasthenia and thymectomy should be considered in all patients other than those who have minimal symptoms. The tumour, thymic remnant, nodes and surrounding fatty tissues are all resected and the procedure is usually carried out through a median sternotomy, although lateral sternotomy and even lateral thoracotomy have been used.

Anaesthetic considerations

Thymectomy is a major surgical procedure, and therefore the usual work-up for such a procedure including haematology, biochemistry, and blood group and cross-match. Patients with thymoma may have symptoms of tracheobronchial compression, and the airway should be fully assessed by plain film radiography, CT scan and fibre optic bronchoscopy. Baseline tests of respiratory function are valuable as a guide to the likely postoperative course and as a means of assessing early postoperative progress. Spirometry (FEV_1 and FVC) and blood gases will be of most benefit. In cases with bulbar involvement, the cough reflex may be impaired and soiling of the lungs may result. Care must be taken to ensure that patients are free from chest infection at the time of surgery.

Myastheniac patients may suffer from associated myocardial degen-erative changes, but generally the condition carries with it little extra cardiac risk. Patients should be evaluated and managed according to their general cardiovascular condition and risk factors.

It should be remembered that patients in the older age group will have the usual incidence of cardiovascular and cerebrovascular disease.

There may also be associated thyroid abnormalities and thyroid function should be checked preoperatively. In addition to lung soiling, patients with chronic bulbar symptoms may suffer from chronic dehydration and nutritional deficiency. Where this is evident, fluid and electrolyte replacement therapy may be necessary.

Anaesthetic management

If the surgical procedure is carried out through a median sternotomy, an endotracheal tube will suffice. In rare circumstances, the thymoma may not be situated in the midline necessitating an endobronchial tube.

Although the relative merits of different anaesthetic techniques have been debated, of more importance is the recognition of the nature of the problems involved in delivering safe anaesthesia. Nonetheless, TIVA techniques have something to offer in this situation.

In general, the following should therefore be noted:

◆ IV induction of anaesthesia is preferable since it is both rapid and smooth. Inhalational agents may cause a reduction in respiratory muscle power at an early stage of anaesthesia, resulting in a partially anaesthetized but hypoventilating patient. Once the patient is anaesthetized, the patients ventilation may need to be assisted immediately if blood gas homeostasis is to be maintained.
◆ Endotracheal intubation may be carried out following IV anaesthesia only, thereby avoiding the use of muscle relaxants. However, the use of muscle relaxants is not contra-indicated providing they are used appropriately.
◆ Patients with myasthenia are resistant to the effects of suxamethonium and an increased dosage should be used (2 mg/kg). This may be followed by a prolonged phase II block.
◆ Patients with myasthenia are sensitive to the effects of non-depolarizing relaxants which should therefore be used in markedly reduced dosage. Between 25 and 50% of the normal dose may be appropriate. Atracurium has the advantage of Hofmann degradation and elimination and may be felt to be the relaxant of choice.
◆ The myorelaxant properties of volatile anaesthetics are enhanced in myasthenia. This may be considered a relative indication for TIVA, since IV anaesthetics do not appear to possess relaxant properties.
◆ The time course of small doses of neuromuscular blocking drugs in myasthenic patients is similar to larger doses given to normals. However, the extent of neuromuscular blockade and the effectiveness of reversal should be tested by a nerve stimulator.
◆ Thoracic epidural anaesthesia has been used as a means of providing intraoperative analgesia with minimal neuromuscular blockade and postoperative analgesia. Ester-type local anaesthetics are best avoided since they are metabolized by plasma pseudocholinesterase.
◆ Although a median sternotomy is one of the least painful thoracic incisions, postoperative analgesia will be necessary. There is no contra-indication to the use of opioids and indeed good analgesia will potentiate postoperative chest physiotherapy. Although the concerns of opioid-induced respiratory depression combined with weak muscular power are understandable, they should not be allowed to result in inadequate postoperative analgesia. Similarly, the use of appropriate continuous intraoperative infusions of opioids should be considered.

◆ The decision to extubate the patient at the end of surgery should be individually based. Some indication of likely success may be given by the patients preoperative history, anticholinesterase dosage and respiratory status (16).

Myasthenic syndrome differs from myasthenia gravis in a number of important ways. The patients are predominately male and frequently have an associated carcinoma of the bronchus, although lung secondary tumors from other primary sources have been described. The proximal limb muscles are most markedly affected and there is an initial increase in muscle power on exercise. Patients are poorly responsive to anticholinesterase therapy and removal of the tumour often leaves the patient's muscle power unaffected.

The anaesthetic dilemma with patients with myasthenia gravis and myasthenic syndrome is whether to make use of the muscle relaxant properties of volatile anaesthetics. In favour is the fact that sufficient muscle relaxation may be achieved without recourse to neuromuscular blocking drugs. However, the relaxant properties of volatile agents cannot be reversed and their effect will last as long as the patients recovery from anaesthesia, which may be prolonged.

Thoracoscopy

Thoracoscopy may be performed relatively easily under local anaesthesia, following anaesthetic infiltration of the lateral chest wall usually at the level of the sixth intercostal space and subsequent infiltration of the parietal pleura. However, if multiple diagnostic procedures are planned it is more usually undertaken under general anaesthesia.

In this circumstance, particularly if it is combined with rigid bronchoscopy, a TIVA technique may not only be an acceptable alternative but the technique of choice. The use of a short-acting opioid plus a propofol infusion allows for good quality anaesthesia despite marked surgical stress, followed by rapid recovery and minimal hangover.

The other main anaesthetic consideration is the value of endobronchial intubation and one-lung anaesthesia. This may be particularly valuable in thoracoscopy, but successful endobronchial tube placement may be difficult if there is compression of the trachea and main bronchii leading to a reduction in diameter of the airways or if there is significant distortion of the carinal angle.

Patients who have seriously impaired lung function may not tolerate one-lung ventilation for any prolonged period and a high FIO_2 may be essential in order to ensure adequate oxygenation. The relative merits of volatile anaesthesia and TIVA are dealt with in the section on lateral thoracotomy below.

Lateral thoracotomy

The majority of major pulmonary and oesophageal surgery is carried out via a lateral or anterolateral thoracotomy. The success of this approach is

Table 10.4   Relative priority for one-lung ventilation

Absolute
  prevention of soiling or contamination from diseased to non-diseased lung
  ◆ infection
  ◆ haemorrhage
  control of the distribution of ventilation
  ◆ broncho-pleural and broncho-pleural cutaneous fistula
  ◆ giant unilateral lung cyst
  unilateral bronchopulmonary lavage
  ◆ pulmonary alveolar proteinosis
Relative
  surgical exposure – high priority
  ◆ thoracic aortic aneurysm
  ◆ pneumonectomy
  surgical exposure – low priority
  ◆ oesophageal resection
  ◆ lobectomy

---

usually dependent on the anaesthetist being able to establish independent ventilation of both lungs, and thus being able to ventilate the dependent (down) lung and discontinue ventilation to the non-dependent (up) lung thereby allowing good surgical access. The relative priority for one-lung ventilation is shown in Table 10.4.

Whatever the strength of the clinical indication for one-lung ventilation, the effect will be to produce a significant increase in V/Q mismatch as blood flows through the lung that is not being ventilated. This intrapulmonary shunting will result in a large reduction in arterial oxygen tension. However, a number of steps may be taken both to reduce the magnitude of the intrapulmonary shunt in the unventilated lung and to improve gas distribution within the dependent ventilated lung. These are shown in Table 10.5.

Table 10.5   Management of hypoxia during one-lung ventilation

---

◆ Check endobronchial tube position
◆ Increase FIO_2
◆ Alter ventilator settings to reduce mean intrathoracic pressure in the
    dependent (ventilated) lung, i.e. tidal volume, respiratory rate, inspiratory
    flow rate, I:E ratio

Consider
◆ PEEP to the dependent lung to improve V/Q in the ventilated lung.
◆ Oxygen insufflation, PEEP or high-frequency jet ventilation to the
    non-dependent lung if shunt and hypoxaemia persist
◆ Clamping the pulmonary artery to the non-dependent lung to minimize
    blood flow to the non-ventilated lung
◆ Two-lung ventilation

Despite these measures, it is not uncommon for relative hypoxia to occur during the period of one-lung anaesthesia to a significant extent and alteration of the inspired oxygen concentration is often required. Indeed, some recommend it as a precautionary measure in all cases.

As described earlier in this section, HPV is a protective reflex whose function is to limit blood flow to unventilated areas of lung thereby limiting V/Q mismatch, intrapulmonary shunting and hypoxia. Inhibition of HPV will tend to maintain blood flow through unventilated lung tissue and thereby worsen hypoxaemia. A number of factors have been noted as influencing HPV (see earlier) and therapeutic strategies have been designed to deal with these. However, of importance in this context is the effect of anaesthetic agents on HPV.

The effects of inhalational and IV anaesthetics have been extensively studied, both in animals and humans. The data generated by these studies is extensive and the reader is advised to consult a standard text for a complete review (17). However, a number of factors are clear:

- The results of studies differ markedly, depending on whether the preparation studied was an experimental vessel strip preparation, an isolated organ preparation or intact and normally perfused. However, halothane ether, enflurane, methoxyflurane, trichlorethylene and N_2O all show a marked inhibition of HPV when administered to experimental animals.
- Inhibition of HPV was substantially less marked in studies in humans with halothane, isoflurane and enflurane. Data on desflurane and sevoflurane are yet substantial, but it is likely that the effects of sevoflurane are similar to those of isoflurane.
- Studies with fentanyl, propofol, morphine, thiopentone, benzodiazepines and ketamine suggest that these agents do not inhibit HPV either in studies in man or in the experimental setting.

These data would suggest that there is a clear theoretical advantage to the use of a TIVA technique. Firstly, there is no inhibition of HPV. Second, if hypoxia does occur during one-lung ventilation, the inspired oxygen concentration can simply be increased without otherwise affecting the delivery of the anaesthetic in any significant way.

Despite the apparent drawbacks of volatile agents during one-lung anaesthesia, it must be stressed that the data implicating volatile anaesthetics in inhibition of HPV is much stronger in the experimental setting than in man. There are, however, few direct comparisons of the effects of inhalational and TIVA techniques for one-lung ventilation. We compared isoflurane with propofol in patients undergoing one-lung ventilation for pulmonary resection and noted a substantial increase in shunt fraction in the isoflurane group compared to those receiving a propofol infusion. However, we also noted that cardiac output was significantly higher in the isoflurane group, such that oxygen flux was greater in the volatile group also, although there was no evidence that tissue oxygen delivery was inadequate in either group (15).

Comparisons of anaesthetic techniques in the clinical environment will always be difficult, and comparisons of volatile and TIVA techniques suffer from difficulties including experimental design and equipotency. However our data would suggest that a TIVA technique with propofol is as good as, but probably not significantly better than, volatile anaesthesia with isoflurane.

Which total intravenous anesthetic technique?

The potential benefits of TIVA in patients undergoing thoracic surgery lies in the following areas:

♦ The comparative effects of volatile anaesthetics and IV agents on aspects of lung function, including airways reactivity, sputum production and the effects on HPV
♦ The effects of volatile and IV anaesthetics on neuromuscular function
♦ The benefits of early recovery, including more active and earlier physiotherapy, deep breaths and cough early after the end of surgery thereby ensuring maximum clearance of secretions

The interest in TIVA has come about in large part with the introduction of drugs which have a rapid onset and relatively short duration of action. The 'titratability' of the drug is also a highly important factor, i.e. the plasma concentration can be increased and decreased with ease, resulting in a rapid alteration of the 'effect site' concentration, thereby ensuring that the change in rate of administration is rapidly mirrored by a change in clinical state, which is usually a change in the depth of anaesthesia. Thus drugs with predictable pharmacokinetics and pharmacodynamics are relatively useful, and drugs which have unpredictable pharmacokinetics and in whom the effects on body systems, particularly the circulation, are unpredictable may be of less use.

Taking these factors into account, how do the currently available IV agents perform, particularly in the context of thoracic surgery.

Thiopentone

Thiopentone has had a long career as an IV anaesthetic agent and is renown for producing a smooth pain-free induction of anaesthesia with relatively small haemodynamic disturbance in healthy patients. In the elderly or haemodynamically compromised, the dose and speed of induction must be reduced, but it is still eminently possible for the sickest of patients to be induced safely with care.

IV anaesthesia may be maintained with thiopentone by either continuous infusion or by repeat IV bolus dosing. However, both these alternatives may be problematic.

We found that repeat bolus dosing with IV thiopentone to be a relatively poor method of anaesthesia for patients undergoing rigid bronchoscopy

(5,13). There was an increased incidence of hypertension and myocardial ischaemia in patients receiving thiopentone alone, in contrast to those patients who received an opioid in addition. However, if thiopentone is given in an attempt at minimizing the response to surgical stimulation, there is a distinct possibility of a relative overdosage resulting in myocardial depression. Hung et al. have shown that the doses or serum concentrations of thiopentone required to remove responses to various stimuli vary from 10 µg/ml to produce no response to verbal commands, to 80 µg/kg to produce no movement response to laryngoscopy and intubation (19). By way of comparison, between 15 and 25 µg/ml are needed to provide clinical anaesthesia in patients in combination with N_2O and an opioid. Rigid bronchoscopy is recognized as being a significantly greater hemodynamic stress than direct laryngoscopy and therefore even higher concentrations of the drug are likely to be required.

Continuous infusions of thiopentone may also be very difficult to manage because of the redistribution and elimination of thiopentone. The hepatic clearance of thiopentone is low (approximately 10% of that of propofol) and therefore the duration of effect is terminated largely by redistribution to peripheral tissues. In fact, if the infusion rate is sufficiently low to maintain a plasma concentration of 15–25 µg/ml, cessation of the infusion will result in rapid patient awakening. If the infusion rate is increased (e.g. to 300 µg/kg/min), plasma thiopentone concentrations will increase exponentially as peripheral storage sites become saturated. Accumulation will therefore occur. Furthermore, metabolic conversion to pentobarbitone will enhance the sedative effect, since pentobarbitone is an active metabolite with a longer elimination half-life (17–50 h) and slower clearance (0.3–0.6 ml/kg/min) than thiopentone. After a 2 h infusion, approximately 20% of the total drug dose will be present as pentobarbitone, leading to prolonged sedation after a thoracic surgical procedure of average duration (20).

The practical consequences of these pharmacokinetic observations are that thiopentone infusions are not appropriate in thoracic surgery patients. The high levels of surgical stress evident in patients undergoing procedures such as rigid bronchoscopy and thoracotomy are such that high infusion rates will be needed to ensure lack of response to surgical stimulation. The resulting high plasma concentrations of thiopentone and its active metabolite pentobarbitone will lead to prolonged sedation postoperatively, with significant reduction in early postoperative physiotherapy.

Methohexitone

Methohexitone is frequently used as an induction agent for short procedures and its use as a constant infusion for longer procedures has been explored (21). Methohexitone is metabolized in the liver and the metabolites are excreted in the urine. The drug has a faster elimination half-life than thiopentone (420–460 min), greater clearance than thiopentone (700–800 ml/min) and the main metabolite is inactive.

Infusions of methohexitone have been described, and the volume of distribution at steady state (4.5–4.7 l/kg), elimination half-life (420–460 min) and clearance (9.6–9.8 ml/kg/min) have been calculated.

Infusion rates of approximately 100–400 µg/kg/min are required for clinical anaesthesia, although this may be effectively lowered to 50–120 µg/kg/min if combined with an opioid and N_2O. In order to avoid a prolonged duration of effect, the total dose administered should be kept below 500 mg. Thus at the upper dose range, the infusion duration is best limited to 1–2 h, which makes it acceptable only for relatively short thoracic surgical procedures.

Etomidate

Etomidate is an imidazole derivative with a marked pharmacokinetic and pharmacodynamic advantage over the barbiturates. The drug shows a high clearance rate (18–24 ml/kg/min) and a shorter elimination half-life (110–320 min), and is metabolized by hepatic esterases to inactive metabolites. There is less haemodynamic depression than with thiopentone or propofol, an indeed we have used etomidate as the induction agent of choice in a TIVA technique in which propofol was used as the maintenance agent (14). However, others have shown that etomidate alone is unable to suppress the haemodynamic responses to instrumentation of the upper respiratory tract (22), and since rigid bronchoscopy and double lumen endobronchial intubation are more stimulating than laryngoscopy and endotracheal intubation this is a relevant observation in thoracic surgery patients.

Etomidate has a number of adverse effect. Despite reformulations, pain on injection remains a significant feature on bolus administration. However, the most significant adverse effect is to cause a dose-related inhibition of adrenal steroidogenesis by interaction with mitochondrial cytochrome P450 (23). Although these effects have been demonstrated, and adverse outcomes documented in patients receiving etomidate infusions in the ICU, there is little data concerning the adverse effects of etomidate infusions in the operative setting. Nonetheless, infusions of etomidate are not licensed for use in the UK and intraoperative maintenance infusions of etomidate should not be used.

Ketamine

In many ways ketamine can be considered a unique and extremely interesting anaesthetic agent. The systemic clearance of the drug is relatively high (1–1.2 l/min) with an elimination half-life of 2.5–4 h. In contrast to other agents, arterial blood pressure is maintained or increased in the presence of an intact sympathetic nervous system, and heart rate and cardiac filling pressures are maintained or increased also. These effects are mediated by blockade of noradrenaline re-uptake centrally and by release of noradrenaline from the sympathetic ganglia. The direct effects of ketamine on the myocardium are depressant.

Nonetheless, these effects may be theoretically valuable in elderly sick patients undergoing thoracic surgery, although the hyperdynamic effect on the circulation would be a potential hazard in patients undergoing bronchoscopy or double lumen endobronchial intubation. he effects on the CNS are also unique, in contrast to other induction agents. Ketamine is an effective analgesic in subanaesthetic concentrations and produces dissociative anaesthesia with little loss of muscle tone at greater concentrations.

Continuous infusions of ketamine have been used both in the operating room and in the ICU. An induction of 2 mg/kg followed by an infusion of 40 µg/kg/min has been shown to produce adequate clinical anaesthesia; corresponding steady-state drug concentrations were between 1.7 and 2.4 µg/ml. However, ketamine metabolites are not inactive, and nor-ketamine has a potency of approximately 30% of ketamine and a longer elimination half-life. Nor-ketamine is detectable in the plasma 5 min after the start of the infusion, and the complex metabolism of ketamine, the production of at least two active metabolites, and the prolonged clinical recovery complicated by postoperative dreams and hallucinations have reduced the use of this agent particularly when early recovery is required. Although benzodiazepines have been used to reduce the adverse hallucinatory aspects of recovery, return of consciousness is prolonged with their use.

The main value of ketamine in thoracic surgery is as an induction agent in the patient who is haemodynamically compromised and particularly those at risk from sudden reduction in cardiac filling pressures. Such patients include those in from haemorrhagic shock, patients with severe constrictive pericarditis and patients with pulmonary artery compression who are dependent on a high right-sided filling pressure. Ketamine will effectively preserve venous tone and ketamine has been used as an induction agent in these situations with no loss of central venous or systemic blood pressure. Once anaesthesia is established, the decision to continue with a suitable TIVA technique or use an additional volatile agent may be made. There is little to chose between the two, provided that vascular tone is well maintained.

Propofol

Propofol is clearly the most frequently used IV anaesthetic for maintenance of anaesthesia and indeed given the lack of other short-acting titratable anaesthetics it might be considered that TIVA in thoracic surgery is virtually dependent on the availability of propofol. Propofol is rapidly metabolized to inactive metabolites, and single-dose kinetics suggest a half life of 226–674 min, high clearance of 1.6–1.9l/min and a high volume of distribution. However, it should be noted that there is considerable variation between different studies that have evaluated the pharmacokinetics of propofol.

The pharmacodynamics of propofol have been extensively studied in different groups, but few studies in thoracic surgery patients have been conducted. We found propofol to be associated with less haemodynamic instability than thiopentone alone, which latter drug we felt should be supplemented with an opioid in order to obtund the initial haemodynamic responses to rigid bronchoscopy (13).

The main advantage to propofol over thiopentone for short thoracic surgical procedures lies in the speed and more importantly the quality of recovery. The two drugs have similar haemodynamic effects, although early comparisons between the two drugs, including our own initial evaluation of the current formulation, were probably hindered by our assumption that both drugs produce anaesthesia in one arm–brain circulation time, thus leading to a relative overdosage of propofol (24).

Details of TIVA techniques in thoracic surgery patients undergoing major procedures are also few, but propofol infusions in combination with opioids, N_2O, and with morphine and benzodiazepine premedication has been extensively studied and details are available elsewhere in this book. We found that propofol compared well with isoflurane in a study of patients undergoing thoracotomy for lung resection. Shunt fraction was markedly less in the propofol group compared to patients receiving isoflurane and although cardiac output was less in the propofol group there was no evidence of inadequate tissue oxygen delivery in either group (18). Equipotency is always difficult to establish between IV and volatile anaesthetics, and was a valid criticism of this study.

However, the ease and titratablilty of propofol-based TIVA makes it a valuable technique for thoracic surgery. Propofol is better able to obtund haemodynamic responses to rigid bronchoscopy than thiopentone, and a TIVA technique allows for ready manipulation of the FIO_2 during one-lung ventilation without unduly lightening the depth of anaesthesia. The above technique combines particularly well with thoracic epidural blockade for intraoperative and postoperative analgesia.

Opioids

Effective analgesia is an essential part of any TIVA technique, and despite attempts to utilize non-steroidals and other analgesics, the opioids remain the drugs of choice. Fentanyl or one of its analogues are commonly used, and the pharmacokinetics and dynamics of these drugs are described elsewhere. Thoracic surgery is not associated with the same level of stress as cardiac surgery and the intraoperative opioid requirements are usually substantially less than in cardiac surgery. By contrast, the postoperative opioid requirements are usually greater. The following should be noted:

◆ Thoracic surgical patients are usually woken and extubated immediately after surgery, in contrast to cardiac surgery where even a short period of IPPV is common
◆ The lateral thoracotomy incision is substantially more painful than a median sternotomy; also, pleurectomy may cause a raw and painful surface inside the chest wall, and even chest drains may be a considerable source of pain

♦ Patients who have undergone pulmonary surgery or prolonged one-lung ventilation for oesophageal surgery will be at greater risk for sputum retention, atalectasis, haemoptysis and clot retention, and pulmonary infection than other patients, particularly cardiac surgery patients

The use of opioids can be profitably continued into the postoperative period, preferably as a continuous infusion. Newer agents may be used in this way, although the ultra-short duration of action of remifentanil may cause some difficulty in management. If remifentanil is to be discontinued after surgery, care must be taken to ensure that an adequate alternative analgesic regime is well established before discontinuing the remifentanil, otherwise severe breakthrough pain will occur. As previously noted, there is considerable value in a combined thoracic epidural/TIVA technique both for intraoperative and postoperative analgesia.

References

1. Munakata M, Huang I, Mitzer W, Menkes H. Protective role of the epithleium in the guinea pig airway. *J Appl Physiol* 1989; **66**: 1547–52.
2. Hirschmann CA, Bergman NA. Factors influencing intrapulmonary airway calibre during anaesthesia. *Br J Anaesth* 1990; **65**: 30–42.
3. West JB, Dollery CT, Naimark A. Distribution of blood flow in isolated lung: relation to vascular and alveolar pressures. *J Appl Physiol* 1964; **19**: 713.
4. Benumof J. Special respiratory physiology of the lateral decubitus position, the open chest, one-lung ventilation. In: Benumof J, ed., *Anesthesia for thoracic surgery*, 2nd edn. Philadelphia, PA: Saunders, 1995: 123–51.
5. Wark KM, Lyons J, Feneck RO. The haemodynamic effects of bronchoscopy. Effect of pretreatment with fentanyl and alfentanil. *Anaesthesia* 1986; **41**: 162–9.
6. Wahi R, McMurtey MJ, De Caro LF, *et al.* Determinants of Perioperative morbidity and mortality after pneumonectomy. *Ann Thor Surg* 1989; **48**: 33–7.
7. Gerson MC, Hurst JM, Hurtzberg VS, Baugham R, Rouan GW, Ellis K. Prediction of cardiac and pulmonary complications related to elective abdominal and non-cardiac thoracic surgery in geriatric patients. *Am J Med* 1990; **88**: 101–7.
8. Mangano DT. Perioperative cardiac morbidity. *Anesthesiology* 1990; **72**: 153–84.
9. Nathan HJ. Coronary physiology. In: Kaplan JA, ed. *Cardiac anesthesia*, 3rd edn. Philadelphia, PA: Saunders 1993: 235–60.
10. Tomori Z, Widdicombe JG. Muscular, bronchomotor and cardiovascular reflexes elicited by mechanical stimulation of the respiratory tract. *J Physiol* 1969; **200**: 25–49.
11. Fox E, Sklar GS, Hill CH, *et al.* Complications related to the pressor response of endotracheal intubation. *Anesthesiology* 1977; **47**: 524–5.
12. Roizen MF, Horrigan RW, Frazer BM. Anaesthetic doses blocking adrenergic (stress) and cardiovascular responses to incision – MAC BAR. *Anesthesiology* 1981; **54**: 390–8.

13. Hill AJ, Feneck RO, Underwood SM, Davis ME, Marsh A, Bromley L. The haemodyamic effects of bronchscopy. *Anaestheia* 1991; **46**: 266–74.
14. George PJM, Pattison JM, Al Jarad N, et al. Preliminary experience with the 1.32 um Nd-YAG laser in the treatment of tracheobronchial malignancy. *Lasers Med Sci* 1991; **6**: 407–14.
15. George RJM, Garrett CPO, Nixon C, Hetzel MR, Nanson E, Millard FJC. Laser treatment of tracheobroncial tumours; local or general anaesthesia? *Thorax* 1987; **42**: 656–60.
16. Leventhal SR, Orkin FK, Hirsh RA. Prediction of the need for postoperative mechanical ventilation in myasthenia gravis. *Anesthesiology* 1980; **53**: 26–30.
17. Benumof J. Choice of anaesthetic drugs and techniques. In: Benumof J, ed. *Anesthesia for thoracic surgery*, 2nd edn. Philadelphia, PA: Saunders 1995: 301–29.
18. Kellow NH, Scott AD, White SA, Feneck RO. Comparison of the effects of propofol and isoflurane anaestheia on right ventricular function and shunt fraction during thoracic surgery. *Br J Anaesth* 1995; **75**: 578.
19. Hung OR, Varvel JR, Shafer SL and Stanski DR. Thipental pharmacodynamics II. Quantitation of clinical and electroencephalographic depth of anaesthesia. *Anesthesiology* 1992; **77**: 237–44.
20. Chan HNJ, Morgan DJ, Crankshaw DP, Boyd MD. Pentobarbitone formation during thiopentone infusion. *Anaesthesia* 1985; **40**: 1155–9.
21. Le Normand Y, De Villepoix C, Pinaud M, et al. Pharmacokinetics and haemodynamic effects of prolonged methohexitone infusion. *Br J Clin Pharmacol* 1988; **26**: 589–94.
22. Harris CE, Murray AM, Anderson JM, Grounds RM, Morgan M. Effects of thiopentone, etomidate, and propofol on the haemodynamic response to tracheal intubation. *Anaesthesia* 1988; **43** (suppl): 32–6.
23. Watt I, Ledingham I. Mortality amongst multiple trauma patients admitted to an intensive therapy unit. *Anaesthesia* 1989; **39**: 973–81.
24. Patrick M, Blair, I. Feneck RO, Sebel PS. Comparison of the haemodynamic effects of propofol and thipentone in patients with coronary artery disease. *Postgrad Med J* 1985; **61**: 23–31.

11

Neurosurgery

C. R. Bailey and M. Sinden

- Neurophysiology
- Cerebral protection
- Effects of anaesthetic agents
- Prerequisites for successful application of total intravenous anaesthesia (TIVA) techniques to neurosurgery
- Spotlight on propofol
- Other anaesthetic agents
- A suggested technique
- TIVA applications

The application of total intravenous anaesthesia (TIVA) in neurosurgical practice represents an opportunity for the anaesthetist to provide excellent surgical conditions, influence neurophysiological changes and minimize adverse neurological sequelae.

Neurophysiology

It is impossible to consider neuroanaesthetic practice without reviewing the pertinent aspects of neurophysiology. Some of the factors mentioned are under the control of, and may be modified by, the anaesthetist and by the various anaesthetic agents used. It is only through a thorough understanding of neurophysiology that an appropriate anaesthetic technique may be chosen. For a more complete description of neurophysiology the reader should refer to a specialized text.

Intracranial pressure

The skull or cranium is a rigid box. The intracranial pressure (ICP) is determined by the intracranial contents, which are essentially incompressible. The intracranial components in a normal adult are listed in Table 11.1.

Table 11.1 Intracranial components in a normal adult

Component	Volume/weight	Percentage of total
Blood	50–70 ml	5–7
Brain	1400 g	80–85
CSF	50–120 ml	5–12

Normal ICP is between 7 and 15 mmHg (1–2 kPa) when supine. When the intracranial volume begins to rise due to an increase in one or other of the components, e.g. brain tissue in the case of cerebral tumour, the ICP does not immediately increase because compensatory mechanisms come into play; cerebrospinal fluid (CSF) is pushed out of the skull into the spinal column, there is increased absorption of CSF into the venous circulation and the venous sinuses become compressed. Eventually the compensatory mechanisms become exhausted and at this point any further increase in intracranial volume is associated with a severe increase in ICP (Figure 11.1).

The increase in ICP will jeopardize the cerebral perfusion pressure (CPP) and reduce the blood supply to the brain. This, together with oedema due to venous outflow obstruction, eventually leads to ischaemia and if the ICP continues to rise structural damage and coning may result.

The anaesthetist has several available strategies for reducing raised ICP. Moderate hyperventilation to a P_aCO_2 of between 3.5 and 4 kPa (27–30 mmHg) produces vasoconstriction and a reduction in cerebral blood volume, but the effect is limited to no more than 48 h. Adequate patient positioning with slight head-up tilt will facilitate venous drainage, whilst adequate sedation and relaxation minimize coughing or straining. Fluid restriction may attenuate further increases in ICP. Diuretics and steroids may be employed to reduce oedema. In addition to these methods surgical decompression may be used and/or CSF may be drained via ventricular shunts.

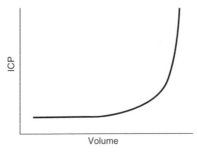

Figure 11.1 ICP plotted agianst intracranial volume.

Cerebral metabolism

The brain is a dynamic organ with high energy requirements, the main substrate for brain metabolism being glucose. In health approximately 90% is metabolized aerobically to produce the necessary energy to maintain transmembrane electrical potentials, facilitate ionic pumping, molecular transport processes and general cellular metabolism.

Cerebral metabolic rate for oxygen

$$\text{Cerebral metabolic rate for oxygen } (CMR_{O_2}) = \frac{\text{cerebral blood flow (CBF)} \times}{\text{arterio-venous oxygen content difference}}$$

The CMR_{O_2} is the volume of oxygen consumed by the brain per unit time and represents *global* cerebral metabolism, which in health remains fairly constant. It should be remembered, however, that there are considerable regional variations dependent upon activity; neurones consume more oxygen than glial cells and grey matter more than white matter. Neural activity is associated with an increased metabolic rate. For adults CMR_{O_2} approximates to 3.5 ml O_2/100 g brain tissue/min. Allowing for an average adult brain mass of 1400 g, this equates to approximately 20% of whole body oxygen consumption. Children have higher rates of CMR_{O_2} (5.2 ml/100 g brain tissue/min). CMR_{O_2} is reduced by approximately 5% per 1°C drop in core temperature and is reduced in old age. Drugs may have significant influences on CMR_{O_2}; it is reduced by barbiturates, benzodiazepines, propofol, etomidate and volatile anaesthetic agents, but is increased by ketamine and nitrous oxide (N_2O).

Cerebral blood flow

Cerebral blood flow (CBF) is high in order to supply sufficient oxygen and glucose to serve the high energy requirements of the brain; approximately 15% of the total cardiac output is directed to the brain (50 ml/100 g brain tissue/min). The areas of greatest metabolism receive preferentially more blood, e.g. grey matter receives more than white matter. In infants and children the global CBF is greater than in adults (approximately 65 ml/100 g brain tissue/min). In parallel with regional metabolism, regional blood flow varies considerably and, although methods of measuring CBF have improved in sophistication, true regional blood flow remains difficult to measure. Pain, anxiety and seizure activity all produce significant increases in metabolism and CBF, and are important considerations in neuroanaesthetic practice.

Control of CBF is complex and multiple factors interact to safeguard blood supply to the brain. These factors may be affected by pathological processes as well as drugs. CBF is tightly coupled to metabolism but the exact mechanism explaining this process remains to be fully elucidated. The traditional theory is that the build up of extracellular fluid concentrations of various ions (H^+, K^+, Ca^{2+}) and metabolic products (prostaglandins, thromboxanes, adenosine) probably result in local vasoregulation. Nitric oxide (NO) has been implicated as playing a major role in control of CBF both in health and pathological conditions. It is also thought to play a role in the vascular action of certain anaesthetic drugs. Endothelium-derived NO under resting conditions is thought to produce a tonic dilatory influence on cerebral blood vessels and inhibition of nitric oxide synthase (NOS), the enzyme responsible for production of NO from its amino acid precursor L-arginine, results in decreased CBF and dose-related cerebral vasoconstriction.

The partial pressure of arterial oxygen (P_aO_2) and CO_2 (P_aCO_2) both have significant effects on CBF control (Figure 11.2).

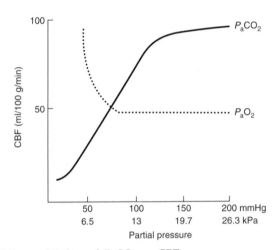

Figure 11.2   Effects of P_aO_2 and P_aCO_2 on CBF.

Little change occurs until P_aO_2 has fallen to less than 6.5 kPa (50 mmHg), but below this partial pressure CBF increases rapidly, although a normal mean arterial pressure (MAP) is required for the changes to occur. Mechanisms suggested to explain the vasodilatory effects of hypoxia include adenosine release, increased tissue concentrations of H^+ and K^+ ions, and amino acid release.

CO_2 reactivity

There is an approximately linear change in CBF to changes in P_aCO_2 between partial pressures of 3.2 kPa (25 mmHg) and 9.8 kPa (75 mmHg); increasing P_aCO_2 results in vasodilatation and increased CBF with the opposite occurring when P_aCO_2 decreases. The acidosis associated with hypercarbia appears to have a critical influence on cerebral blood vessels. NO-related mechanisms may be important in the response to hypercapnia but do not seem to be involved with the CBF response to hypoxia.

Cerebral perfusion pressure

$$\text{Cerebral perfusion pressure (CPP)} = \begin{array}{l}\text{mean arterial pressure (MAP)} - \\ \text{intracranial pressure (ICP)} + \\ \text{central venous pressure (CVP)}\end{array}$$

CVP is usually taken as zero unless greater than ICP.

The determinants of CPP are as described in the above equation. As previously discussed, raised ICP may compromise perfusion unless there is an associated increase in MAP.

Autoregulation

Autoregulation describes the maintenance of relatively constant CBF despite wide variations in MAP. CBF remains constant in health between MAP values of 50 and 150 mmHg by either arteriolar constriction or dilatation as appropriate (Figure 11.3).

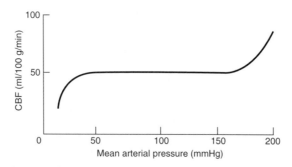

Figure 11.3   Autoregulation.

At low values of MAP, CBF is directly proportional to perfusion pressure, whilst at very high levels of MAP there is damage to fragile blood vessels resulting in potential disruption of the blood–brain barrier, plasma leakage, haemorrhage and cerebral oedema. Autoregulation also maintains spinal cord blood flow. Whilst the exact mechanisms explaining autoregulation are unknown, two popular theories are 'myogenic' and 'metabolic'. The myogenic theory suggests that autoregulation occurs due to the intrinsic properties of smooth muscle cells in arteriolar walls, i.e. increased arterial pressure produces stretching of the smooth muscle with resultant constriction, whereas decreased pressure produces less distension and leads to smooth muscle relaxation and subsequent vasodilatation. The metabolic theory suggests that decreased oxygen and substrate delivery secondary to reduced perfusion produces reflex arteriolar dilatation.

The autoregulation curve may be shifted to the left or right; factors associated with a left shift include hypoxia, hypercarbia and vasodilating drugs, whilst a right shift occurs with chronic hypertension and increased sympathetic activity. Following appropriate treatment of hypertension the curve may return towards its normal position. Autoregulation may be affected by cerebral disease processes and abolished by trauma, hypoxia and drugs (including some anaesthetic agents).

Cerebral steal and inverse steal

Cerebral steal is the diversion of blood away from abnormal areas of the brain. In such abnormal areas, e.g. ischaemia or space-occupying lesions, cerebral vessels are already maximally dilated and autoregulation does not occur. Vasodilatation of the cerebral vasculature in the remaining normal areas of the brain results in a reduction of blood flow to the abnormal areas. Inverse steal is essentially the opposite of the above. Cerebral vasoconstriction of normal cerebral vessels from whatever cause results in proportionally more blood being diverted to the maximally dilated vessels in the abnormal areas.

Cerebral protection

Cerebral protection involves physiological or pharmacological inter-ventions prior to the onset of cerebral ischaemia with the aim of reducing the incidence of cerebral deficit. The cellular mechanisms underlying neuronal injury and cell death post ischaemia still remain to be fully elucidated. Ischaemia results in loss of cellular membrane integrity secondary to calcium influx via agonist-sensitive ion channels, together with the leak of excitatory amino acids, particularly glutamate and glycine. Oxygen radicals are produced following ischaemia and reperfu-sion injury, which prevent NO function.

Principles of management include either reduction in metabolic oxygen consumption or increase in oxygen delivery.

Hypothermia

CMR_{O_2} decreases by approximately 5% for each 1°C reduction in body temperature and this together with the evidence that there is a reduction in release of neurotransmitters during hypothermia is the main basis for its use. However, deep hypothermia and circulatory arrest utilized to clip giant aneurysms requires cardiopulmonary bypass techniques, and may lead to cardiac arrhythmias and coagulation disturbances.

Barbiturates

The benefits of barbiturates such as thiopentone include:

- Decrease in cerebral metabolic requirements, ICP and CSF secretion
- Scavenging of free radicals
- Suppression of convulsions

◆ Anaesthesia
◆ Stabilization of membranes
◆ Calcium channel blockade
◆ Alteration of fatty acid metabolism
◆ Suppression of catecholamine-induced hyperactivity
◆ Impairment of thermoregulation

Mannitol

Mannitol is hyperosmolar, drawing free water from intracellular and interstitial compartments into the vascular space, resulting in diuresis and consequent reduction in ICP. It is also reputed to scavenge oxygen free radicals.

Steroids

The benefits of steroids include:

◆ Stabilization of membranes
◆ Reduction in cerebral oedema
◆ Scavenging of free radicals
◆ Reduction in CSF production
◆ Increasing the threshold for convulsions

Phenytoin

Phenytoin decreases CBF but has no effect on cerebral metabolism. It stabilizes membranes and slows the release of potassium from ischaemic neurones. Increases in extracellular potassium concentration cause contraction of vascular smooth muscle, thereby reducing CBF and increasing the water content of glia; these effects are prevented by phenytoin. Furthermore, phenytoin reduces the accumulation of free fatty acids during ischaemia and thus the cascade leading to free radical production.

Ketamine

Considerable interest has focused upon the role of the N-methyl-D-aspartate (NMDA) receptors in the pathophysiology of ischaemic neuronal secondary injury. Ketamine, an NMDA antagonist, may provide a useful source of cerebral protection following ischaemic injury by minimizing calcium influx, although further studies need to be undertaken (1). Research regarding the use of glutamate and glycine antagonists as neuroprotective agents shows promise.

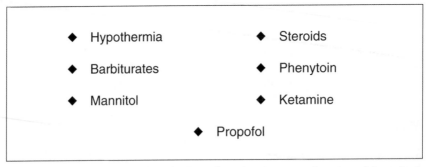

Figure 11.4   Intraoperative methods and medications employed to aid cerebral protection

Prerequisistes for successful application of TIVA techniques in neurosurgery

We believe that anaesthesia for neurosurgery should provide the following:

- Safety and effectiveness
- Cost-efficiency
- Easy administration
- Favourable pharmacokinetic profile
- Maintenance of CBF
- Reduction of metabolic demands
- Neuroprotection against ischaemia and cerebral oedema
- Optimal operating conditions
- No adverse effects on neurological monitoring
- Clear-headed recovery and few postoperative sequelae such as vomiting
- Early assessment of neurological function following surgery

Although the specific effects of anaesthetic agents can be demonstrated and usefully employed in neuroanaesthetic practice, successful outcomes also depend upon the following factors:

- Co-administration of other agents
- Physiological interventions
- Positioning of the patient
- Ventilatory adjustments
- Drainage of CSF

Propofol

Propofol, at the time of writing, is the most suitable agent available around which to base a TIVA technique (2).

Safety and effectiveness

Propofol is an aqueous isotonic emulsion administered in a vehicle containing glycerol, purified egg phosphatide, sodium hydroxide, soybean oil and water. An amount of 1 ml of 1% propofol contains 0.1 g fat and blood lipid levels should be monitored in patients thought to be at particular risk of fat overload. One study noted an increase in total lipid concentrations and triglycerides but reduction in cholesterol levels during propofol use for 3 h and, although no causal relationship was established, serious adverse events (including deaths) have been noted, usually in children with respiratory tract infections given high doses of propofol. Propofol contains no antimicrobial preservatives and supports growth of microorganisms and asepsis must be maintained at all times. Propofol is now an established IV anaesthetic agent, but possesses little amnesic or analgesic properties and, as a sole agent, does not prevent intraoperative recall; for these reasons we believe it should never be the sole anaesthetic agent.

Propofol and convulsions

Evidence for a proconvulsant action of propofol

- Case reports of convulsions
- Epileptiform movements reported as propofol levels decreased abruptly at the termination of an infusion
- Dystonic or choreiform reactions which may occur on induction of anaesthesia with propofol and have been interpreted as convulsions

Evidence for anticonvulsant activity

- Animal experiments
- Reduction in convulsion activity during electroconvulsive therapy (ECT) in patients given propofol
- High doses of propofol causing burst suppression on the electrocorticogram (ECoG) during epilepsy surgery

Cost

Propofol is more expensive to administer than volatile agents; one of the authors has calculated that an hour long anaesthetic using 0.76% isoflurane (1 MAC), oxygen/N_2O at 6 l/min fresh gas flow, following induction with thiopentone and pancuronium cost £9.69 in 1992 (3), and Rowe (4) calculated the cost of 1 h long anaesthetic using 2% isoflurane and 6 l/min fresh gas flow as £14.32. If a circle system with a 2 l/min fresh gas flow and 2% isoflurane is used this is reduced to £4.77. This is in comparison with a propofol infusion run at 6 mg/kg/h which costs £8.15/h for an average adult (£13.58/h if run at 10 mg/kg/h in the same patient). However, anaesthetic drugs account for a small percentage of the overall cost of surgery and the reduction in postoperative complications such as vomiting and clearer-headed recovery makes the use of propofol, in our opinion, a justifiable expense.

Ease of administration

Propofol is presented in already constituted syringes in concentrations of both 1 and 2%, and does not need to be kept refrigerated. It is easily prepared for infusion by placing in 'Diprifusor' syringe drivers and attached to the patient via an IV line. There may be pain on injection and we therefore attach the infusion to a large bore venous cannula (18G) placed in an area easily visible during surgery in order to check for extravasation. Syringes are easily replaced during the operation.

Favourable pharmacokinetic profile

The pharmacokinetics of propofol are discussed in detail elsewhere. With regard to neuroanaesthesia, there is some evidence that the concomitant chronic administration of anticonvulsants (such as phenytoin) induces liver enzymes and reduces serum levels of propofol during infusion after the steady state is achieved, perhaps requiring a slightly increased target serum level to be set than would be first thought. Interestingly, in one study tissue concentrations of propofol within the brain following an infusion were found to be highest in the medulla compared with the cortex, which in turn was higher than in the hippocampus.

Maintenance of cerebral blood flow and reduction of metabolic demands

Although the neurophysiological effects of propofol are in general favourable (Table 11.2), an undesirable reduction in systemic blood pressure and consequently CPP may occur if the induction dose is too high or too quickly administered. Also, one study found that the combination of propofol with hypocarbia caused undesirable neurophysiological changes, including a reduction in jugular bulb venous oxygen saturation and increase in arterio-venous oxygen difference.

Neuroprotection against ischaemia and cerebral oedema

Most molecules have paired electrons in their electron orbits. The two electrons spin in opposite directions and cancel out each others magnetic field, resulting in a low energy state. Free radicals are formed by homolytic fission of a covalent bond which splits symmetrically and both fragments retain a single electron. This unpaired electron in the outer orbital has a magnetic field that produces a high energy state, making the

Table 11.2 Relative neurophysiological effects of anaesthetic agents

Drug	Direct cerebral vasodilation	Hypercarbic vasodilation	CMR_{O_2}	CBF	Neuroprotection	CSF formation	ICP
Halothane	+	+	-	+++	0	-	+
Enflurane	+	+	-	++	0	+	+
Isoflurane	+	+	--	+	0	0	0
Sevoflurane	+	+	--	+	0	?	0
Desflurane	+	+	--	+	0	+	0
N_2O	+	0	+	+	0	0	+
Thiopentone	-	-	--	--	+++	-	-
Etomidate	-	0	--	--	++	?	-
Propofol	-	-	--	--	++	-	-
Midazolam	-	+	--	--	0	-	-
Ketamine	+	0	+	++	? ?+	0	+
Morphine	0	0	0	0	0	?	0
Fentanyl	0	0	-	-	0	0	?+
Sufentanil	?+	0	?	?+	0	?	?+
Alfentanil	?+	0	?	?+	0	?	?+
Remifentanil	?0	0	?	?+	0	?	?+
Vasodilators	+	+	?+	+	0	0	+
Suxamethonium	0	0	+	-	0	0	+

Key: 0 = no change; +, + +, + + + = mild, moderate, significant increase; −, − −, − − − = mild, moderate, significant decrease; ? = uncertain effect.

molecule highly reactive and unstable with a very short half-life. Free radicals exist in low concentrations and do not travel far from their site of formation; they act to remove electrons from adjacent non-radical molecules, resulting in a chain reaction of free radical generation until a scavenger molecule is met. During ischaemia hypoxanthine is produced which is converted by xanthine oxidase to xanthine, reducing $O_2{}^{.-}$ to the superoxide radical, $O_2{}^{.-}$. During anoxia or complete cerebral ischaemia free radical generation is limited because of the absence of oxygen, but during reperfusion the cells are exposed to oxygen and in the presence of inadequately functioning mitochondria that were damaged during the ischaemia, a high free radical load results. Propofol has been shown to scavenge free radicals.

Optimal operating conditions

Depth of anaesthesia is easily adjusted using an infusion technique in much the same way as for volatile agents and it has been successfully employed, for example, to reduce blood pressure acutely before applying clips to cerebral aneurysms.

Interactions with monitoring equipment

Propofol in high doses causes burst suppression on the electroencephalogram and will affect surface ECoG readings performed during epilepsy surgery. Monitoring of sensory evoked responses in supratentorial and spinal surgery is probably accurate (if N_2O is omitted), but there are reports that motor evoked responses recorded during spinal surgery are inaccurate and this is certainly our observation if propofol is administered during surgery on children with spinal cord tethering.

Early assessment of neurological function following surgery

Before the introduction of target-controlled infusion (TCI), the concentrations of propofol following termination of infusions were unpredictable but one study found that patients were opening their eyes on command at serum levels of 1 mg/l (about 10 min after the end of an infusion) following a mean dose of 4.14 mg/kg/h for between 330 and 1440 min. With the introduction of TCI, following termination of a propofol infusion there is a more predictable decrease in serum levels. A quick, clear-headed recovery is possible together with a reduction in previously reported adverse effects such as vomiting which, as well as being unpleasant for the patient, increases intracranial and arterial pressures postoperatively, and may result in the development of subdural bleeding.

Other advantages of propofol pertaining to neurosurgery

◆ Reduction in the vasoconstrictor sympathetic response to laryngoscopy, intubation and extubation

- Synergism with other drugs, including alfentanil
- Obviating the need for N_2O; N_2O causes an increase in CBF (although this can be counteracted by other maneouvres, e.g. hyperventilation), as well as increasing the volume of air-filled cavities
- Propofol is applicable to patients with conditions such as malignant hyperthermia (MH) and acute intermittent porphyria (AIP)

Other anaesthetic agents

Thiopentone

Thiopentone is a dose-dependent cerebral vasoconstrictor and during anaesthesia CMR_{O_2} is reduced in proportion to the depth of anaesthesia. CBF appears to follow these changes in metabolic rate and the greatest reduction in flow is with the deepest anaesthesia. Thiopentone attenuates the vasodilatation produced by N_2O (and ketamine) and continuous infusions have been employed for neurosurgical procedures. However, notwithstanding its effects as a cerebral protective agent, the use of thiopentone infusions have been largely surpassed following the introduction of propofol.

Etomidate

Etomidate produces little cardiovascular depression in healthy patients and may have advantages for poor-risk patients when preservation of normal arterial pressure is necessary. Etomidate induces parallel reductions in CBF, CMR_{O_2} and ICP without decreasing CPP as well as preserving CO_2 reactivity, but enthusiasm for its use is tempered by the knowledge that there is involuntary muscular activity and suppression of adrenocortical function.

Ketamine

Ketamine increases CBF and reduces cerebrovascular resistance, but CMR_{O_2} does not change significantly; it also increases ICP although such increases are attenuated by hypocarbia. Despite possible advantages due to its effects on NMDA receptors, available evidence suggests that ketamine should not be used during anaesthesia for neurosurgery in patients with elevated ICP or reduced intracranial compliance.

Benzodiazepines

Because they are receptor-specific, benzodiazepines have unique cerebral effects; midazolam, a water-soluble compound, reduces CBF and CMR_{O_2} to a maximum effect (of 25%) due to receptor saturation. It causes relatively little reduction in ICP and less metabolic suppression than thiopentone. All these effects are antagonized by flumazenil and care must be taken when administering this agent to patients with impaired intracranial compliance. In our view midazolam is better employed as a sedative rather than an anaesthetic.

Opioids

When used in conjunction with vasodilating agents (e.g. isoflurane) opioids usually cause cerebral vasoconstriction and a reduction in CBF, whereas if used in conjunction with a vasoconstricting agent (e.g. thiopentone) there is no effect.

Remifentanil

Remifentanil is a pure μ opioid receptor agonist, derived from fentanyl and displays similar pharmacodynamic properties (5). The advantages of remifentanil include its favourable pharmacokinetic profile; remifentanil has a volume of distribution of 25–40 l, is 70% plasma protein bound, is metabolized by non-specific esterases (and is unaffected by cholinesterase deficiency, liver or renal disease) to clinically insignificant metabolites, and has a terminal half-life of 10–21 min and a clearance of approximately 5 l/min. It possesses a context-sensitive half-time (the time for the effect site concentration to fall by 50% after terminating an infusion designed to maintain a constant plasma concentration) of 3.6 min following a 3 h infusion. In neuroanaesthetic practice this effectively means that following cessation of an infusion neurological assessment is possible within minutes following an operation and abnormal signs need not be attributed to the effects of anaesthesia. Following a bolus dose of 1 μg/kg and infusion rate of 0–0.25 μg/kg/min, the TCI of propofol can be reduced by up to 50% when compared with other analgesic regimens, thus offering some cost savings.

The disadvantages of remifentanil include:

♦ Chest wall rigidity and apnoea
♦ Nausea and vomiting
♦ Bradycardia and hypotension
♦ Pain following discontinuation of use

Chest wall rigidity and apnoea follow large bolus doses of remifentanil, and are not a problem in neuroanaesthetic practice whereby patients are paralysed and intubated, whilst the incidence of nausea and vomiting (similar to that with other opioids) is reduced by propofol and anti-emetics. Bradycardia and hypotension are dose-related and easily managed by concomitant administration of colloid infusions and/or small doses of anticholinergics. In neurosurgery postoperative pain is not usually a major problem and most pain is relieved by codeine phosphate; this can be administered intramuscularly 30 min before the end of surgery to provide analgesia in the immediate postoperative period.

Inhalational agents

The inhalational agents are cerebral vasodilators (but reduce CMR_{O_2}) and may increase ICP when intracranial compliance is reduced, although hyperventilation may blunt this response. Enflurane may cause convulsions and should be avoided in neurosurgical anaesthesia, whilst isoflurane may induce cerebral steal as mentioned earlier. Both of the newer inhalational agents desflurane and sevoflurane have similar effects to isoflurane, the slight advantage being that their low blood:gas solubility and pharmacokinetics favour a more rapid cerebral wash in and wash out than previous inhalational agents resulting in a more rapid recovery from anaesthesia.

Nitrous oxide

N_2O causes an increase in CBF and CMR_{O_2}, especially when co-administered with inhalational agents. Although N_2O provides some amnesic and analgesic effects, the increase in CBF, the potential to increase air-filled cavities and suspicions regarding bone marrow suppression following long-term use may lead to its abandonment in favour of a TIVA technique employing an oxygen/air mixture.

Supplementary agents

Neuromuscular blockers

Suxamethonium causes modest, transient increases in ICP and CBF, while the newer non-depolarizing agents have no clinical effect on ICP. A non-paretic limb must be monitored for neuromuscular function because paretic limbs are resistant to the effects of these agents, which may result in relative overdosage. Chronic administration of phenytoin and/or carbamzepine increases the dose requirements of these agents.

A suggested technique for supratentorial tumour surgery

A suggested technique for supratentorial tumour surgery is given in Table 11.3.

Situations in which total intravenous anasthesia is applicable

◆ Supratentorial and posterior fossa surgery
◆ Neuroradiological procedures such as magnetic resonance imaging
◆ Intensive care sedation
◆ Interhospital patient transfer
◆ Carotid endarterectomy
◆ Aneurysm clipping
◆ Spinal cord surgery

Table 11.3 Suggested technique for supratentorial tumour surgery

Full monitoring (including that of neuromuscular function) should be applied before induction of anaesthesia. Venous cannulation should be performed at a site that will be visible during surgery.

Induction

Following preoxygenation, fentanyl 1 μg/kg is given as a bolus and TCI of propofol is commenced aiming for serum levels of 6–8 μg/ml depending on the physical status of the patient. Following loss of consciousness, vecuronium 0.15 mg/kg is administered and the patient is ventilated via a mask to maintain a P_aCO_2 of approximately 5 kPa until full neuromuscular paralysis occurs. At this point give a further fentanyl bolus of 1 μg/kg (to help reduce the sympathetic response to laryngoscopy and intubation), wait 2 min and then perform endotracheal intubation. Ventilate the patients lungs with a mixture of oxygen and air to maintain a P_aCO_2 of 4 kPa.

Maintenance

♦ Propofol TCI (2–4 μg/ml).
♦ Vecuronium infusion to maintain single twitch following a train of four stimulus (TOF).
♦ Boluses of fentanyl at stimulating times, e.g application of head pins, incision of pericranium, opening of dura, traction on brain tissue.
♦ The patient is kept warm with a warm air convection blanket to avoid coagulation problems and arrhythmias.
♦ Other drugs given include dexamethasone, ranitidine, phenytoin and antibiotics.
♦ When closure of the dura takes place give intramuscular codeine phosphate (1 mg/kg) and an IV antiemetic.

Reversal and recovery

♦ Stop propofol infusion as the surgeon is closing the skin wound, reverse neuromuscular blockade and establish spontaneous respiration. Extubate patient while propofol is still clinically active.

Unfortunately, propofol has been reported to cause muscle spasm in children with spastic cerebral palsy having dorsal rhizotomies and the use of propofol impairs the accuracy of motor evoked responses (MEPs), although sensory evoked responses (SEPs) are accurate.

'Awake' procedures

Craniotomies

Huggins (6) used a TCI of propofol to obtain conditions whereby a spontaneously breathing patient was unresponsive to scalp infiltration of local anaesthetic for a field block to turn a flap and perform a craniotomy to excise epileptic foci in the dominant hemisphere. Despite hypercarbia and what we would consider high target propofol concentrations (up to 7 µg/ml) outcomes were satisfactory in the 20 patients studied.

Other procedures

Using a TCI technique and aiming for serum levels of 4 µg/ml, both trigeminal rhizotomies and stereotactic burrhole biopsies can be performed if supplementary analgesia and oxygen are administered.

Conclusion

The relatively recent introduction of TIVA into neuroanaesthetic practice has produced distinct advantages as compared with established inhalational agent-based anaesthetics. Propofol, in combination with remifentanil and a neuromuscular blocking agent, is easy to administer, provides superb operating conditions and rapid recovery, allowing accurate postoperative neurological assessment.

References

1. Ravussin P, Wilder-Smith OHG. Intravenous anaesthetics in neurosurgery. *Curr Opin Anaesthesiol* 1996; **9**: 381–4.
2. van Hemelrijck J, van Aken H, Merckx L, Mulier J. Anesthesia for craniotomy: total intravenous anesthesia with propofol and alfentanil compared to anesthesia with thiopental sodium, isoflurane, fentanyl and nitrous oxide. *J Clin Anesth* 1991; **3**: 131–6.
3. Bailey CR, Ruggier R, Cashman JN. Anaesthesia: cheap at twice the price. *Anaesthesia* 1993; **48**: 906–9.
4. Rowe WL. Economics and anaesthesia. *Anaesthesia* 1998; **53**: 782–8.
5. Thompson JP, Rowbotham DJ. Remifentanil – an opioid for the 21st century. *Br J Anaesth* 1996; **76**: 341–3.
6. Huggins NJ. Reversible anaesthesia for awake craniotomy. Presented at *11th World Congress of Anaesthesia*, Sydney, Australia 1996: abstr 265.

12

Maxillofacial, plastic and ear, nose and throat (ENT) surgery

N. L. Padfield

- Functional anatomy of the larynx
- Major head and neck surgery
- Facial injuries
- Intraoral surgery
- Free tissue transfer
- Burns
- Microlaryngoscopy
- Laser surgery
- Tonsil surgery
- Ear surgery

These three branches of specialist surgery have been grouped together because anaesthesia for them shares many common features.

- ◆ Recovery must be rapid and of good quality with rapid return of protective pharyngeal reflexes
- ◆ Induction should be smooth and agreeable, with minimal coughing to reduce incidence and degree of haemorrhage
- ◆ The airway must be protected with an inflated tracheal cuff to prevent aspiration
- ◆ The widespread use of reverse trendelberg to prevent venous oozing may have significant cardiovascular consequences
- ◆ Suspected laryngeal narrowing requires the best radiological imaging possible
- ◆ Long operations make the maintenance of the patient's core temperature difficult; there is a need for extra precautions with warming devices in patients with vasodilatory anaesthetics
- ◆ There are cases where muscle relaxants are best avoided such as tympanoplasty, stapedectomy and meringoplasty where the facial nerve is monitored

- Laser surgery can proceed more safely with total intravenous anaesthesia (TIVA) as the gases used do not so readily support combustion
- In pharyngeal pouch surgery, packing the pouch and pharyngeal 'toilet' is much easier with TIVA than with inhalational anaesthesia

Anaesthesia for ENT, plastic and faciomaxillary surgery requires close cooperation with the surgeon as there is often a shared airway. The length of surgery can sometimes be long, which brings its own special challenges. Blood pressure and blood flow are often manipulated to reduce intraoperative blood loss. Conversely, blood flow in the micro circulation has to be optimized for the survival of free tissue transfer grafts, which requires maintaining or augmenting venous filling pressure of the heart whilst encouraging venous drainage by special positioning of the patient.

The anaesthetist may frequently be confronted with decisions regarding difficult airway management. A detailed knowledge of the anatomy and the functioning of the airway is therefore essential.

Functional anatomy of the larynx

The function of the larynx is to protect the airway, to allow ingress and egress of gasses for respiration, and to alter the shape and tension of the vocal cords for phonation (1,2).

The larynx comprises, from above downwards, of the rima glottidis consisting of the epiglottis in front, the false cords at the sides and the arytenoid cartilages at the back. The pyriform fossae are situated lateral to the false cords, and curve backwards and downwards behind the arytenoid cartilages to enter the superior third (under voluntary motor control) of the oesophagus. Below the false cords are lateral out pouchings called the ventricles, and below these lie the true cords attached to the thyroid cartilage in the front and the arytenoids at the back.

The cricothyroid membrane lies below the cords, which is an important consideration when the need for emergency cricothyroidotomy arises to restore an obstructed airway. The false cords can act as a muscular flap which can close to prevent the egress of air from below, whereas the true cords when closed will prevent the entry of air into the trachea – an important reason why positive pressure ventilation alone will not overcome laryngeal spasm.

The sensory innervation to the larynx is supplied by the superior laryngeal nerve that arises from the inferior ganglion of the vagus nerve. It also supplies a motor branch to the arytenoid muscles. Sensory innervation below the true cords and to the upper tracheal rings is supplied by the recurrent laryngeal nerves which also supply the motor fibres to the intrinsic laryngeal muscles, except the cricothyroid and inferior pharyngeal constrictors which derive their motor supply from the external branch of the superior laryngeal nerve.

The recurrent laryngeal nerves can be injured by endotracheal intubation, neck surgery (especially thyroid surgery) or by stretching the neck during surgery. If the lesion is unilateral the true cord on the affected side will lie in the para median position because of the unopposed action of cricothyroid muscle which causes adduction of the cord. If the external branch of the superior laryngeal nerve is also injured then the true cord will be less medial and less tense. Clinically the patient will be hoarse, the voice will be weak and there will be an increased risk of aspiration. If the duration of the palsy is prolonged a degree of compensation occurs within the muscles and the cord will lie more medially.

The sensory components of the internal branch of the superior laryngeal nerve also include joint, pressure and muscular stretch receptors. This highly sensitive structure then will on occasion respond in an exaggerated way to irritating glottic or supraglottic stimuli such as food, blood, vomit, saliva or a foreign body to cause laryngeal spasm. This often persists long after the original mucosal irritation has ceased. Hypercarbia and hypoxia reverse it by decreasing the post-synaptic potentials and brain stem output to the superior laryngeal nerve and thus cause less strenuous glottic closure. Because, if untreated, laryngeal spasm is potentially lethal anaesthesia is geared to avoid it or minimize it.

Specific local anaesthetic blocks

There are a few specific local anaesthetic blocks (3,4) that may be employed in special circumstances. However, their use should be limited to the experienced practitioner who has weighed the risk versus the benefit of their employment.

♦ The *glossopharyngeal nerve* can be blocked by infiltration of local anaesthetic just posterior to the palatopharyngeal fold at its midpoint, 1 cm deep to the mucosa of the lateral pharyngeal wall. Since this abolishes the gag reflex it also increases the risk of aspiration. The concomitant paralysis of the pharyngeal muscles and the floor of the tongue can cause respiratory obstruction so if awake intubation is planned this should be effected first.

♦ The *superior laryngeal nerve* in the absence of infection can be blocked by introducing a 23G needle 1 cm medial to the superior cornu of the hyoid bone aiming caudally to pierce the thyrohyoid membrane. After negative aspiration 2 ml of local anaesthetic solution is injected. This anaesthetizes all the structures above the rima glottidis and attenuates the protective reflexes, and so increases the risk of aspiration in patients with a full stomach.

♦ Topical lignocaine can be applied to the mucosa of the larynx and pharynx very effectively in a cooperative patient to allow awake nasal or oral intubation. However, because of the rapid absorption of the lignocaine into the systemic circulation, the upper safe limit in order to avoid toxicity is 4 mg/kg body weight.

Intubation

ENT and faciomaxillary surgery require endotracheal intubation frequently as laryngeal masks do not guarantee airway patency and protection. The anatomy may often be abnormal adding to the morbidity of this kind of surgery (5). If there is the possibility of an awake intubation prior to anaesthesia this can be very satisfactorily followed with TIVA as induction is smooth and pleasant, provokes very little airway irritation, and will allow intermittent positive pressure ventilation with little or no need for muscle relaxation. This may have obvious advantages on recovery where a rapid return to normal airway protective reflexes will lessen the risk of aspiration in these debilitated patients.

Patients with bulbar palsies requiring general anaesthesia are best managed by awake intubation. Patients with muscular dystrophies that cannot be managed by regional anaesthesia alone and who therefore require airway protection during general anaesthesia need intubation. TIVA with propofol causes reversible depression of laryngeal reflexes, thus the necessity of concomitant muscle relaxants can be greatly reduced and often avoided altogether.

Attenuation of cardiovascular reflexes to intubation is frequently achieved with propofol induction and maintenance. There are definite advantages over inhalational agents, which can often stimulate pharyngeal and laryngeal reflexes causing considerable morbidity in patients with concomitant raised intracranial pressure (see Chapter 11) or ischaemic heart disease (see Chapter 9).

Major head and neck surgery

These patients are often having palliative surgery for cancer. The operations include laryngectomy, radical neck block dissection, hemi-mandibulectomy, radical sinus surgery and orbital exenteration, and can be undertaken by any of these three surgical disciplines.

The patients are frequently heavy drinkers and smokers with poor health and oral hygiene. They may therefore have concomitant chronic bronchitis, emphysema and/or cardiovascular disease such as hypertension, arrhythmia and myocardial ischaemia. If the tumour interferes with eating then weight loss, malnutrition, vitamin deficiency, dehydration, electrolyte imbalance, and haematological disorders such as anaemia and clotting disorders may be a significant source of morbidity.

The use of TIVA with propofol often permits a smooth induction in patients with chronic pulmonary disease and allows bronchial toilet for the removal of excessive secretions at any stage of the anaesthesia/surgery. This advantage has to be weighed against exacerbating the management of a difficult airway by producing the rapid loss of protective pharyngeal and laryngeal reflexes. Caution must be exercised in patients with myocardial ischaemia as TIVA with propofol can result in bradycardia and low diastolic pressure, thus aggravating myocardial ischaemia.

The use of the head-up position reduces venous oozing and also venous return by encouraging pooling of blood in the legs (6). This may be exaggerated by the use of propofol TIVA, which though may reduce blood loss without resorting to hypotensive drugs. Careful physiological monitoring is therefore mandatory.

This form of major surgery also has other unique sources of morbidity, i.e. air embolism and carotid sinus-induced vasovagal episodes. Because the jugular vein is higher than the heart in the head-up position, if it is opened it has the opportunity to entrain air and therefore penetrating injuries to the neck along with operative mishap can lead to fatalities. During dissection for radical lymph node clearance the stellate ganglion may be damaged causing a Horner's syndrome and the carotid sinus may be stimulated causing bradycardia, hypotension or even cardiac arrest. TIVA does provide excellent anaesthesia without the need for the inhalation of nitrous oxide (N_2O). It is often the equilibration of this gas in the middle ear, in the gut and in air emboli that causes so much morbidity. Thus using TIVA and avoiding N_2O altogether can reduce the fatalities following air embolism.

Patients may already have a tracheostomy *in situ*. TIVA is a very pleasant method of induction and avoids difficulties in administering volatile agents in these circumstances because of difficulties in making an air-tight seal between the anaesthetic circuit and the tracheostomy.

Facial injuries

The commonest fractures of the face involve the maxilla and the mandible (le Fort 1, 11 and 111). Because of the presence of loose teeth, blood and bone fragments, all these fractures may be accompanied by a compromised airway. It is striking how quickly the soft tissues of the oro-/naso-pharynx can swell, and how a patient with a clear airway can become obstructed and require emergency measures to relieve the obstructed airway.

There may also be concomitant damage to the cervical vertebrae and traumatic injury to the head. Unilateral fracture of the mandible tends to be stable but bilateral fracture is unstable and by the unopposed action of the pterygoids the base of the tongue is pulled medially and upwards causing trismus and pharyngeal obstruction. Lingual oedema may develop rapidly to cause life threatening obstruction.

Management of facial fractures

Management of these patients requires securing the airway as a top priority (7). If there is no trismus or mechanical problem to the airway then a rapid sequence induction will suffice, and TIVA and a rapidly acting muscle relaxant is ideal.

If, however, there is mechanical instability then a decision has to made either to perform an awake intubation, try a gaseous induction with a suitably qualified surgeon scrubbed and ready to perform an emergency tracheostomy or perform an awake elective tracheostomy. These last choices require an experienced competent anaesthetist and an experienced surgeon. Fibre optic laryngoscopy/bronchoscopy is not easy, and these are not the circumstances to try and learn how it is done!

The fracture will be reduced and immobilized by interdental fixation. Therefore any anaesthetic that will produce a rapid return of consciousness and pharyngeal reflexes with minimal postoperative nausea and vomiting is the ideal in these circumstances. This is currently best provided by TIVA with propofol (see Chapter 7).

Intraoral surgery

Anaesthesia for advancement/reduction osteotomies requires nasal intubation to guarantee airway patency, packing of the pharynx to avoid soiling of the airway, good venous drainage, 'bloodless' field, rapid return to consciousness, and freedom from nausea and vomiting. Because the mandible will be fixed by arch wires to the maxilla the patient will have difficult coughing, spitting, ingestion of food and fluids initially, so nausea and vomiting would be particularly distressing. TIVA with propofol is particularly suitable therefore because of the rapid return of consciousness on cessation of infusion and because of its proven track record of being the method least likely to promote postoperative nausea and vomiting. It also provides a good surgical field in conjunction with 1% prilocaine and 1:80 000 adrenaline, thus the need for deliberate hypotension is frequently avoided. Because propofol tends, if anything, to be vagotonic the arrhythmias seen with halothane anaesthesia in these circumstances just do not occur. Instillation of cocaine prior to nasal intubation provided the toxic dose of 3 mg/kg body weight is not exceeded rarely causes any problems from hypertension, arrhythmia let alone stroke or myocardial infarction. In practice I limit the dose to about 1.5 mg/kg body weight as for the average adult I instill 1 ml of 10% (100 mg). This provides topical anaesthesia and vasoconstriction of the nasal mucosa, and lasts for at least 2 h. Further addition of adrenaline as a vasoconstrictor to the mixture, as in Moffat's solution, is not only unnecessary it is also dangerous.

Intubation for these cases and also for shorter cases of surgical extraction of impacted third molars can be achieved easily without the use of muscle relaxants under the influence of the induction dose of propofol. The avoidance of suxamethonium is a great benefit to this young fit population who mobilize rapidly after surgery and who were prone to severe myalgia following the administration of suxamethonium.

Plastic surgical procedures

Many plastic surgical procedures that have traditionally been performed under general endotracheal anaesthesia may safely be undertaken using combinations or regional anaesthesia and IV sedation. In situations before target-controlled infusion propofol for patient sedation became available ketamine had been used. (8). The refinement of the laryngeal mask and methods of sedation (see Chapter 14) have now rendered sedation techniques based on ketamine obsolescent.

Free tissue transfer

The greatest challenge to the anaesthetist of this relatively non-invasive body surface surgery is the length of time of the operation. Temperature regulation and fluid balance require invasive monitoring and skill. Positioning is very important to avoid neuropraxias, ischaemic pressure point damage. It may be necessary to start the surgery in the prone position and then change to the supine position at a later stage of the operation, thus endangering airway, IV access and monitoring. Regional anaesthesia is only useful if the area innervated can be satisfactorily blocked by an infusion technique, i.e. axillary brachial plexus cannula, because a single shot block will not last long enough. At the end of the procedure the patient should be warm so that shivering is avoided which greatly increases local oxygen demand and therefore may determine success or failure of the graft. Under-patient warming blankets alone are insufficient to achieve this, and an over-patient Bair® hugger which can cover part or all of the patient and be heated to 32/38 or 42°C is essential along with fluid and respiratory gas warming. Extremities that are likely to lose heat that cannot be reached by the Bair hugger I wrap in an exposure blanket and as bipolar diathermy is used there is virtually no risk of diathermy burns.

The patient's haematocrit should have been reduced by plasma volume expansion to about 30% or an haemoglobin content of 10 g/dl. This is the best compromise value between reducing the blood viscosity to encourage flow in the micro circulation while not impairing oxygen delivery by reducing the oxygen content (1.34 ml O_2/g haemoglobin) too much. Because of this fluid expansion and the dilatation caused by the propofol, patients will have a large diuresis postoperatively and so it is therefore necessary to insert an urinary catheter.

TIVA with propofol is ideal for these cases as it is a vasodilator so the plasma volume can be expanded readily whilst monitoring haematocrit and central venous pressure or even capillary wedge pressure if the patient's cardiac state dictates this more invasive monitoring.

All anaesthetic agents will accumulate after long anaesthetics lasting upward of 10 h and propofol is no exception. However, it appears to be relatively safe as it does not directly depress the myocardium at anaesthetic doses. The target values of the 'Diprifusor' are often 1.6–2 µg/ml at the end of a 10 h procedure.

It is very important that analgesia is effective as pain will cause vasoconstriction, and therefore can compromise the micro circulation and microanastomoses to the new graft. This can be achieved by generous intraoperative opiate administration and continuation with a patient-controlled analgesia (PCA) system postoperatively. Remifentanil is the opiate of choice for these long anaesthetics as it does not accumulate and has a context independent half-life. However, there is evidence that the conversion to morphine for PCA requires a higher than expected loading dose initially of morphine and recovery staff must be warned about this as it is vital to avoid severe pain at this stage.

Anaesthesia for burned patients

In the initial acute stage there are numerous practical difficulties which face the anaesthetist. Routine non-invasive physiological monitoring may be difficult or even impossible if there is nowhere suitable to apply a blood pressure cuff or site electrocardiograph (ECG) electrodes. Burned patients often need several anaesthetics within a short space of time. This precludes the use of halothane because of the 6 week rule to avoid hepatotoxicity. Propofol is ideal as it can be used in varying levels from sedation to full general anaesthesia. Because IV access in these patients can be a problem, central venous cannulation is often undertaken to secure it. Central venous access is often required as well for physiological monitoring or the administration of large quantities of plasma and blood. Applying a face mask for oxygenation may be difficult when there are burns to the head and neck. The airway may be compromised because of oedema due to smoke inhalation and it must be secured early because rapid progression of intrapharyngeal oedema can result in complete airway occlusion and asphyxia if not relieved.

Nasal intubation is probably a better alternative to tracheostomy in these circumstances because of the likelihood of infection in these severely immunocompromised patients. TIVA with propofol whilst delivering 100% oxygen with a face mask, monitoring oxygen saturation, has the advantage that muscle relaxants can be avoided. The administration of suxamethonium in these circumstances has lead to fatalities by causing a catastrophic rise in serum potassium from a massive release of potassium by burned tissue. There is also resistance to non-depolarizing muscle relaxants so the dosage required, and hence the length of duration of action, is increased or even doubled.

Whilst direct burn damage is rare below the glottis because of protective glottic closure inhalation of aldehydes from wood smoke, HCl from PVC, SO_2 and NO_2, and CO, etc., will cause pulmonary oedema requiring ventilation. Propofol TIVA can then seamlessly continue to provide sedation in the intensive care. It has also been shown to have antioxidant properties and thus may help resolution of pulmonary dysfunction by oxygen radical scavenging.

Analgesia is very important in burned patients to reduce the stress on an already hypermetabolic and hypercatabolic patient. In addition to opiates a sub-anaesthetic infusion of ketamine at 10–25 mg/h for an adult has been shown to reduce the secondary hyperaesthesia by action on N-methyl-D-aspartate (NMDA) receptors and thus may have a beneficial morphine sparing effect. Because of the attendant risk of renal failure as a result of myoglobinuria non-steroidal anti-inflammatory drugs are probably best avoided in severe burns.

Microlaryngoscopy

In order to undertake microlaryngeal endoscopic surgery the surgeon needs a clear view, immobile field and space to work in. The anaesthetist, ideally, would like not only a protected trachea, minimal secretions, minimal laryngeal reflexes, and good ventilation and oxygenation, but also rapid recovery and return of protective reflexes with minimal nausea and vomiting.

The nature of the lesion to be examined/treated will determine the choice of intubation and anaesthetic. A small localized vocal cord tumour is a totally different proposition from a large friable supraglottic lesion that could easily cause complete obstruction of the glottis. If there is any question about the safety of the airway then direct laryngoscopy with topical anaesthesia must be performed to determine the nature of the pathology in relation to the airway.

Only 5% of patients presenting for endoscopic examination have pathology involving the vocal cords or the posterior commissure. Thus 95% of microlaryngoscopic procedures will be suitable for a 5 mm microlaryngoscopy endotracheal tube that allows tracheal protection by the soft large cuff but allows the surgeon room to work in because of the smaller than normal tube diameter (9). TIVA with propofol is ideal in these circumstances with the added advantage that jet ventilation can also be employed with air oxygen mixtures without perturbation of depth of anaesthesia.

Occasionally direct laryngoscopy and rigid oesophagoscopy require venturi jet ventilation with oxygen and air entrainment. TIVA is ideal in these circumstances (10) as it difficult to maintain adequate levels of inhalational anaesthesia and there is also a lot of theatre pollution when it is attempted. This jet technique cannot be employed in children, obese patients or adults with bullous emphysema because of the risk of barotrauma. It is also essential that there be free egress of air with minimal gastric distension by ensuring the tip of the jet lies within the laryngoscope.

The rapid recovery and minimal nausea and vomiting are again a great advantage of TIVA in these circumstances.

Laser surgery

Neodymium yttrium aluminium garnet (Nd-YAG) and CO_2 lasers are frequently used for microsurgery of the upper airway and trachea. Light amplification by the stimulated emission of radiation produces a monochromatic beam and depending on the emission medium can be focused into an extremely small point of very high-power density. This beam is capable of vaporizing biological tissue and depending on its wavelength has a different depth of penetration. CO_2 lasers are strongly absorbed by water and will damage tissue surfaces to a depth of $200\,\mu m$. It is thus suitable for surface surgery to lesions on the larynx and vocal cords. The Nd-YAG laser by contrast is absorbed preferentially by haemoglobin and pigmented tissue, has deep penetrating effects, and is used in treating detached retinas.

Reflection or scatter of laser beams can cause immediate damage or delayed injury to biological tissues. To minimize the risk the patients, eyes and exposed areas must be covered with moist gauze, the operating department personnel must wear goggles to absorb the wavelength emitted by the laser in use and instruments used with lasers should have a dull matt finish to reduce reflection.

Combustion of anaesthetic tubing can lead to severe burns to the oro pharynx, the subglottic and epiglottis areas. The CO_2 laser will ignite PVC tubes to release HCl, a pulmonary toxin, and it will cause red rubber tubes to char, melt and burn to produce CO gas. To reduce this fire hazard it is now recommended that the gas mixture should be 30% oxygen in nitrogen or helium, thus avoiding N_2O which supports combustion. The benefits of jet ventilation and IV anaesthesia have been recognized since the early 1980s which was facilitated by the development of short-acting high-potency opioids and short-acting muscle relaxants (11,12).

TIVA with propofol in these circumstances is now the method of choice. There is no interruption of delivery at any stage of the induction or procedure, and recovery is rapid and least likely to result in postoperative nausea and vomiting. Double-cuffed silicon-coated metal endotracheal tubes are the gold standard, if rather expensive. However, in practice ordinary tubes are wrapped with metallic tape as this increases the ignition time from 4 to 60 s (13). Alternately a jet ventilation technique using a rigid laryngoscope with a venturi attachment may be employed to avoid the risk of tube fire.

Treatment of airway fires requires removal of the burning endotracheal tube, re-intubation of the trachea and flushing the pharynx with cold saline. A rigid bronchoscopy should then be performed to check the bronchial mucosa for damage and the presence of detritus from the burned tube. Further management may require steroids continuous positive airway pressure ventilation, antibiotics and even tracheostomy. All of which can be carried under TIVA.

Tonsil surgery

The perioperative mortality for this procedure has been reduced to virtually zero with the introduction of safe anaesthetic practice. As the airway is shared with the surgeon who may soil it with tissue, pus or blood, it has to be protected. Since many of the patients will be children one has to add loose teeth to this list! Therefore premedication with an antisialogogue is useful, but heavy sedation is best avoided because return to consciousness should be as rapid as possible.

Induction and maintenance with TIVA is ideal as IV access has to be established to permit the administration of muscle relaxants. In children preformed oral endotracheal tubes which can be held by the Boyle Davis gag are fine, but adults are probably more easily managed with a soft cuffed nasal tube. Extubation once the patient has regained consciousness will ensure that protective airway reflexes have returned, and positioning in the lateral position with the pillow under the chest and shoulder allows for easy suction and removal or secretions. Some surgeons will try to argue that head-up is better as this reduces venous pressure and encourages better venous drainage. Obviously each case had to stand on its individual and particular merits. Personally I feel more comfortable if the patient is recovered in the 'tonsil' position.

The bleeding tonsil

Occasionally it is necessary to return to theatre because of bleeding. This can be a difficult anaesthetic management problem as there may be a considerable amount of swallowed blood which is very emetic – usually at induction. It is easy to underestimate the amount of blood already lost and thus not to appreciate how hypovolaemic the patient is. There may be considerable mucosal swelling making it necessary to employ a smaller diameter endotracheal tube, which may be technically more difficult to place within the trachea. The patient will also be very apprehensive. Thus it is mandatory to have a good, established IV infusion to restore normovolaemia, and blood should be cross-matched and checked for any clotting disorder. A rapid sequence induction with cricoid pressure, even positioning the patient in the left lateral position with plenty of trained assistance is essential in these circumstances. TIVA is very useful in these circumstances as inhalational agents can irritate the larynx to cause coughing and further bleeding at the worst possible time for the anaesthetist.

Peritonsillar abscess

A peritonsillar abscess may require surgical drainage. There may be considerable oedema and distortion of the normal pharyngeal anatomy, making visualization of the cords difficult or even impossible. Often the abscess can be drained by needle aspiration or incision under local anaesthesia first. There is a serious risk of soiling the airway by spontaneous rupture during rough instrumentation. Therefore management should be directed towards a gentle induction and gentle intubation under direct vision if possible. If the abscess is large and indurated, elective tracheostomy under local anaesthesia may have to be considered. Cellulitis of the mandible, Ludwig's angina, often renders visualization of the glottic opening impossible and elective tracheostomy through the cellulitis is probably the safest way to secure the airway.

Ear surgery

Anaesthesia for ear surgery has specific factors that make TIVA an ideal choice. It will provide a smooth adjustable depth of anaesthesia without the need for N_2O that, if the Eustachian tube is blocked, can cause pressure changes within the middle ear of plus 375 mmH$_2$O after 30 min inhalation to minus 285 mmH$_2$O on withdrawal. Such pressure changes can cause serous otitis, disarticulation of the stapes and impaired hearing (14). By its reversible depression of airway reflexes it can greatly reduce the need for muscle relaxation so that assessment of facial nerve function can be undertaken intraoperatively.

Patients are often placed in the head-up position in order to reduce venous oozing; this can introduce an increased risk of air embolism but the elimination of N_2O from the anaesthetic will minimize the consequences provided it is detected early from a fall in end-tidal CO_2 or from Doppler sound changes.

Deliberate hypotension can also be easily employed in patients anaesthetized with a TIVA technique. In practice though I find head-up positioning with the vasodilatory effects of propofol TIVA produce a good surgical field that rarely requires additional measures to lower the blood pressure further. Remember to use a separate IV infusion if using sodium nitroprusside and/or glyceryl trinitrate infusions.

References

1. Sasaki CT, Isaacson G. Dynamic anatomy of the larynx in physiology and consequences of intubation. In: Bishop MJ, ed. *Problems in anaesthesia.* Philadelphia, PA: Lippincott 1988; **2**: 163.
2. Morrison JD, Mirakhur RK, Craig HJL. The larynx. In: *Anaesthesia for eye, ear, nose and throat surgery,* 2nd edn. Edinburgh: Churchill Livingstone 1985: 21.
3. Gotta AW, Sullivan CA. Anaesthesia of the upper airway using topical anaesthetic and superior laryngeal nerve block. *Br J Anaesth* 1981; **53**: 1055.
4. Barton S, William JD. Glossopharyngeal nerve block. *Arch Otolaryngol* 1971; **93**: 186.
5. Blanc V, Tremblay N. Complications of tracheal intubation. A new classification and review of the literature. *Anaesth Analg* 1974; **53**: 202.
6. Washburn MC, Hyer RL. Deliberate hypotension for elective major maxillofacial surgery. *J Maxillofac Surg* 1982; **10**: 50.
7. Benumof JL. Management of the difficult airway: a review. *Anaesthesiology* 1991; **75**: 1087.
8. Pennant Jh, White PF . The laryngeal mask airway: its uses in anaesthesiology: a review. *Anaesthesiology* 1993; **79**: 144.
9. Gates LE, Hamacher EN, Simonson D. Reducing the need for intubation in plastic surgery. *Am Assoc Nurse Anesthet J* 1991; **59**: 298.
10. Torres LE, Reynolds RC. Experience with a new endotracheal tube for micro laryngeal surgery. *Anaesthesiology* 1980; **52**: 347.
11. Ewalenko P, Deloof T, Gerin M, *et al.* Propofol infusion with fentanyl supplementation for microlaryngoscopy. *Acta Anaesth Belg* 1990; **41**: 297.

12. Gussack GS, Evans RF, Tacchi EJ. Intravenous anaesthesia and jet ventilation for laser micro laryngeal surgery. *Ann Otol Rhinol Laryngol* 1987; **96**: 29.
13. Blomquist S, Algotsson L, Karlsson SE. Anaesthesia for resection of tumours in the trachea and central bronchi using the Nd-YAG-laser technique. *Acta Anaesthesiol Scand* 1990; **34**: 506.
14. Patel KF, Hicks JN. Prevention of fire hazard associated with the use of carbon dioxide lasers. *Anaesth Analg* 1981; **60**: 885.
15. Patterson ME, Bartlett PC. Hearing impairment caused by intratympanic pressure changes during general anaesthesia. *Laryngoscope* 1976; **85**: 399.

13

Anaesthesia for the elderly

J. Peacock

- Physiological changes
- Pharmacology
- Specific drugs
- Disease
- Anaesthesia

As we are frequently being made aware within medicine and society in general, the population is getting increasingly older. This not only has implications of funding and provision of services for medicine as a whole, but also for how we manage each specific, individual patient. As a patient's age increases in years the likelihood of the need for surgery also increases because of disease – cancer in particular. The problem relates not only to the fact that surgery is more likely in a given patient but we must also recognize two additional factors: the problem of age-associated disease and the actual process of ageing. Nor can we simply recognize that the average age of the population is getting higher as mortality rates fall. There is also the appearance of the so-called elderly elderly (i.e. 85 years and older) who respond in a significantly different way to younger patients and who need to be treated as totally different entities. The issues are further highlighted by the appearance of societies and journals relating specifically to anaesthesia and the elderly patient.

We must therefore be prepared to provide for the specific anaesthetic needs of this portion of the population, and understand how both the elderly patients' physiology and disease states affect the pharmacokinetic and pharmacodynamic responses to the drugs we administer (Table 13.1). In addition, although beyond the remit of this chapter, we need to recognize that the likelihood of polypharmacy is significantly increased in the older patient and thus the possibility for drug interactions, which may also have an important bearing on how an older patient responds.

Table 13.1 General principles affecting drug response in elderly patients

Physiology	Reduced function and reserve; altered drug delivery with increased drug concentrations
Pharmacology	Changes in pharmacokinetics and dynamics – increased drug concentrations and reduced metabolism/clearance with greater response and slower recovery
Disease	Altered pharmacokinetics and pharmacodynamics

Physiology

As age increases, so physiological function declines in all systems, and these changes relate specifically to both how the body handles the drug we administer and how the body responds to those drugs. At what particular age a specific patient or function starts to decline will vary between individuals, with additional deterioration as a result of disease. We therefore cannot generalize as to the degree of impairment, which may have taken place just because the patient has reached a particular age, but we must recognize that potentially the function of systems may be impaired. We must also recognize that function may be maintained but with the functional *reserve* significantly reduced.

Since intravenous (IV) drugs are distributed via the circulation, one of the more important systems is the cardiovascular system, with the respiratory system obviously having less effect on IV anaesthetics compared to the inhalation agents. As the central nervous system deteriorates so the patient's response to the drug increases, and as hepatic and renal function decline so metabolism and excretion are reduced with changes in duration and intensity of effect.

Cardiovascular system

Cardiac output at rest reduces with age by up to 30% at 75–80 years compared to 30 years – by a reduction in both resting heart rate and stroke volume. Although cardiac output can still be increased in the elderly, this is primarily by an increase in stroke volume rather than by an increase in heart rate as in the younger patient. It is of considerable importance therefore to ensure that adequate fluids are administered to elderly patients so that they can maintain their cardiac output. Since these changes are also associated with an increase in peripheral vascular resistance, this requires a fine balance between an adequate fluid volume that will maintain cardiac output and excess fluid volume that may result in congestive cardiac failure.

These changes, even in the absence of disease, will cause a decrease in the delivery of drug throughout the body to the various organs. Of importance during induction in the elderly patient, the reduced cardiac output results in an increased circulation time that increases the time for drug to be delivered to the brain. Also the redistribution of the drug may be altered so that higher concentrations result. During maintenance of anaesthesia, responses to changes in infusion rates may be manifest more slowly and to a different degree compared with younger patients.

Nervous system

Brain weight and blood flow are both decreased in the elderly with loss of neurones and a reduction in neurotransmitter synthesis. However, these are not necessarily associated with intellectual impairment and many elderly patients have normal responses. Intuitively one would expect a greater response to anaesthetics in individuals where such changes have occurred but it is uncertain whether the loss of neurones and neurotransmitter synthesis alters the responses to anaesthetics *per se*. Initial reductions in loading dose are primarily attributable to pharmaco-kinetic changes. Clinical observation, as will be seen later, would indicate that lower maintenance infusion rates are required in the elderly population. However, autonomic impairment is a well-recognized component of the ageing process, leading to changes in control of the cardiovascular system. This will cause reductions in venous return, and further impairment of the homeostasis of arterial pressure and also temperature. Such changes will further exaggerate the potential effects of anaesthesia described above.

Renal and hepatic systems

Ageing also affects the kidneys, and is associated with a reduction in renal mass with fewer glomeruli and a decreased volume of proximal tubules. These, along with reductions in renal plasma flow, will result in a decreased glomerular filtration rate, impaired concentrating ability and lower capacity to conserve sodium. These may not be superficially apparent on clinical examination but will be evident by a significant reduction in creatinine clearance in the majority of, although not necessarily all, elderly patients. This will constitute a significant decline in renal function, which will result in impaired excretion of drugs cleared by renal mechanisms.

Liver mass and blood flow may decline significantly with age but due to the relatively large hepatic reserve may not be clinically apparent preoperatively. A reduction of liver blood flow, however, may significantly reduce clearance of certain drugs with high hepatic extraction ratios (e.g. pethidine). Changes in enzyme function are less important where there is a greater reserve, and where it is also thought that disease and environmental factors (e.g. smoking and alcohol) primarily affect changes in enzyme activity rather than age itself.

Associated with the changes in renal and hepatic function there are also changes in fluid balance and protein synthesis. Although these changes will be significantly greater in the presence of disease such as cirrhosis, renal failure or rheumatoid arthritis, there will be reductions in total body water and plasma proteins that will alter protein binding and the volumes of distribution of drugs. The extent and importance of these changes will depend upon the characteristics of the drug.

Pharmacology

The physiological changes described above result in significant alterations in the pharmacology of IV anaesthetic agents in the elderly.

Pharmacokinetics

The initial volume of distribution is affected by cardiac function, with reduced vascular volume and cardiac output leading to diminished distribution of blood flow to some organs. As a result there is a higher initial concentration of drug in the circulation. Initially thought to be due to a smaller initial volume of distribution, it is now thought this higher drug concentration is due to a reduced initial redistribution of drug from the circulation to other organs. However, the initial delivery of drug into the primary compartment is slower due to an increased circulation time in the elderly and this may also affect the concentrations of drug measured. This may explain why Schnider et al. (1) found that there were differences in the pharmacokinetics of propofol following bolus or infusion. Using parameters available from infusion data, there was a significant under prediction of the concentrations measured following bolus administration.

As age increases there is a reduction in lean body mass and therefore total body water since any increase in total body mass will be due to fat which contains relatively less water. Overall this will result in a decrease in the volume of distribution for water-soluble drugs and a relative increase in total body fat which will result in an increase in the volume of distribution of lipid-soluble drugs. These effects will cause an increase in the elimination half-life of lipid-soluble drugs including many anaesthetics and an increased duration of effect although the clearance itself may not be affected. Thus the lean body mass rather than the total body weight may better predict the initial volume of distribution, peak concentration and therefore initial loading dose for water-soluble drugs. Conversely, total body weight may give an indication of recovery with lipid-soluble drugs.

Protein synthesis is also altered in the elderly with reduced concentrations of plasma albumin and increased concentrations of plasma globulin, and this may result in altered protein binding. In disease states α_1-acid glycoprotein is also produced, and the relative changes in protein concentrations and therefore protein binding of the relevant drugs are much larger. The change in unbound fraction and therefore active proportion of a drug will vary between individual drugs and whether binding is increased or reduced. With reductions in protein binding for highly bound drugs small increases in the free fraction will be of far greater significance than for poorly bound drugs where a small change in the free fraction will not significantly alter the active concentration of drug. Although the changes are unlikely to be significant in the absence of disease, the unbound fraction of pethidine was significantly higher in older patients than in younger patients.

Pharmacodynamics

The pharmacodynamics of IV agents in any patient are difficult to interpret accurately since the pharmacokinetic changes and ideally the concentration of drug at the active site also have to be taken into consideration, and the elderly are no exception. Although it is clear that lower doses of IV agents at induction are needed to induce anaesthesia the pharmacokinetic changes may account for the majority of these differences rather than an increased pharmacodynamic response. Combined studies recording the pharmacodynamic effects on the electroencephalogram (EEG) using a pharmacokinetic model to administer the drug have suggested that there is no significant difference in sensitivity between the young and the elderly. However, most pharmacokinetic models do not necessarily take account of the pharmacokinetic changes in the elderly. The widespread clinical impression that the elderly are more sensitive to the depressant effects of centrally acting agents has recently been confirmed by Schnider *et al.* (2). At steady state they identified that the propofol concentrations at which 50% of individuals lost consciousness were significantly reduced in those aged 75 years and older. It is well documented that they need lower infusion rates of IV drugs to maintain anaesthesia.

Specific drugs

Anaesthesia involves different elements, which can be fulfilled by separate drugs via the IV route. Hypnosis or loss of consciousness and analgesia or lack of response are separate effects and both must be met, the former by hypnotics and the latter by opioids and/or high-dose hypnotics. Although frequently not referred to within the context of IV anaesthesia, muscle relaxants and the responses to them should also be included.

Hypnotics

Hypnotics have traditionally been barbiturates or benzodiazepines, with thiopentone the agent against which most comparisons were originally made. Increasingly propofol, a hindered phenol, is the standard agent in view of the fact that it is most suitable for administration by infusion for maintenance.

Thiopentone

Thiopentone was first introduced in 1934 as an induction agent of ultra-short duration since its effect was rapidly terminated. This short duration of action is primarily by redistribution of the drug away from the site of action and is not related to rapid metabolism of the drug. It was recognized as an ideal agent since it has a rapid onset with minimal side effects, even in the elderly, but such patients require a significantly lower dose than younger patients do. However, the variability within different patient groups is such that some elderly individuals require higher doses than younger patients do, due to a variability of 30–70% in distribution pharmacokinetics. Attempts at repeat administration or continuous infusion resulted in prolonged recovery due to accumulation of drug within the lipid tissues and redistribution from them to significantly slow the rate of decline of drug concentration. This effect was significantly exacerbated in the elderly due to the increased total body fat and volume of distribution for lipid-soluble drugs that further delayed recovery.

Methohexitone

The alternative barbiturate methohexitone has a much shorter elimination half-life than thiopentone and was recommended as the agent of choice for repeat administration. However, methohexitone has a high hepatic extraction ratio which is largely dependent upon liver blood flow and which may significantly decline with age, resulting in reduced clearance and slower recovery, and it never reached favour because of the unwanted movements it can cause.

Etomidate

Etomidate is an imidazole derivative with similar pharmacokinetics changes to the other agents. Due to the wide variation between individuals in steady-state volume of distribution there is no demonstrable difference with age and the elimination half-life therefore does not change despite the clearance decreasing with age. It has favour in the elderly since it is meant to be cardiovascularly stable; however, this will be discussed in greater depth under induction of anaesthesia. Due to its effects on steroid synthesis during maintenance of sedation on ITU its use for maintenance of anaesthesia has been curtailed.

Midazolam

Midazolam is the most commonly used benzodiazepine with significant changes in the pharmacokinetics between the young and elderly (3). Although the volumes of distribution were not significantly changed, the elimination half-life was significantly increased in the elderly and may indicate that a more prolonged recovery is likely. Despite the minimal changes in the volume of distribution, the dose required is reduced by

50% in the elderly, suggesting an increased intrinsic sensitivity of the elderly CNS. The greatest use of midazolam is for co-induction with other hypnotic agents to reduce the dose and side effects of the other agents used, although the reduced clearance and prolonged recovery with midazolam may nullify some of the advantages of co-induction in the elderly.

Ketamine

Ketamine is a phencyclidine derivative which was used in 'dissociative anaesthesia' and it has increased risks of hallucinations in the elderly which may be attenuated by midazolam. Its sympathomimetic effects may help maintain arterial pressure but these same effects cause concern in patients with ischaemic heart disease. Also the changes in the autonomic nervous system in the elderly may minimize these cardiovascular effects where upon its myocardial depressant effects may become apparent. It is currently receiving increased interest due to its N-methyl-D-aspartate (NMDA) antagonist effects that may provide significant analgesia.

Propofol

Propofol is a phenol derivative that also has rapid recovery due to redistribution but also a much faster metabolism and this has made it the new standard for maintenance of anaesthesia by infusion. The pharmacokinetics are also altered in the elderly, resulting in higher initial concentrations due to a smaller volume of distribution or a slower initial redistribution and longer recovery due to reduced hepatic metabolism.

Opioids

Opioid analgesics are an essential part of the picture as they provide suppression of noxious stimuli. This is more important in the elderly with the likely presence of cardiac disease than in the young. Attempts to produce adequate surgical anaesthesia are difficult with a single agent without resorting to high doses of hypnotics which will frequently induce unwanted side-effects and produce a delay in recovery, especially in the elderly patient. The only reasonable alternative to the profound analgesia which adequate doses of opioids can produce is the use of local anaesthetic techniques. The particular choice of opioid will depend upon the circumstances in which it is being used so that the drug with the appropriate characteristics can be selected.

Morphine

Morphine is a long-acting drug with reduced clearance in the elderly. This tends to limit its usefulness in the anaesthetic context since it is not easily adjustable without the risk of delayed recovery and respiratory depression. However, it is still the most commonly used agent for postoperative analgesia.

Fentanyl

Fentanyl is probably the opioid most commonly used intraoperatively and produces similar effects to any of the other opioids. It also has the same pharmacokinetic changes associated with the elderly with a reduced initial volume of distribution or intercompartmental clearance depending upon the particular study. Unlike the hypnotics, the elderly have been identified as having increased sensitivity to fentanyl. After administration of larger doses it also has a longer duration of action and optimal control of noxious stimuli may not be achieved due to concern about recovery. Again this may be more noticeable in the elderly.

Alfentanil

Alfentanil was until recently the most appropriate opioid for IV infusion. It has rapid equilibration between the blood and the brain, and a relatively short elimination half-life but primarily due to redistribution and this may result in delayed recovery after prolonged infusions. These characteristics have been eloquently described by the introduction of the concept of context-sensitive half-time. In the elderly there is again reduced clearance and an increased elimination half-life suggesting a need to reduce infusion rates. Although changes in protein binding may be expected in the elderly there was no direct relationship between the free fraction and age although variability of response was related to protein binding. This may be more important in the elderly with associated disease than in the elderly who are otherwise healthy.

Remifentanil

Remifentanil is the newest addition to the opioid family and is different because of its rapid metabolism by non-specific tissue esterases. Its opioid effects are identical to the other drugs except that its rapid metabolism allows it to be given in higher doses without significantly affecting recovery and therefore the responses seen are greater. The rapid metabolism also means that it has an extremely short elimination half-life which results in rapid and predictable recovery, and makes it ideal (if not essential) for administration by IV infusion.

Initially it was reported that there was no difference in the pharmacokinetics of remifentanil in the elderly; however, more recent research (4) has identified that the initial volume of distribution and the clearance are both decreased by approximately 30% from 20 to 85 years. In terms of the pharmacodynamic response, there was also a 50% decrease in the concentration that produced a 50% response (EC_{50}), and the equilibration constant (k_{eo}). Due to these differences there is therefore a recommendation that the doses are reduced by 50% in the elderly to avoid side effects from excessive responses.

Muscle relaxants

Just as the opioids have different characteristics, so the non-depolarizing muscle relaxants are not all alike. The pharmacokinetic changes follow the general pattern previously described but with the clear addition that, despite there being no changes in the pharmacodynamic response in the elderly, there is a clear loss of muscle mass with age which would indicate a need to significantly reduce the dose administered.

Pancuronium

Pancuronium as a long-acting drug has reduced urinary excretion in the elderly with a potential doubling of its duration of action. Its cardiovascular effects may minimize the overall hypotensive effect of anaesthesia but may similarly be a potential disadvantage in the elderly patient with cardiovascular disease.

Vecuronium

Vecuronium is excreted by the liver, which due to the decline in liver blood flow in the older patient may again have a longer duration of action than normal.

Atracurium

Atracurium metabolism is contingent upon the pH- and temperature-dependent Hoffman elimination and not hepatic or renal excretion. Therefore metabolism is more reliable except that changes in the volumes of distribution may indicate the need for a larger loading dose and increase the elimination half-life, and still extend its duration of effect.

Disease

It is important to recognize that the elderly are more likely to have disease processes which will significantly alter the response to IV agents compared to the effects of age alone. These effects may be mediated via pharmacokinetic changes as a result of the disease process and/or an altered sensitivity to the drug effect.

Christensen et al. (5) reported that patients with cardiac disease on long-term digoxin therapy had reduced dose requirements for thiopentone for induction. On further investigation, in comparison with matched controls of elderly patients, there were no differences in the pharmacokinetics of thiopentone between the two groups and they proposed increased cerebral sensitivity to the drug in the cardiac patients.

Other studies have investigated the effects of specific disease processes on anaesthesia and individual drugs, and these will be relevant to the elderly patient with such diseases.

Anaesthesia

Perhaps the most important aspect of IV anaesthesia in the elderly is the variable response which has been highlighted throughout the chapter. The need to adjust drug administration at all stages of a surgical procedure, from induction to recovery, to the requirements of the individual patient cannot be over-emphasized. Dundee in the 1950s (6) reported reductions in the dose of thiopentone required for induction and maintenance in elderly patients, recognizing both the importance of age and disease. However, although he later reported lower mean doses of propofol for induction in the elderly (7), the variability between individual patients was high, with some older patients requiring more than some younger patients.

An unfortunate aspect of research is that elderly patients are often excluded from early studies of new drugs, although licensing authorities are increasingly requesting information on the use of drugs in older patients. This often means that there is little practical guidance on the doses and combinations of drugs which should be used in the elderly population, although it does prevent information being used as a recipe which must be strictly adhered to. As a result, the general principles which need to be applied are based on the changes in pharmacology due to age and disease rather than specific information based on randomized controlled trials of the specific drug in particular circumstances.

Although it may produce an artificial distinction, it is worth considering the changes that are required at different stages of anaesthesia.

Induction

The first detail of induction which must be recognized is that the cardiovascular changes in the elderly reduce the mean loading dose required to induce anaesthesia. The reason for this reduction is the pharmacokinetic changes that may reduce the initial volume of distribution so that the same concentration can be achieved with a smaller dose. In addition there is a reduction in the redistribution of drug from the blood to the tissues that will reduce the rate of decline of drug and again minimize the dose required. This pattern of results has been reported for thiopentone (8), propofol (9) and the majority of IV agents (10).

In addition the reduction in cardiac output will also slow the circulation time, and increase the time required for drug to be delivered from the point of injection and to reach the brain. Therefore in order to titrate the dose of drug administered with reasonable accuracy to the reduced amount which is actually required, the rate of administration should be slowed in the elderly. The rate of administration should be sufficiently slow so that there is a minimal amount of drug 'unused' in the circulation when loss of consciousness is achieved without unnecessarily increasing the time for induction of anaesthesia to take place. Veal (11), using a model which injected fluoresceine in the arm that appeared as fluorescence in the retina when viewed by indirect ophthalmoscopy, identified a significant and consistent increase in the circulation time between the antecubital fossa and the retina in the elderly compared with the young. Rapid administration of drug for induction will therefore tend to increase the amount of drug administered and increase the possibility of a relative overdose of drug, and therefore risk an exaggerated response and unwanted side effects.

The most commonly reported unwanted effect is hypotension. Dundee *et al.* (7) reported the reduced dose requirements in the elderly and emphasized the increased risk of hypotension in the elderly with the introduction of propofol, especially if administered more quickly and in larger doses. However, at this time other work (12) emphasized the importance of rate of administration in identifying the smallest effective dose which would induce loss of consciousness. Initial work in the elderly, with temazepam premedication and fentanyl before induction, showed that a reduction in the rate of administration of propofol from 200 to 50 mg/min reduced the degree of hypotension. This was associated with a lengthening of the induction time from 51 to 104 s but a reduction in the induction dose of propofol from 2.5 to 1.2 mg/kg. Further work compared slower rates of infusion and identified 0.8 mg/kg in the elderly and 1.4 mg/kg in the young as smallest effective doses with no significant differences in the degree of hypotension whether the drug was given by infusion or rapid injection. These doses are markedly lower than the earlier recommended doses, which were associated with noticeable reductions in arterial pressure in the elderly patient when the drug was first introduced.

Due to a lack of cardiovascular effects when etomidate is used to induce anaesthesia in healthy subjects, it is often proposed as the agent of choice for elderly patients. Larsen *et al.* (13) compared the effects of fixed doses of propofol or etomidate for induction and maintenance of anaesthesia in patients older than 65 years who had no evidence of significant cardiac disease other than hypertension. They compared changes in heart rate, systolic, mean and diastolic pressures, cardiac index and myocardial blood flow as the lowest value after induction, the highest after intubation, and at 5 and 30 min after intubation with the awake values. Although arterial pressure and heart rate declined with time following administration of both drugs, they found no significant differences in the lowest values after induction between the two drugs. However, they did find that the incidence of hypertension following intubation was significantly higher with etomidate and suggested that propofol may be preferable to prevent such responses, although counseling caution with both drugs in older patients with cardiac disease.

An alternative method of induction is to use a target-controlled infusion (TCI) system for propofol which will calculate a loading dose based on a selected target concentration. Suggested target concentrations have been 3 and 6 µg/ml with induction occurring more rapidly at the higher concentrations. In an open study to compare manual infusion techniques with TCI, Servin (14) reported a significant reduction in propofol requirements for induction within the TCI group with increasing age. No evidence is available as to the most appropriate concentrations for induction in elderly patients, but reduced dose requirements of IV agents in general would suggest that lower concentrations should be selected which may be increased if inadequate.

Induction using a TCI has also been reported to result in a lower incidence of hypotension and is probably due to the fact that administration of the initial loading dose is at 600 ml/h. Depending upon the initial target concentration, the loading dose approximates to 1 mg/kg rather than the 2 mg/kg which is often administered manually. This is similar to the manual infusion scheme described by Roberts *et al.* (15) who administered a loading dose of 1 mg/kg before commencing a maintenance infusion and also reported a more gradual decline in arterial pressure. Although there is no specific evidence for this in the elderly, it would appear to have potential advantages.

None of the above schemes, however, have addressed the issue of what effect there may be from the co-administration of other drugs and what doses of both drugs should be used. Co-induction has become a popular technique with administration of midazolam and propofol the most common agents. Again, however, there is no published evidence as to the most appropriate doses of the agents for use in the elderly. Application of general principles suggests that 1–2 mg of midazolam will significantly reduce the induction requirement of propofol and potentially therefore minimize any hypotensive changes following induction.

It is unusual to administer an induction agent without an opioid and the interactions of different opioids with the induction agents in the elderly have not been completely explored. Vuyk *et al.* (16) has produced a clear picture of the interaction between propofol and alfentanil in the younger patient but no such research has been published for the elderly.

Maintenance

In addition to the choice of agent(s) to use for the maintenance of IV anaesthesia, just as in the young there is also the choice of method to use, i.e. manual or TCI systems. Similarly there are the same variables to take into consideration when determining the dose of drug to be administered. In 1954, Dundee (6) published the results of a study which identified that the dose of thiopentone required to maintain anaesthesia was reduced in the elderly, even taking into consideration the potential effect of disease.

The present choice of drug is most commonly propofol for the IV maintenance of hypnosis, which may be administered by manual or computer controlled systems. Since the introduction of a commercial TCI system ('Diprifusor') there has been greater acceptance of the computer and TCIs. This is primarily because the system automatically adjusts the infusion rate to take account of the effect of time on the required rate of administration as the drug is distributed throughout the body. Manual infusion schemes such as the 'Bristol' regimen can also approximate this when a single target has been selected but provide no guidance once the concentration is adjusted to alter the depth of anaesthesia. However, both the manual system and TCI involve the use of a pharmacokinetic algorithm to calculate the infusion rate. The effect of age on the pharmacokinetics of the drug, and how it affects the calculated parameters and the accuracy of control may be an important source of inter-individual variability.

From one perspective it does not matter whether the control is as accurate in the elderly as in the young since the drug should be adjusted to the response it produces as the procedure progresses. Swinhoe et al. (17) compared the predictive performance of the 'Diprifusor' TCI system in three age groups, i.e. 18–40, 41–55 and 56–80 years, and compared the target concentrations required to maintain adequate anaesthesia in the elderly. Measured arterial concentrations of propofol were compared with the calculated values from the TCI system during major surgery. The performance indices of the system, median performance error (MDPE) and median absolute performance error (MDAPE) were similar in all three groups, indicating no difference in the degree of accuracy between the age groups. These are shown in Table 13.2 and show that the measured concentrations tended to be higher than the predicted concentrations throughout the study as indicated by the overall MDPE of 16.2%. However, this positive error was more marked after induction or increases in the target concentration. The overall mean target concentrations with an infusion of alfentanil were higher in the younger age groups than in the older age group and varied from 4.2 (SD 0.6) and 4.3 (0.7) to 3.5 (0.7) µg/ml. This pattern is similar to that reported in other studies although instead of a target concentration being quoted it is usual for a mean infusion rate to be used as the measure.

As indicated earlier in this section there is little published data on the doses of combinations of anaesthetic drugs in the elderly. The above study used alfentanil at 30 µg/kg and 0.5–2.0 µg/kg/min. By comparison a lower dose of alfentanil at 0.25 µg/kg/min resulted in a mean utilization of propofol which reduced from approximately 170 µg/kg/min at 20 years of age to 120 µg/kg/min at 65 years of age (18). Following fentanyl 1.5 µg/kg, the mean propofol infusion rate was 166 µg/kg/min at 25–40 years and 143 µg/kg/min at 65–80 years in patients paralysed with vecuronium (19). Despite these lower infusion rates and lower doses of fentanyl there was a delayed recovery in the elderly patients. Neither of these studies takes account of the varied duration of anaesthesia and the exponential changes in drug concentration or infusion rate with time.

Table 13.2 Drug concentrations and performance indicators of 'Diprifusor' [data from Swinhoe et al. (17)]

	18–40 years	41–55 years	56–80 years	All patients
Mean induction dose (mg/kg) (SD)	1.10 (0.05)	1.15 (0.23)	0.84 (0.18)	
Mean maintenance target concentration (µg/ml) (SD)	4.2 (0.6)	4.3 (0.7)	3.5 (0.7)	
Mean infusion rates (mg/kg/h) (SD)	8.9 (1.4)	9.1 (1.6)	7.3 (1.5)	
MDPE (%) (range)	13 (–21–64)	18 (–16–46)	16 (–11–84)	16 (–21–84)
MDAPE (%) (range)	23 (6–64)	25 (14–48)	24 (11–84)	24 (6–84)

In combination with remifentanil, there is no specific data as to the dose of propofol required in elderly patients, although the dose of remifentanil should be reduced by 50%. Although some of the studies have included older patients and contain comments about their relative sensitivity to the drugs, there has been no published data as to the most appropriate infusion rates. Despite the increased sensitivity to remifentanil there is no evidence that there is any increase in the mean recovery times in the elderly, although there may be increased variability in the rate of decline of remifentanil concentrations in a small number (1%) of older patients.

The actual combination of drugs and the infusion rates that will be used will be dependent upon the case in question and will also be a matter of personal choice. However, inter-individual variability will require the doses to be titrated to the patient response. Further research is required as to the most effective combinations and doses in the elderly patient in particular circumstances.

Relaxants

Although the choice of muscle relaxants is not always included within a discussion of IV anaesthesia, the drugs fit into the broader concept as they are administered via the IV route and their use may have a significant impact on the outcome of anaesthesia. Viby-Mogensen et al. published the outcome of two studies and identified various risk factors for the development of pulmonary complications following surgery (20). These included increasing age, abdominal surgery, prolonged surgery and the presence of residual neuromuscular block on arrival in the recovery room. The second also identified that the use of pancuronium with a train of four below 0.7 in recovery increased the likelihood of pulmonary complications. The use of long-acting neuromuscular blocking agents in the elderly may produce adverse effects since their metabolism may be altered.

Conclusion

Anaesthesia of any type in any patient requires vigilance. Due to the changes in physiology and pharmacology in the otherwise healthy elderly patient, variation between patients is potentially greater. For some this may mean larger doses than 'normal' not just dose reductions. If the significant changes associated with disease are also added to this scenario then even greater caution is required. Perhaps the changes in pharmacokinetics may have a greater effect on variability within IV anaesthesia, but the ability to adjust the dose of drug to the response of the patient means that IV anaesthesia is an entirely reasonable form of anaesthesia. The advent of TCI and drugs which are more reliably titrated will ensure that the potential benefits of IV anaesthesia are also available for the elderly patient.

References

1. Schnider TW, Minto CF, Gambus PL, *et al.* The influence of method of administration and covariates on the pharmacokinetics of propofol in adult volunteers. *Anesthesiology* 1998; **88**: 1170–82.
2. Schnider TW, Minto CF, Shafer SL, *et al.* The influence of age on propofol pharmacokinetics. *Anesthesiology* 1999; **90**: 1502–16.
3. Greenblatt DJ, Abernethy DR, Locniskar A, Harmatz JS, Limjuco RA, Shader RI. Effect of age, gender and obesity on midazolam kinetics. *Anesthesiology* 1984; **61**: 27–35.
4. Minto CF, Schnider TW, Egan TD, *et al.* Influence of age and gender on the pharmacokinetics and pharmacodynamics of remifentanil. I. Model development. *Anesthesiology* 1997; **86**: 10–23.
5. Christensen JH, Andreasen F, Jansen JA. Increased thiopental sensitivity in cardiac patients. *Acta Anaesthesiol Scand* 1985; **29**: 702–5.
6. Dundee JW. The influence of body weight, sex and age on the dosage of thiopentone. *Br J Anaesth* 1954; **26**: 164–73.
7. Dundee JW, Robinson FP, McCollum JSC, Patterson CC. Sensitivity to propofol in the elderly. *Anaesthesia* 1986; **41**: 482–5.
8. Stanski DR, Maitre PO. Population pharmacokinetics and pharmacodynamics of thiopental: the effect of age revisited. *Anesthesiology* 1990; **72**: 412–22.
9. Kirkpatrick T, Cockshott ID, Douglas EJ, Nimmo WS. Pharmacokinetics of propofol (Diprivan) in elderly patients. *Br J Anaesth* 1988; **60**: 146–50.
10. Arden JR, Holley FO, Stanski DR. Increased sensitivity to etomidate in the elderly: initial distribution versus altered brain response. *Anesthesiology* 1986; **65**: 19–27.
11. Veal GRQ, Peacock JE. Influence of circulation time on the onset of i.v. anaesthesia. *Br J Anaesth* 1994; **73**: 272.
12. Peacock JE, Spiers SPW, McLaughlan GA, Edmondson WC, Berthoud M, Reilly CS. Infusion of propofol to identify smallest effective doses for induction of anaesthesia in young and elderly patients. *Br J Anaesth* 1992; **69**: 363–7.
13. Larsen R, Rathgeber J, Bagdahn A, Lange H, Rieke H. Effects of propofol on cardiovascular dynamics and coronary blood flow in geriatric patients. A comparison with etomidate. *Anaesthesia* 1998; **43** (suppl): 25–31.

14. Servin FS. TCI compared with manually controlled infusion of propofol: a multicentre study. *Anaesthesia* 1998; **53** (suppl 1): 82–6.
15. Roberts FL, Dixon J, Lewis GTR, Tackley RM, Prys-Roberts C. Induction and maintenance of propofol anaesthesia. *Anaesthesia* 1988; **43** (suppl): 14–7.
16. Vuyk J, Lim T, Engbers FH, Burm AG, Vletter AA, Bovill JG. The pharmacodynamic interaction of propofol and alfentanil during lower abdominal surgery in women. *Anesthesiology* 1995; **83**: 8–22.
17. Swinhoe CF, Peacock JE, Glenn JB, Reilly CS. Evaluation of the predictive performance of a 'Diprifusor' TCI system. *Anaesthesia* 1998; **53** (suppl 1): 61–7.
18. Hilton P, Dev VJ, Major E. Intravenous anaesthesia with propofol and alfentanil. The influence of age and weight. *Anaesthesia* 1986; **41**: 640–3.
19. Scheepstra GL, Booij LHDJ, Rutten CLG, Coenen LGJ. Propofol for induction and maintenance of anaesthesia: comparison between younger and older patients. *Br J Anaesth* 1989; **62**: 54–60.
20. Viby-Mogenssen J, Roed J, Mortensen CR, Engbaek J, Skovgaard LT, Krintel JJ. Residual neuromuscular block is a risk factor for postoperative pulmonary complications. A prospective, randomised and blinded study of postoperative pulmonary complications after atracurium, vecuronium and pancuronium. *Acta Anaesthesiol Scand* 1997; **41**: 1095–103.

14

Sedation for regional anaesthesia

N. L. Padfield

- Merits of regional anaesthesia
- Reduction in sympathetic response to surgery
- Postoperative pain relief
- Pharmacology of propofol relevant to regional anaesthesia
- Patient assessment and preoperative risk factor
- Current clinical experience of sedation combined with regional anaesthesia

The anaesthetist may decide to employ regional anaesthesia alone to enable surgery to proceed. This will also depend on the preference of the patient and the cooperation of the surgeon. Not every surgeon feels happy to have an awake patient for complicated surgery and many patients in the UK would prefer to know nothing about their surgical procedure. Often a compromise is reached when the patient receives either sedation in order to allay anxiety or full general anaesthesia.

The case for regional anaesthesia is supported by a good body of evidence in the medical literature demonstrating the benefits of its employment. These lie in three areas:

- Reduction of sympathetic response to the painful stimulation of surgery
- The reduction in the neurohumoral 'stress' response postoperatively
- Provision of immediate postoperative pain relief

Reduction in sympathetic response

Increased sympathetic tone may not cause any permanent harm to young ASA grade 1 patients undergoing body surface surgery. However, even in such patients the situation alters, e.g. if they undergo a depressant general anaesthetic with a concomitant rise in P_aCO_2 and an increased level of circulating catecholamines irrespective of origin. Runs of multifocal ventricular ectopics or even supraventricular tachycardias may occur and cause concern, especially in previously asymptomatic patients who have the potential for fatal cardiac arrhythmias when exposed to high levels of adrenaline for the first time, and any procedure that causes increased heart rate will increase myocardial oxygen consumption.

The patients who are particularly at risk may have:

- Ischaemic heart disease and/or hypertension
- Diabetes mellitus and complications, particularly peripheral and autonomic neuropathies
- Peripheral vascular disease, especially since there may be other atherormatous disease in other microvascular beds, i.e. cerebrovascular disease
- Endocrine disease like thyrotoxicosis
- Apudomas and other hormone-secreting tumours like oat cell carcinoma of the lung

Regional anaesthesia benefits patients undergoing repair of aortic aneurysms – in addition to a judiciously administered general anaesthetic and appropriate after care.

Reduction in neurohumoral 'stress' response

The increase neurohumoral output can precipitate acute adrenal insufficiency, especially in:

- Severely traumatized patients with multiple fractures and extensive tissue damage
- Burned patients with a greatly raised basal metabolic rate
- Septic patients with or on the edge of multiple organ failure

The evidence is conflicting about the precise role of regional anaesthesia in attenuating such a response. Epidural block may well block the hyperglycaemic response by prolonged sympathetic blockade (1), but it is less successful in blocking the adrenocortical response to the stress of surgery (2).

It is generally agreed that by employing regional anaesthesia other techniques can be avoided or modified that are known to be deleterious to such critical patients. We know, for example, that etomidate blocks 11-β-hydroxylase involved in the synthesis of gluco- and mineralocorticoids in the adrenal cortex thus blocking the effect of adrenocorticotrophic hormone (ACTH). It has been implicated in the demise of septic ITU patients sedated with an infusion of it. In a study of patients with Addison's disease, both propofol and thiopentone when compared with etomidate appeared to preserve the response to ACTH (3). By extrapolation in a comparative study of healthy women undergoing hysterectomy, both propofol–alfentanil and methohexitone–alfentanil groups showed less intraoperative production of catecholamines and cortisol compared with an isoflurane group. Plasma production of glucose, fatty acids and lactate were lower in the total intravenous anaesthesia (TIVA) groups (4).

Provision of postoperative pain relief

The provision of postoperative pain relief can be very difficult in the first hour by opiates alone. Regional anaesthesia should provide immediate postoperative pain relief and by employing catheter techniques can prolong this for as long as desired. They can also eliminate the need for opiate or non-steroidal anti-inflammatory drugs. Thus patients at risk from haemorrhage or ventilatory depression can be better managed perioperatively. There has been an increasing use of the α_2-blocker clonidine in combination epidural conduction anaesthesia. In a comparative study of IV versus epidural clonidine with propofol/nitrous oxide (N_2O) sedation/anaesthesia, the epidural clonidine significantly reduced the intraoperative alfentanil requirements for 'rescue' analgesia as well as the postoperative morphine requirements for the first 6 h. However, also there was no difference in the sedation scores or changes (reduction) in heart rate or blood pressure. No other adverse occurrences were reported either (5).

Some of the same authors also published a report comparing epidural clonidine with epidural sufentanil under propofol hypnosis. The clonidine group required significantly less rescue injections during surgery of initially propofol and then, if deemed necessary, of sufentanil to treat intraoperative rises of blood pressure and heart rate. Also, less sufentanil via a PCA was required postoperatively in the clonidine group (6).

In order to select the most suitable agents and techniques one must consider what it is that is required to complement the regional anaesthesia. Having made an executive decision, taking into account the needs of the surgeon, the patient and the procedure, to provide sedation or general anaesthesia, the anaesthetist will find that a target-controlled infusion of propofol is ideal for this. The level of anxiolysis and sedation can be deepened or lightened at the touch of a button and one can even let the patient control their own level of sedation.

Because with effective and appropriate regional anaesthesia there should be no increased sensory input, only a very light level of anaesthesia is all that is necessary. However, excessive theatre noise should be discouraged. From the author's personal experience this can lead to arousal. During a total hip replacement with morphine and bupivacaine spinal conduction anaesthesia a patient opened her eyes, because of the noise of the saw, just scratched her nose and after a bolus of 5 ml of propofol settled down again – in recovery she had no recall whatsoever of the event. This would bear out the statement in Chapter 5 that muscular movement does not indicate conscious awareness.

Relevant pharmacology of propofol: in combination with regional anaesthesia

Vascular

If regional anaesthesia has been chosen because of the presence of ischaemic heart disease, then light levels of propofol infusion should be quite safe. In rats, propofol has a direct coronary artery vasodilatory effect which appears to be mediated by multiple substances including nitric oxide. However, the effect is not mediated by the opening of K^+ (ATP) channels (7). It should also be remembered that these channels are blocked by chlorpropamide so diabetic patients on oral hypoglycaemics may be better for changing to metformin prior to surgery.

In pigs, propofol attenuated the constrictor effect on vascular smooth muscle mediated by noradrenaline, 5-hydroxytryptamine or carbachol. The authors went on to conclude that this effect might be due to an antagonism of calcium channels (8). In dogs, the coronary sinus blood flow and myocardial oxygen consumption decreased in parallel along with a decrease in left ventricular work index without producing lactate (9).

In another experiment with dogs, where the left anterior descending branch of the left coronary artery was selectively perfused with either propofol 5–10 µg/ml or thiopentone 40 µg/ml (with the area supplied by the circumflex coronary artery acting as control), thiopentone produced a significant systolic shortening compared with propofol (10).

Thus one would conclude that propofol does not have an effect on myocardial contractility and that the hypotensive effect due to propofol is due to a direct vascular or a central effect. However, in the ischaemic myocardium propofol caused significant increases in heart rate and decreases in left ventricular contractility with a decrease in diastolic perfusion pressure compared with normal or collateral-dependant myocardium in chronically instrumented mongrel dogs (11). Propofol does not appear to cause significant problems in other vascular beds. One investigation in normal rats studied the effects of a continuous infusion of propofol on systemic and splanchnic haemodynamics using a new method of measuring liver oxygen consumption after cannulation of the hepatic artery, the portal and hepatic veins. The authors concluded that the maintenance of anaesthesia using an infusion of propofol resulted in an increased liver oxygen consumption that was fully compensated for by an increase in oxygen delivery to the liver. Splanchnic haemodynamics and liver oxygenation are not adversely affected during maintenance of anaesthesia with propofol in the normal rat (12). Propofol has been shown to attenuate the sympathetically mediated baroreceptor response to hypotension by sodium nitroprusside infusion but not the response to phenylephrine in normal healthy volunteers. The authors also noted that reflex regulation of sympathetic nervous activity was nearly abolished during propofol anaesthesia during normocarbic conditions but restored to conscious levels during hypercarbia and during N_2O administration (13).

However, what of its effects in humans with either myocardial insufficiency due to either valvular or coronary causes? In one study of 42 patients presenting for coronary artery bypass and 22 patients for valvular surgery, Isoflurane was compared with propofol. After 15 min there was a significant fall in mean arterial pressure, left ventricular stroke work index and systemic vascular resistance in the propofol group (14).

In another study using propofol–fentanyl TIVA, 23 CABG patients were compared with 16 valve surgery patients. Despite differences in baseline haemodynamic parameters, overall, propofol and moderate dose fentanyl anaesthesia was deemed to be no more detrimental to the haemodynamics in patients undergoing valve surgery when compared with those undergoing coronary artery surgery (15). Does this matter? In one study of propofol and regional anaesthesia in patients with myocardial ischaemia the conclusion was that the use of propofol was justified but that it was imperative to prevent a fall in blood pressure as a result of the regional anaesthesia itself otherwise the vasodilatory effects of propofol would reduce the diastolic pressure to values below which severe myocardial ischaemia and decompensation, if untreated, would occur.

Neurological

Propofol, like the benzodiazepines, activates the γ-amino butyric acid (GABA) receptor chloride ionophore complex. However, its effect does not appear to antagonized by flumazenil (16). In an investigation of cultured hippocampal neurones in the mouse propofol produced a dose dependent reversible inhibition of whole cell currents activated by the N-methyl-D-aspartate (NMDA) subtype of the glutamate receptor, possibly through an allosteric modulation of channel gating rather than by blocking the open channel. The authors concluded that depression of the NMDA-mediated excitatory neurotransmission may contribute to the anaesthetic, amnesic and anti-convulsant properties of propofol (17).

There is *in vitro* evidence that high concentrations of propofol attenuate NMDA receptor-mediated glutamate neurotoxicity but further studies are needed to confirm this beneficial effect *in vivo*, and to evaluate propofol as a neuroprotective anaesthetic agent in pathologies involving glutamate release and NMDA-mediated toxicity (18).

Another benefit that has been reported is that low doses of propofol can relieve spinal-morphine-induced pruritis as effectively as naloxone but because it does not reverse any analgesia the postoperative pain scores were significantly lower in the propofol group (19,20).

Haematological

As of 1994 (21) there have been no reports of adverse effects of the lipid formulation or indeed of propofol itself on blood clotting or platelet aggregation, thus its use with regional anaesthesia should cause no extra concern in patients having extradural conduction anaesthesia.

Respiratory

In a study of the sedative/hypnotic effects of low-dose propofol administration on central respiratory drive in 10 ASA patients, undergoing carpal tunnel decompression, there were no significant changes relative to basal values of respiratory rate, minute volume, tidal volume inspiratory and expiratory time, T_i/T_{tot}, TV/T_i, E_tCO_2 and blood gas analysis (22).

In one study of healthy volunteers the effects of TIVA with propofol on thermoregulation was found to decrease the threshold to vasoconstriction like the inhalational anaesthetics but *not* to increase the threshold to sweating (23).

Patient assessment and preoperative risk factors

Because of the cardiovascular factors just mentioned, if regional anaesthesia is contemplated then it must be optimally managed. If planning a spinal conduction block, it is imperative in the elderly patient with suspected ischaemic cardiac or cerebrovascular disease that they be fully hydrated prior to starting the block and that the blood pressure never be allowed to fall significantly. This means that immediately after the intrathecal injection of bupivacaine the patient should be given an intramuscular (IM) injection of ephedrine 30 mg. This, I find, is effective in preventing a fall in blood pressure which this group of patients are particularly unable to tolerate and will show ischaemic changes on the electrocardiogram (ECG) if it is allowed to persist.

Patients can have a serious perturbations on cardiac function if the diastolic falls below a value critical to them because restoration of diastolic pressure requires treatment with drugs that increase myocardial oxygen consumption. Thus by ensuring full hydration, prior to the block, monitored by central venous pressure (CVP) and administering IM ephedrine after the block any consequent fall in blood pressure is minimal without causing a significant rise in cardiac oxygen consumption. If patient assessment suggests a particular risk of post block hypotension then it is probably better to avoid TIVA or sedation with propofol and to select the more cardiostable etomidate. These 'at-risk' patients may have had huge reductions in blood pressure following previous propofol administration or they may have exhibited exaggerated lability in their blood pressure on the ward.

Poorly controlled hypertensive patients will undergo a dramatic fall in blood pressure as a result of a subarachnoid conduction block. If they were to be anaesthetized with propofol as well, the resulting vasodilatation would almost certainly jeopardize myocardial oxygen delivery, resulting in subendocardial ischaemia. This, in turn, if not promptly and adequately corrected would lead to arrhythmia or even infarction.

If it is not possible or practical to 'stabilize' their hypertension preoperatively then epidural/spinal anaesthesia and TIVA with propofol should be avoided.

Current clinical experience of regional anaesthesia combined with sedation/total intravenous anaesthesia

Sedation

Sedation has advantages and disadvantages. Traditionally benzodiaze-pines were the mainstay of sedation, often combined with an analgesic such as pentazocine or, better, pethidine. It is technically difficult to judge the appropriate level of sedation that will sufficiently reduce the patient's anxiety but will not so obtund their protective reflexes that more physical airway management becomes mandatory.

Whilst this will be annoying to the operator when the site of intervention, be it surgical or radiological, is peripheral, it becomes a nightmare if such a site be in the head or neck.

Age and position must also be taken into account. The elderly arthritic patient for ophthalmic procedures may have excellent anaesthesia but finds lying still on the operating table very uncomfortable. It is unrealistic to expect such patients to stay still for the length of the procedure without some pharmacological intervention. Benzodiazepines, however, may further compound the problem by their disinhibiting effect, thus converting an uncomfortable but cooperative patient into a confused and highly mobile one!

Quite understandably the temptation to 'deepen' the sedation becomes irresistible, but the patient may as a result lose their airway or even start to cough, which can cause a catastrophic rise in intraocular pressure with extrusion of the contents of the anterior chamber of the eye. Such a situation is avoided in the first place by giving a general anaesthetic with a protected airway. With explanation, both patient and operator can see the sense in such a course and, as with all good anaesthetic practice, a successful outcome starts with good planning.

However, there are many situations where, with an appropriate patient undergoing a suitable intervention, sedation and regional anaesthesia will lead to a successful outcome. Sedation can be provided by a computer driven target-controlled infusion (TCI) of propofol to aim for a plasma concentration of around $1\,\mu g/ml$ reasonably accurately (24). Propofol has been successfully used in patient-controlled sedation techniques (25).

The first use of propofol TCI was reported in 1991 (26). This study reported 20 patients with a mean age of 52.1 years undergoing upper GI endoscopy. The median blood propofol concentration for the insertion of the endoscope was $2.5\,\mu g/ml$ (range 1.5–4.0 $\mu g/ml$). Conditions were described as good in 15 patients and fair in the remaining five. Patient cooperation was good in 16 patients and fair in four. There was a significant reduction in S_pO_2 during the procedure from a mean of 94.2 to 89.3%. Satisfactory sedation was also reported with propofol TCI in patients undergoing orthopaedic procedures under regional neural blockade. Here the median blood propofol concentration was $0.93\,\mu g/ml$ (range 0.15–2.63 $\mu g/ml$). The lower dose in this study illustrates the effect of adequate analgesia on the sedation requirements. The patients in the regional block study spent 88% of the time at a satisfactory level of sedation with sedation scores of 3 or 4. Undesirable oversedation, corresponding to a sedation score of 5 occurred for an average of 2.5% of the total time and was quickly reversed by selecting a lower target concentration.

There is also the advantage that the level of sedation can be suitably controlled by a cooperative patient, thus leaving the operator free to undertake the procedure. The likelihood of loss of airway reflexes is greatly reduced, and can be minimized by careful and appropriate programming of the syringe driver delivering the propofol. However, there is increasing peer pressure for stopping the practice of single-handed procedures on sedated patients.

One study compared propofol sedation using three techniques, all administered by an anaesthetist. The groups received intermittent bolus administration, conventional infusion following a bolus or a TCI. The overall quality of sedation, operating conditions and clinical recovery profiles were the same in all three groups (27). However, the anaesthetist had to intervene more often in the bolus dose group compared with the conventional infusion and TCI groups.

TCI sedation had been used satisfactorily for 21 h in a patient undergoing gynaecological radiotherapy (28). Oversedation was not reported although the patient required assisted ventilation by mask for 5 min following the administration of 0.75 mg of alfentanil.

Assessment of snoring has been undertaken using TCI propofol sedation (29). Patients were sedated until they began to snore and the degree of airway obstruction was then assessed by nasal endoscopy. The technique could reliably produce snoring in the 25 patients studied.

In a study of propofol (6 mg/kg for 10 min then 3 mg/kg) and midazolam (initial bolus of 0.06 mg/kg followed by an infusion of 0.05 mg/kg) sedation, 40 patients were contrasted for changes in intra-operative haemodynamics, respiration, sedation scores and plasma biochemistry compared with baseline values.

No significant differences were reported between the two groups for any of those parameters. However, there was significantly greater amnesia in the midazolam group (30).

In a comparative study of 30 female patients undergoing regional anaesthesia for lower abdominal surgery all had established epidural conduction anaesthesia before sedation with either propofol 2.8 mg/kg/h or midazolam 0.08 mg/kg/h and there was a control group who received no sedation additional to the epidural blockade. All groups had excellent haemodynamic stability. In the recovery room all three sedation groups showed significantly impaired vigilance but this lasted for 24 h in the methohexitone group, who also showed significant impairment of their ability to concentrate. Patients treated with midazolam or methohexitone needed longer to recall their date of birth than those sedated with propofol (31).

Patient-controlled sedation

Patients can titrate their own level of sedation in a manner similar to patient-controlled analgesia by requesting bolus doses. Use of this technique substantially increases the anaesthetist's responsibilities compared with the standard bolus administration (32). In addition to the safety and well-being of the patient, the anaesthetist must also explain the control system and is responsible for its satisfactory operation during the procedure. However, patient-controlled sedation affords several advantages over physician-controlled techniques. Patients titrate the level of sedation to suit their own anxiety, thus overcoming inter-individual variations both in pharmacokinetics and pharmacodynamics. Many patients also prefer the control which the technique allows, and oversedation is prevented because the patient is involved in the control loop and no drug is administered if the patient is asleep.

One study used a randomized crossover design to compare a patient-controlled bolus of 18 mg propofol delivered over 5.4 s (lockout time of 1 min) with a physician set continuous infusion at 3.6 mg/kg/h (33). Both groups received 0.7 µg/kg of fentanyl and were given supplementary oxygen. Patients used less propofol with the patient-controlled sedation (mean 2.39 mg/kg) compared with the infusion (mean 2.58 mg/kg) group but the difference was not statistically significant. Patient-controlled sedation was preferred by 19 patients, continuous infusion by 10 and nine were indifferent to the technique employed. No patients experienced cardiovascular instability and S_pO_2 was at least 97% in all patients.

Hamid et al. compared patient-controlled sedation using propofol with patient-controlled sedation using methohexitone in 42 patients having dental extractions under local anaesthesia (34). Patients in both groups achieved their desired levels of sedation, but those who received methohexitone reported that they felt more drowsy immediately after the procedure. More patients in the methohexitone group had wisdom teeth extracted and may have used more sedation. There were no differences 15 min following the procedure. The main disadvantage of patient-controlled bolus dosing is that the blood concentration of drug is not at a steady state but changes continually, resulting in periods of relatively high and low sedation. It also takes time for adequate sedation to be achieved. One study reported a sedation score of 3 being reached at approximately 9 min, making the technique unsuitable for very short procedures.

Patient-controlled/target-controlled infusion sedation

Recently, TCI and patient control of sedation have been combined (35). In this study TCI propofol was started at a target concentration of 1 µg/ml. The patient was able to increase the target propofol concentration in 0.2 µg/ml increments by double pressing a demand button. There was a lockout interval of 2 min and a maximum permissible target concentration of 3 µg/ml. If no demands were made for 6 min the system reduced the target concentration by 0.2 µg/ml. There was considerable inter-individual variability in propofol consumption with a mean of 39 µg/kg/min (range 3–131 µg/kg/min). Optimum sedation was provided with a median target concentration of 0.8–0.9 µg/ml and 89% of patients were happy to use the technique again. Reasons cited were comfort, self-titration, anxiolysis and clear-headed recovery. One patient would not use the system again because of pain in the infusion arm.

A patient-controlled sedation system, similar to the one described above, is currently undergoing assessment at Glasgow Royal Infirmary for preoperative sedation in day surgery patients (36) Twenty patients were studied. There was a highly significant reduction in anxiety scores 15 min after sedation was started. The technique was safe and there was a high degree of patient satisfaction.

The advantages of a patient-controlled TCI sedation system include:

◆ Rapid onset and offset of sedation
◆ Ability to rapidly titrate the level of sedation to degree of anxiety experienced
◆ Patient control adds to patient satisfaction and improves safety

In developing a patient-controlled TCI sedation system, the initial target concentration, the incremental target concentration achieved by patient demand, the lockout interval and the time before the target concentration is decreased are all important in ensuring that the system is safe but also flexible enough to provide additional sedation when required.

Neuroleptanalgesia

Neuroleptanalgesia has enjoyed more popularity abroad than in the UK. Whilst it was thought to minimize cardiovascular perturbations, in a recent comparative study in 1318 patients with cardiac disease there were more reported incidents, events and complications after neuroleptanaes-thesia compared with balanced anaesthesia or TIVA. The incidence of postoperative nausea and vomiting was lower in the TIVA groups who also had a better recovery profile (37). Neuroleptanaesthesia almost always causes significant psychomimetic effects that rule out its use for day surgery because of the prolonged time taken to the return of street fitness. It is also unpopular with patients. In one study of patients undergoing elective gynaecological laparotomy 20 had propofol–fentanyl TIVA + pancuronium and 20 had droperidol, fentanyl pancuronium. At 24 h post operation significantly more patients judged their recovery good in the propofol group than the neurolept group who reported significantly more 'locked-in' feelings and impairment of memory (38). Propofol has been successfully combined with ketamine and produced far fewer of the common ketamine recovery dysphoric effects. It was postulated that propofol's GABA receptors agonist properties were responsible (39).

Total intravenous anaesthesia

In practise, TIVA with propofol combined with regional anaesthesia is found to be versatile and widely applicable. Examples of the types of suitable procedures would include:

♦ *General surgery.* Inguinal hernia repair, colonic surgery, varicose vein surgery, inguinal node block dissection, carpal tunnel decompression, removal of ganglion, etc.
♦ *Gynaecology.* Hysterectomy abdominal and vaginal, colposuspension, vaginal repairs, etc.
♦ *Ophthalmology.* Cataract correction, trabeculectomy, etc.
♦ *Orthopaedics.* I find that spinal conduction anaesthesia quicker and more consistently effective than epidural blockade for hip and knee arthroplasty. This agrees with a Canadian study in hip replacement arthroplasty where the two techniques were compared in 65 patients (32 spinal and 30 epidurals plus two epidural failures) with regard to sensory blockade degree of hypotension and perioperative haemorrhage. Interestingly, the amount of propofol required to maintain adequate hypnosis was significantly lower in the spinal group (40).
♦ *Urology.* Transurethral resection of prostate, retropubic excision of prostate, etc.

There are miscellaneous examples in the literature. For example, it has been successfully used in combination with cervical epidural conduction anaesthesia for the surgical correction of a mycotic aneurysm of the right carotid artery in a 75-year-old patient with a concomitant 75% stenosis of the left carotid artery (41).

Complications

Full cardiovascular monitoring during regional anaesthesia is mandatory. The threat of toxic doses is particularly prevalent amongst big volume caudal blocks in children and in large volume infiltrations of vascular areas such as intrapleural blocks. These examples are in addition to the large volume epidural where there has been undetected catheter migration IV or lack of aspiration of blood prior to an unsuspected IV injection into an epidural vein. Failure of double cuffs for Bier's blocks can cause sudden and catastrophic rises in plasma local anaesthetic concentrations. This is of course a valid reason for not employing bupivacaine for Bier's blocks. Ropivacaine, which is 16 times less likely to cause malignant ventricular fibrillation than bupivacaine, may well supplant bupivacaine as the long-acting local anaesthetic of choice. The risk of using air in loss of resistance to injection techniques for space localization can lead to air embolism. Thus the technique is gradually being outlawed.

If the regional blockade does actually cause toxic plasma levels of local anaesthetic, the presence of propofol rather than other general anaesthetics probably does not place the patient at any further risk since sedative doses are known to be less depressant to the myocardium than thiopentone. Since the first clinical signs of toxicity in a situation of rising plasma local anaesthetic concentrations are neurological rather than cardiac, the anticonvulsant properties of propofol theoretically make it a more desirable agent than methohexitone or etomidate in such circumstances.

References

1. Licker M, Suter PM, Krauer F, Rifat NK. Metabolic response to lower abdominal surgery: analgesia by epidural blockade compared with intravenous opiate infusion. *Eur J Anaesthesiol* 1994; **11**: 193–9.
2. Trayner C, Paterson J, Ward ID, Morgan M, Hall GM. Effects of extradural analgesia and vagal blockade on the metabolic and endocrine response to upper abdominal surgery. *Br J Anaesth* 1982; **54**: 319–23.
3. Fragen RJ, Weiss HW, Motteni A. The effect of propofol on adenocorticois steroidogenesis: a comparative study with etomidate and thiopental. *Anaesthesiology* 1987; **66**: 839–42.
4. Crozier TA, Muler JE, Quittkat D, Sydow M, Wuttke W, Kettler D. TIVA with Meth–alf or propofol–alf in hypogastric laparotomy. Clinical aspects and the effects of stress reaction. *Anaesthesist* 1994; **43**: 594–604.
5. De Kock M, Crochet B, Morimont C, Scholtes JL. Intravenous or epidural clonidine for intra- and postoperative analgesia. *Anaesthesiology* 1993; **79**: 525–31.
6. De Kock M, Famenne F, Deckers G, Scholtes JL. Epidural clonidine and sufentanil for intraoperative and postoperative analgesia. *Anaesth Analg* 1995; **81**: 1154–62.
7. Park KW, Dai HB, Lowenstein EW, Selke FW. Propofol-associated dilation of rat distal coronary arteries is mediated by multiple substances, including endothelium-derived nitric oxide. *Anaesth Analg* 1995; **81**: 1191–6.
8. Yamanoue T, Brum JM, Estafanous FG. Vasodilation and mechanism of action of propofol in porcine coronary artery. *Anaesthesiology* 1994; **81**: 443–51.
9. Nakaigawa Y, Akazawa S, Shimizu R, Ishii R, Yamato R. Effects of graded infusion rates of propofol on cardiovascular haemodynamics, coronary circulation and myocardial metabolism in dogs. *Br J Anaesth* 1995; **75**: 616–21.
10. Belo SE, Kolesar R, Mazer CD. Intracoronary propofol does not decrease myocardial contractile function in the dog. *Can J Anaesth* 1994; **41**: 43–9.
11. Mayer N, Legat K, Weinstabl C, Zimpfer M. Effects of propofol; on the function of normal, collateral-dependent, and ischaemic myocardium. *Anaesth Analg* 1993; **76**: 33–9.
12. Carmichael FJ, Crawford MW, Khayyam N, Saldivia V. Effect of propofol infusion on splanchnic haemodynamics and liver oxygen consumption in the rat. A dose–response study. *Anaesthesiology* 1993; **79**: 1051–60.
13. Ebert TJ, Muzi M. Propofol and autonomic reflex function in humans. *Anaesth Analg* 1994; **78**: 369–75
14. Phillips AS, McMurray TJ, Mirakhur RK, Gibson FM, Elliott P. Propofol–fentanyl anaesthesia: a comparison with isoflurane–fentanyl anaesthesia in coronary artery bypass grafting and valve replacement surgery. *J Cardiothorac Vasc Anaesth* 1994; **8**: 289–96.

15. Bell J, Sartain J, Wilkinson GA, Sherry KM. Comparison of propofol and fentanyl in coronary artery versus valve surgery. *Anaesthesia* 1995; **50**: 644–8.
16. Fan SZ, Liu CC, Yu HY, Chao CC, Lim SM. Lack of effect of flumazenil on the reversal of propofol anaesthesia. *Acta Anaesthesiol Scand* 1995: **39**: 299–301.
17. Orser BA, Bertik M, Wang LY, MacDonald JF. Inhibition by propofol (2,6-di-isopropylphenol) of the *N*-methyl-D-aspartate subtype of glutamate receptor in cultured hippocampal neurones. *Br J Pharmacol* 1995; **116**: 1761–8.
18. Hans P, Bonhomme V, Collette J, Albert A, Moonen G. Propofol protects cultured rat hippocampal neurons against *N*-methyl-D-aspartate receptor-mediated glutamate toxicity. *J Neurosurg Anaesthesiol* 1994; **6**: 249–53.
19. BorgeatA, Wilder-Smith OH, Saiah M, Rifat K. Subhypnotic doses of propofol relieve pruritis induced by epidural and intrathecal morphine *Anaesthesiology* 1992; **76**: 510–2.
20. Salah M, Borgeat A, Wilder-Smith OH, Rifat K, Suter PM. Epidural-morphine-induced pruritis: propofol versus naloxone. *Anaesth Analg* 1994; **78**: 1110–3.
21. Haberer JP Does the lipid content of Diprivan explain some pharmacological effects? *Ann Franc d'anesth Reanimat* 1994; **13**: 460–4.
22. Rosa G, Conti G, Orsi P, *et al.* Effects of low dose propofol administration on central respiratory drive, gas exchanges and respiratory pattern. *Acta Anaesthesiol Scand* 1992; **36**: 128–31.
23. Leslie K, Sessler DI, Bjorksten AR, *et al.* Propofol causes a dose-dependent decrease in the thermoregulatory threshold for vasoconstriction but has little effect on sweating. *Anaesthesiology* 1994; **81**: 353–60.
24. Skipsey IG, Colvin JR, McKenzie N, Kenny GN. Sedation with propofol during surgery under local blockade. Assessment of a target-controlled infusion system. *Anaesthesia* 1993; **48**: 210–3.
25. Bryson HM, Fulton BR, Faulds D. Propofol: an update of its use in anaesthesia and conscious sedation. *Drugs* 1995; **50**: 513–59.
26. Church JA, Stanton PD, Kenny GNC, Anderson JR. Propofol for sedation during endoscopy: assessment of a computer controlled infusion system. *Gastrointest Endosc* 1991; **37**: 175–9.
27. Newson C, Joshi G, Victory R, White PF. Comparison of propofol administration techniques for sedation during monitored anaesthesia care. *Anaesth Analg* 1995: **81**: 486–91.
28. Oei-Lim VLB, Kalkman CJ, Van Tienhoven G, Engbers FHM. Remote controlled prolonged conscious sedation for gynaecological radiotherapy. *Anaesthesia* 1996; **51**: 866–8.
29. Connolly AAP, Martin J, White P. Sedation with a target-controlled propofol infusion system during assessment of the upper airway in snorers. *J Laryngol Otol* 1994; **108**: 865–7.
30. De Andres J, Bolinches R. Comparative study of propofol and midazolam for sedation in regional anaesthesia. *Rev Esp Anestesiol Reanimac* 1993; **40**: 354–9.
31. Atanassoff PG, Alon E, Pasch T. Recovery after propofol, midazolam, and methohexitone as an adjunct to epidural anaesthesia for lower abdominal surgery. *Eur J Anaesthesiol* 1993; **10**: 313–8.
32. Osbourne GA. Monitored patient-controlled sedation: practical technique or academic research tool? *Eur J Anaesthesiol* 1996; **13** (suppl 13): 13–7.
33. Osbourne GA, Rudkin GE, Jarvis DA, Young G, Barlow J, Leppard PI. Intraoperative patient-controlled sedation and patient attitude to control. *Anaesthesia* 1994; **49**: 287–92.

34. Hamid SK, McCann N, McArdle L, Asbury AJ. Comparison of patient-controlled sedation with either methohexitone or propofol. *Br J Anaesth* 1996; **77**: 727–30.
35. Irwin MG, Thompson N, Kenny GNC. Patient-maintained propofol sedation. Assessment of a target-controlled infusion system. *Anaesthesia* 1997; **52**: 525–30.
36. Murdoch JAC. Patient-maintained propofol sedation for premedication in day case anaesthesia. *Br J Anaesth* 1998; **80** (suppl 1): A58.
37. Harke H, Schmidt K, Gretenkort P, *et al.* Qualitative comparison of modified neurolept-balanced and intravenous anaesthesia. 2. Results of a clinical study *Anaesthesist* 1995; **44**: 687–94.
38. Linneman MU, Guldager H, Nielsen J, Ibsen M, Hansen RW. Psychomimetic reactions after neurolept and propofol anaesthesia. *Acta Anesthesiol Scand* 1993; **37**: 29–32.
39. Guit JB, Koning HM, Coster ML, Niemeijer RP, Mackie DP. Ketamine as analgesic for total intravenous anaesthesia with propofol. *Anaesthesia* 1991; **46**: 24–7.
40. Davis S, Erskine R, James MF. A comparison of spinal and epidural anaesthesia for hip arthroplasty. *Can J Anaesth* 1992; **39**: 551–4.
41. Llorente A, Bronte E, Ramos G Carpentero M, Gimenez C. Cervical epidural anaesthesia for carotid mycotic aneurysms. *Rev Esp Anestesiol Reanimac* 1995; **42**: 341–3.

15

Endocrine surgery

N. L. Padfield

- Pituitary physiology, pathophysiology and anaesthesia
- Thyroid physiology, pathophysiology and anaesthesia
- Parathyroid physiology, pathophysiology and anaesthesia
- Endocrine pancreas physiology, pathophysiology and anaesthesia
- Adrenal cortex physiology, pathophysiology and anaesthesia
- Adrenal medulla physiology, pathophysiology and anaesthesia

Anaesthesia for endocrine surgery can offer the anaesthetist some of the greatest challenges. A thorough understanding of the physiology and pathophysiology along with a knowledge of the pharmacodynamics of the commonly used intravenous (IV) agents is essential.

This chapter will deal with each major endocrine system individually, and describe the interaction between disease and the requirements of surgery and anaesthesia.

Pituitary

Physiology and pathophysiology

The pituitary is morphologically divided into two halves with quite different functions. The anterior pituitary produces the thyroid stimulating hormone (TSH), growth hormone, the gonadotrophic hormones (follicle stimulating hormone and interstitial cell stimulating hormone), luteinizing hormone and the adrenocorticotrophic hormone (ACTH). The release of these hormones is essentially under a negative feedback control by hypothalamic regulatory hormones.

There are three common disorders of pituitary overproduction: excessive production of prolactin (amenorrhoea, galactorrhoea and infertility), ACTH (Cushing's syndrome) and growth hormone (acromegaly). Acromegaly is associated with weakness, enlargement of hands and feet, and a widened mandible. Also these patients may have abnormal glucose tolerance, osteoporosis and appear myxoedematous. There may also be retention of sodium and potassium, diabetes mellitus, and premature atherosclerosis and cardiomegaly. Of anaesthetic significance is thickening of the mucosa of the pharynx, enlarged larynx and even calcification of the cords, and paralysis of the recurrent laryngeal nerve and laryngeal stenosis has been known for a long time (1).

Excessive prolactin production causes galactorrhoea in females and impotence in males. It has little surgical relevance. Excessive ACTH production leads to Cushing's syndrome and the management is described later on in the chapter.

Insufficiency of anterior pituitary hormones is usually the result of bleeding into a tumour. When this occurs patients may present with headache, visual loss, nausea and vomiting, ocular palsies, disturbances of consciousness, fever, vertigo or hemiparesis.

The posterior pituitary produces anti-diuretic hormone (ADH) and oxytocin, and these are controlled by the hypothalamus via a neuro-humoral pathway. In addition to the production of the trophic hormones, the hypothalamus is also affected by temperature via hot and cold peripheral and central thermoreceptors, blood volume via natriuretic hormone and volume receptors in the great veins, season via melatonin, and emotion via input from the limbic system. Excessive production of ADH (2) causes hyponatraemia and fluid retention, and can arise from numerous central nervous system lesions. It can also arise from treatment with nicotine, narcotics, chlorpropamide, clofibrate, vincristine and vinblastine, cyclophosphamide, pulmonary infections, pulmonary tumours, and other endocrine disorders such as hypothyroidism and adrenal insufficiency.

Lack of ADH which presents as diabetes insipidus is less of a problem to deal with as patients readily respond to intravascular fluid and electrolyte correction and DDAVP (Desmopressin). However, care has to be taken in the pregnant patient because of the oxytocic qualities of DDAVP and in the patient with ischaemic heart disease as DDAVP is a vasoconstrictor of the coronary arteries (3).

Surgery for tumours of the pituitary is rare. Pituitary adenomas present with disturbances to vision by pressure effects on the optic chiasm before manifesting endocrine disturbances (see Chapter 11). Pituitary infarction though can manifest itself as an endocrine emergency following a complicated labour and delivery, as in Sheehan's syndrome (4), which initially presents as alactorrhoea but rapidly progresses to Addison's syndrome with fatal results if not diagnosed and treated immediately. Meningiomas and giant aneurysms are rare, and may occasionally manifest by endocrine disorders, although these tumours more commonly manifest as space-occupying lesions and thus the anaesthetic considerations are also dealt with in Chapter 11.

Anaesthesia

The principles of protected airway, judicious IV fluid management and reliable appropriate physiological monitoring ensure the optimum anaesthetic outcome.

The pathophysiology that is likely to affect the conduct of anaesthesia is usually from the secondary endocrine organ effects, i.e. hypothyroid or Addison's syndrome mediated by dysfunction of the anterior pituitary caused by an adenoma.

The indication for surgery tends to be compromise to the optic nerves rather than endocrine problems *per se*. However, if the posterior pituitary is also dysfunctional because of compromise to its vasculature by the enlarging adenoma then fluid homeostasis may be adversely affected due to altered ADH production. Too little ADH results in diabetes insipidus which manifests as hypotension, a contracted intravascular volume, electrolyte disturbance and muscular weakness. Such patients if untreated with DDAVP and fluid and electrolyte correction are extremely intolerant of the vasodilating effects of anaesthesia with propofol and have an increased sensitivity to muscle relaxants. If surgery has to be performed to save life or limb then propofol is best avoided and etomidate possibly combined with ketamine makes a wise choice (see Chapter 5). In such circumstances fluid balance is critical and this will require invasive physiological monitoring, i.e. pulmonary capillary wedge pressure (PCWP), central venous pressure (CVP), continuous blood pressure, etc.

Tumours of the posterior pituitary are extremely rare but there are some other rare malignant tumours that secrete ADH directly into the systemic circulation and thus by by-passing the liver exert an unpredictable effect. For example, oat cell carcinoma of the lung can cause water retention with hyponatraemia which does not respond predictably to loop diuretics. Thus patients presenting for thoracotomy/mediastinotomy/open lung biopsy may have fluid and electrolyte imbalance which affects the anaesthesia for a relatively minor surgical procedure (see Chapter 10).

Thyroid

Physiology and pathophysiology

The thyroid plays a pivotal role in the body's metabolism mediated by the two hormones, i.e. triiodothyronine (T3) and tetraiodothyronine (T4). Eighty percent of T3 is produced outside the thyroid gland. Their release is under a negative feedback control of TSH produced by the anterior pituitary and this is in turn under control of thyrotropin releasing factor produced by the hypothalamus.

The conversion of T3 to T4 is blocked by propranolol, glucocorticoids and amiodarone, thus elevating T3 levels. Levels of TSH are often high when conversion of T3 to T4 is blocked. Cardiac function and responses to stress are abnormal in hyperthyroidism, and return of cardiac function to normal parallels the return of TSH to normal values.

The effects of T3 are by binding to high-affinity nuclear receptors and the resultant activation of DNA-directed mRNA synthesis may account for its anabolic growth and developmental effects, plus some calorigenic effect. T3 also causes an increased concentration of adrenergic receptors which may account for some of its cardiovascular effects (5).

Hyperthyroidism can exist in a number of forms where either one or both of the hormones can be raised. The clinical effects are weight loss, diarrhoea, warm moist skin, weakness of large muscle groups, menstrual disturbances, nervousness, intolerance to heat, tremor, tachycardia and atrial fibrillation which can exacerbate pre-existing heart disease. In most clinical situations this can be treated medically first before undertaking partial or total thyroidectomy. β-Blockade for tachycardia is fraught with problems as its employment can precipitate patients into frank cardiac failure. If surgery must proceed in a seriously toxic patient, full physiological monitoring must be in place and only then can an infusion of a short acting β-blocker like Esmolol be started. Intravascular fluid and electrolyte balance must be restored as well but even these measures will not necessarily prevent a 'thyroid storm' (6). This is manifested by hyperpyrexia, tachycardia and impressive alterations of consciousness. The differential diagnosis is malignant hyperthermia, phaeochromocytoma and neuroleptic malignant syndrome. Treatment consists of using anti-thyroid drugs like carbimazole, treatment with iodine to prevent release of preformed T4, correcting the precipitating cause and judicious treatment of hypovolaemia, and electrolyte imbalance.

Hypothyroidism is under diagnosed because of its insidious onset. However, it can have devastating results during major (even unrelated) surgery. Not every case of anaesthetically significant hypothyroidism will have the florid symptoms and signs of myxoedema, such as thickening of facial features, macroglossia, coarsening of the hair, deepening of the voice, bradycardia, cold intolerance and constipation.

If confirmed by lowered T3 and T4 it must be treated by thyroxine first though this will take some days to accomplish. The dangers with hypothyroidism are the unresponsiveness of the cardiovascular system to inotropes, both endogenous and exogenous. This can pose particular problems for patients with ischaemic heart disease presenting for myocardial revascularization and the need for thyroid therapy must be balanced against aggravation of angina (7).

Anaesthesia

The majority of thyroid surgery is performed in the euthyroid state, where single or multiple discreet nodules or lobules may be removed or the entire gland be partially or totally removed. In the cases of carcinoma or retrosternal external there may be airway compromise visible on computed tomography (CT) scan which will alert the anaesthetist to the necessity of formulating a difficult intubation plan. However, the operations which form the bulk of thyroid surgery do not indicate or contraindicate a particular method of general anaesthesia providing there is a protected airway. This will require intubation and the use of muscle relaxants.

Untreated florid hyperthyroid states that require emergency surgery, i.e. because of airway compromise, provide a great challenge to the anaesthetist. There is a short therapeutic window of a few days where pretreatment with Lugol's iodine may control the hyperactive gland. Otherwise, in addition to invasive physiological monitoring, the patient should be given high-dose steroids prior to induction. A plan for difficult intubation should have been made and a bed booked on the intensive care unit for the postoperative period. Suitable drugs such as β-blockers and vasodilators should be immediately available. The use of digoxin is controversial but should be considered as an uncontrolled ventricular rate is associated with greater intraoperative morbidity and mortality.

The choice of agents for TIVA will be indicated by the individual cardiovascular disturbance. Etomidate has the advantage that it *per se* causes the least cardiovascular perturbation but has the disadvantage that it inhibits α_{11}-hydroxylase, and thus reduces the production of gluco- and mineralocorticoids in the adrenal cortex in response to the stress of surgery. Propofol is both an arterial and a venous dilator. In anaesthetic doses it does not have any direct affect on ventricular contractility, but if diastolic pressure is reduced and the time of diastole is reduced because of tachycardia its vasodilating effects could be secondarily deleterious and thus it may be better avoided. However, the tonic effects on the vagus may exert a useful counter effect on the tachycardia. Thus each case has to be judged on its individual merits.

Hypothyroid states requiring emergency surgery pose one of the greatest risks in anaesthesia. Apart from airway problems associated with the macroglossia, the relative and unpredictable responsiveness of the cardiovascular system poses the greatest threat. Profound hypotension and bradycardia can follow induction if injudiciously administered and this may be refractory to the effects of β and α stimulants. Very tight control of fluid balance is essential in these patients, which require full invasive monitoring as their ability to compensate for changes in blood volume is severely compromised. TIVA with vasodilating drugs such as propofol should be avoided. Etomidate is the agent of choice.

Parathyroids

Physiology and pathophysiology

These four small glands produce parathormone which raises serum calcium by encouraging osteoclastic activity causing bone resorption. Serum calcium is lowered by the action of calcitonin produced by the thyroid gland which increases the uptake of calcium by osteoblasts. Primary adenomas causing primary hypercalcaemia are rare. Secondary hyperparathyroidism is more common, whereby because of calcium losing nephropathies in an attempt to compensate and maintain calcium homeostasis there is an excessive production of parathormone. If untreated typical lytic lesions of osteitis fibrosa develop and frequently the parathyroid glands undergo adenomatous change resulting in tertiary hyperparathyroidism which does not respond to correction of serum calcium.

Hyperparathyroidism presents with anorexia, vomiting constipation, thirst, polydipsia, renal calculi, pancreatitis, lethargy, confusion and psychiatric disturbance, and characteristic changes of shortened QT intervals on the ECG. There may also be a relative hypovolaemia and one-third of hypercalcaemic patients are hypertensive.

Hypocalcaemia is due to hypoparathyroidism, hypomagnesaemia, hypoalbuminaemia and chronic renal disease. The clinical signs are clumsiness, convulsions, laryngeal stridor, muscle stiffness, paraesthesia (circumoral) parkinsonism and tetany, Chvostek and Trousseau signs, dry flaky skin, brittle nails, and coarse hair. Pure hypoparathyroidism is seen most commonly occurs after thyroid surgery where tingling and muscular tetany develop within 6 h of surgery. There are also typical electrocardiogram (EEG) changes of prolonged QT intervals.

Anaesthesia

Hyperparathyroidism

Patients who are moderately hypercalcaemic with normal cardiac and renal function do not present any special problems for TIVA. If the calcium is very raised then treatment with rehydration, diuretics such as frusemide and IV phosphate administration will reduce serum calcium and encourage bone uptake of calcium. If this is still not enough then treatment with corticosteroids will inhibit gastric calcium absorption and thus reduce the serum calcium level.

Hypoparathyroidisim

Because there may be cardiac and muscular dysfunction, the serum calcium, magnesium and phosphate must be corrected first before anaesthesia and surgery is undertaken. Because there is no specific surgery for parathyroid deficiency, in practice therefore anaesthesia for hypoparathyroid patients will be for unrelated surgery.

The choice of agent for TIVA will be indicated by the stability of the cardiovascular system since in some cases hypocalcaemia can cause bradycardia.

Propofol is vagotonic, but this is usually overcome with glycopyrrolate.

Endocrine pancreas

Physiology and pathophysiology

Failure of the endocrine pancreas causes diabetes mellitus. This occurs either in childhood and tends to be associated with insulin dependence. There is either a lack of or a resistance to insulin, the major anabolic hormone. It can be linked with hyperlipidaemia, and can lead to eye problems (retinopathy, new vessels, haemorrhages and exudates), renal problems, cardiovascular problems and neurological problems, mono-neuropathies, and even autonomic neuropathy. These in turn can lead to cadiorespiratory arrest, gastroparesis, postural hypotension, postoper-ative urinary retention and sleep apnoea (8–10). All these complications need to assessed in their own right as it is these that cause the problems rather than the hyperglycaemia *per se* (11–13).

It also occurs in maturity where there is a partial failure of the gland and there is a need for oral hypoglycaemic agents, although older patients can develop an insulin-dependent type of diabetes (14). Efficacy of glucose homeostasis can be indicated by the percentage of glycosylated haemoglobin.

Anaesthesia

In practice it is the cardiac problems of ischaemia coupled with autonomic neuropathy that pose the greatest challenge to the anaesthetist in addition to maintaining glucose homeostasis. Painless myocardial infarction (15) can lead to unexpected and potentially fatal complications. If the patient is hypertensive then there is a 50% chance of concurrent autonomic neuropathy. Renal problems and the increased susceptibility to infection along with bone marrow suppression can also cause significant delayed operative morbidity.

If the heart rate is slow it is probably better to avoid propofol because of the vagotonic effects since there is unpredictable response to glycopyrrolate and inotropes. Ideally if the surgery is suitable for regional anaesthesia then this should be employed. If the patient is insistent on general anaesthesia then etomidate is probably the induction and maintenance agent of choice. Great care must be taken at the induction of anaesthesia as it is at this stage that the rate of administration of induction agent can be too rapid and thus cause profound perturbation of heart rate and blood pressure. Once this has occurred it is very difficult to correct in some circumstances and can even be fatal; therefore, it is much better to avoid it if possible by a slow rate of induction with fully invasive arterial monitoring.

Hyperglycaemia causes problems by dehydration and changes in osmotic load. Too rapid correction by the administration of insulin can cause profound changes in plasma potassium, and therefore cardiac function and neuromuscular function. Hyperglycaemia in association with maturity-onset diabetes responds well to rehydration first then if refractory conversion to an infusion of a sliding scale of insulin. The CVP must be monitored during rehydration and there may be concomitant cardiac disease so over transfusion must be avoided to avoid tipping the patient into cardiac failure. The selection of agent for TIVA, provided that plasma volume, glucose and potassium are optimized, will depend on the cardiac status of the patient. In most cases propofol will be ideal combined if possible with regional anaesthesia to minimize the cardiac perturbation.

Insulinoma

Occasionally the β cells of the islets of Langerhans become adenomatous and secrete excessive amounts of insulin. This presents as hypoglycaemia with neurological disturbances and sympathetic overactivity. Anaesthesia needs to include regular monitoring of blood sugar every 15 min and infusion of 25–50% dextrose via a central vein. TIVA is quite suitable.

Adrenal cortex

Physiology and pathophysiology

The adrenal cortex produces androgens (16), mineralocorticoids (17) and glucocorticoids (18).

The normal adrenals produce 166–185 mg of cortisol/24 h in the unstressed state, which can increase to 200–500 mg/24 h in times of maximum stress. Tumours can arise which secrete excess amounts of mineralocorticoids (Conn's syndrome) or glucocorticoids (Cushing's syndrome). Occasionally the cortex may fail to produce both types of corticosteroids and cause Addison's syndrome. This is characterized by hypotension (19) and can lead to fatalities as measures to restore blood pressure prove ineffective, e.g. there can be an unpredictable response to inotropes.

Anaesthesia

In situations of glucocorticoid excess (Cushing's syndrome), thin skin and striae may cause problems with healing and venipuncture, but fluid retention and hypertension coupled with diabetes mellitus need the most careful evaluation as these pose the main problems for the anaesthetist. Osteoporosis (20) will require extra care in positioning a patient for surgery to avoid fracture. Spontaneous Cushing's syndrome is caused in 60–70% of cases by the overproduction of pituitary ACTH (21).

Tumours responsible for ectopic ACTH secretion may cause hypokalaemic alkalosis which will require correction with spironolactone prior to anaesthesia.

Bilateral adrenalectomy for Cushing's disease has a high surgical mortality rate of 5–10% (22) and many patients require permanent adrenocorticoid replacement therapy.

Also, 10% of patients presenting for bilateral adrenalectomies have an undiagnosed pituitary tumour and this can then subsequently enlarge. It is often invasive and, by excessive production of ACTH and melanocyte stimulating hormone, causes pigmentation and ophthalmic symptoms by pressure effects on the optic chiasm.

Excessive mineralocorticoid activity leads to hypokalaemia and sodium retention, muscle weakness hypertension tetany, polyuria with inability to concentrate urine, and hypokalaemic alkalosis (23). Primary hyperaldosteronism (Conn's syndrome) is present in 0.5–1% of hypertensive patients who have no other known cause of hypertension. These patients may have a normal serum potassium, but will have a reduced body potassium; they also have a high incidence of myocardial ischaemia. Anaesthetic management is optimal when preoperative hypertension, hypokalaemia and hypovolaemia are corrected.

TIVA with propofol should be uneventful if the induction rate of administration is slow and the total induction dose is not excessive provided the patient has been treated preoperatively. Full physiological monitoring must be *in situ* to warn against excessive perturbations in cardiovascular parameters.

Adrenocorticoid underproduction is far more hazardous to the patient and is most frequently the result of withdrawal of steroid therapy or suppression of synthesis by steroid treatment. Anaesthesia for patients in Addisonian crisis has been well described by Smith *et al.* (24). Other important but less common causes include defects in ACTH secretion, and destruction of the adrenals themselves by cancer, tuberculosis, haemorrhage (Waterhouse–Friederickson syndrome), auto-immune disease and cytotoxic drugs. Primary adrenal insufficiency Addison's disease is autoimmune and involves all zones of the adrenal cortex. It is associated with high levels of ACTH, and because it develops slowly these patients develop marked pigmentation and cardiopenia probably secondary to chronic hypotension.

If unstressed glucocorticoid-deficient patients have little to no preoperative problems. However, even minor stress will tip them into Addisonian crisis of hypotension, hyperkalaemia and hyponatraemia, and this is particularly refractory to treatment if allowed to develop. Therefore the pre-anaesthetic management not only includes steroid pretreatment but also correction of hypotension, hyponatraemia and hyperkalaemia. Traditionally this would be by stress doses, 200 mg, of cortisone given over 24 h on the day of operation but it would seem that a smaller dose of 25 mg IV at induction followed 100 mg in divided doses over the next 24 h is even more desirable as it is closer to physiological requirements.

Pure mineralocorticoid deficiency is rare and is most likely to occur with concomitant renal disease (25) with long-standing diabetes, nonsteroidal anti-inflammatory treatment, heparin administration or following unilateral adrenalectomy. Plasma renin levels are low and do not increase appropriately in response to sodium restriction or diuretic drugs. The problems in these patients arise from electrolyte disturbances which can cause myocardial conduction defects.

Anaesthetic management requires correction of these electrolyte disturbances with fludrocortisone 0.5–1 mg/24 h.

TIVA with propofol is the method of choice in these patients. As has already been described in Chapter 2, etomidate is contraindicated in these patients. It causes a dose- and time-related adrenal suppression acting on 11-β-hydroxylase and cholesterol side-chain cleavage enzyme (26).

Adrenal medulla

Physiology and pathophysiology

Although rare, less than 0.1% of causes of hypertension (27), phaeochromocytomas, catecholamine-producing tumours of chromaffin tissue, are the cause of significant anaesthetic morbidity and mortality. These vascular tumours usually are found in the adrenal medulla but can occur in the right atrium, spleen, the broad ligament of ovary and the organs of Zucherkandl at bifurcation of the aorta. They may be part of the multiple endocrine adenoma type IIa or type IIb. Type IIa consists of medullary carcinoma of the thyroid, parathyroid adenoma or hyperplasia and phaeochromocytoma.

Symptoms and signs that suggest the diagnosis are excessive sweating, headache, hypertension, orthostatic hypotension, glucose intolerance, polycythaemia, weight loss and psychological disturbance. Tumour location is facilitated by magnetic resonance imaging, CT scan, metaiodobenzylguanidine nuclear scan, ultrasound and IV urography. In fact, the combined occurrence of paroxysmal headache, sweating and hypertension is probably a more sensitive and specific indicator than any biochemical test.

Anaesthesia

Anaesthesia is as trouble free as α- and β-blockade is effective (28). β-blockade as sole treatment runs the risk of hypotension, and α-blockade alone runs the risk of tachycardia and arrhythmia and even serious ST changes (29). Most patients take 10–14 days to optimize their condition prior to surgery on phenoxybenzamine and propranolol therapy. There are four criteria that ideally will be fulfilled before surgery: no blood pressure reading higher than 165/90, whilst orthostatic hypotension should be present no standing blood pressure should be lower than 85/45, there should be no ST changes on the ECG and finally there should be no more than one premature ventricular ectopic present every 5 min (30,31).

Provided the patient is effectively blocked TIVA can proceed with no particular problems. In fact the cardiac stability of propofol is an advantage in these circumstances. Tumour handling though is critical and unpredictable during the course of surgery, and while there may be an exaggerated response from nerve endings that are loaded by the re-uptake process, plasma catecholamines levels may rise to 20–2000 pg/ml. Even simple stresses though may cause a rise in plasma levels to 2000–20 000 pg/ml. However, if there is infarction of the tumour with release of products onto the peritoneal surface then a massive release may result in plasma levels of 200 000–1 000 000 pg/ml. The anaesthetist should be ready to counter this with an infusion of sodium nitroprusside until the venous drainage is isolated then provided that intravascular volume is normal the blood pressure should return to normal or even lower and some patients then paradoxically require inotropes to support the sagging blood pressure (32).

Tumours producing vasoactive substances

Physiology and pathophysiology

There are a miscellaneous group of neoplastic tumours that can secrete a number of vasoactive substances that can cause serious perturbations during anaesthesia if unrecognized and treated.

Seventy-five percent of carcinoid tumours are sited in the gastro-intestinal tract (33). Tumours rising in the ileocaecal region have the greatest tendency to metastasize and it is only when there is an extra portal site that the features of excessive serotonin production manifest. These are facial flushing, diarrhoea, hypotension, tachycardia and occasionally wheezing. Any handling of the tumour in an unblocked patient may result in catastrophic release of vasoactive substances and result in a fatality. Several neurohumoral agents are excreted, vasoactive intestinal peptide, substance P, neurotensin, somatostatin and dopamine have all been implicated in the flushing and hypotension.

Anaesthesia

Successful management starts with blockade of all the vasoactive effects. Various agents have been employed such as ketanserin, aprotonin, methotrimeprazine, parachloroaminobenzoic acid and cyproheptadine in combination, recognizing that not only serotonin but vasoactive peptides have to be blocked. In practice today with the availability of somatostatin which is the most potent inhibitor of peptide release and inhibitor of peptic effects on receptors cells this agent or its synthetic analog, octreotide (34), is the treatment of choice for pre-, peri- and postoperative management of carcinoid symptoms and crises (35). If the hypotension proves intractable to somatostatin, then angiotensin or vasopressin may be the next best treatment, but care must be taken that the patient has not developed tricuspid incompetence and pulmonary hypertension as these drugs could exacerbate this.

Thus the patient with carcinoid presenting for anaesthesia must be assessed for pulmonary, neurological, nutritional, fluid and electrolyte, and cardiovascular disturbance. The anaesthetist will then be in the best position to gauge the likely response of that particular patient to α- and β-adrenergic blockade, aprotonin, methotrimeprazine, and bronchodilators.

The anaesthetist must also avoid administering drugs known to cause release of vasoactive substances such as morphine and d-tubocurarine, but at the same time provide an adequate level of analgesia to prevent release of catecholamines.

The best compromise is to block the peripheral effects of the vasoactive substances as fully as possible, and to correct fluid and electrolyte disturbances prior to induction. This may take a few days.

The maximum amount of non-invasive monitoring should be attached with a calm and reassuring attitude from the anaesthetist! Every conceivable useful therapeutic agent that might be needed should be drawn up and labelled ready for immediate administration.

IV access must be established and, if indicated by the nature of surgery, regional neural blockade established prior to induction.

TIVA with propofol is a very pleasant way to induce anaesthesia in these circumstances, especially in combination with regional anaesthesia. If muscular relaxation is indicated then vecuronium is recommended. Because propofol can be a vasodilator and can be vagotonic, care should be taken not to select too high an initial plasma target in order to minimize vascular perturbations. This means that induction will take longer and the anaesthetist must reassure the patient at this critical time. Effect-site concentrations should be within the normal range. Once the tumour is resected or embolized it is not uncommon to have to support the circulation with inotropes for a few hours. Therefore postoperative intensive care is mandatory. As each patient is unique in manifestation, treatment and management is expectant. However, by being well prepared and able to recognize and treat disturbances the anaesthetist can play a pivotal role in the management of these very special patients.

References

1. Chappell WF. *J Laryngol* 1896; **10**: 142.
2. Weiss NM, Robertson GL: Water metabolism in endocrine disorders. *Semin Nephrol* 1984; **4**: 303.
3. Corliss RJ, McKenna DH, Sialers S, *et al.* Systemic and coronary haemodynamic effects of vasopressin. *Am J Med Sci* 1968; **256**: 293.
4. Sheehan HL. *Am J Obstet Gynaecol* 1954; **68**: 202
5. Williams LT, Lefkowitz RJ, Watanabe AM, *et al.* Thyroid hormone regulation of beta-adrenergic receptor number. *J Biol Chem* 1977; **252**: 2787.
7. Mackin JF, Canary JJ, Pittman CS. Thyroid storm and its management. *N Engl J Med* 1974; **291**: 1396.
8. Levine HD. Compromise therapy in the patient with angina pectoris and hypothyroidism: a clinical assessment . *Am J Med* 1980; **69**: 411.
9. Fowkes FGR, Lunn JN, Farrow SC, *et al.* Epidemiology in anaesthesia III. Mortality risk in patients with co-existing disease. *Br J Anaesth* 1982; **54**: 819
10. Page MM, Watkins PJ. Cardiopulmonary arrest and diabetic autonomic neuropathy. *Lancet* 1978; **i**: 14
11. Burgos LG, Ebset TJ, Asiddao C, *et al.* Increased intraoperative cardiovascular morbidity in diabetics with autonomic neuropathy. *Anaesthesiology* 1989; **70**: 591.
12. Bilous RW. Diabetic autoimmune neuropathy (Editorial) [See comments]. *Br Med J* 1990; **301**: 565.
13. Rees PJ, Prior JG, Cochrane CM, *et al.* Sleep apnoea in diabetic patients with autoimmune neuropathy. *J R Soc Med* 1981; **74**: 192.
14. Hjortrup A, Sorenson C, Dyremose E, *et al.* Influence of diabetes mellitus on operative risk. *Br J Surg* 1985; **72**: 783.
15. Mackenzie CR, Charlson ME. Assessment of perioperative risk in the patient with dibetes mellitus. *Surg Gynaecol Obstet* 1988; **167**: 293–9.

16. White PC, New MI, Dupont B. Congenital adrenal hyperplasia. *N Engl J Med* 1987; **316**: 1519.
17. Hollenberg NK, Williams GH. Hypertension, the adrenal and the kidney: lessons from the pharmacologic interruption of the renin–angiotensin system. *Adv Intern Med* 1980; **25**: 327.
18. McPartland RP. Metabolic and pharmacologic actions of glucocorticoids. In: Mulrow PJ, ed. *The adrenal gland*. New York: Elsevier 1986: 85.
19. Sampson PA, Brooke BN, Whinstone NE. Biochemical confirmation of collapse due to adrenal failure. *Lancet* 1961; **i**: 1377.
20. Lampe GH, Roizen MF. Anaesthesia for patients with abnormal function at the adrenal cortex. *Anaesthesiol Clin North Am* 1987; **5**: 245.
21. Tyrell JB, Brooks RM, Fitzgerald PA, *et al*. Cushing's disease. Selective trans-sphenoidal resection of pituitary micro-adenomas. *N Engl J Med* 1978; **298**: 753.
22. Ernest I, Exkman H. Adrenalectomy in Cushing's disease: a long term follow-up. *Acta Endocrinol* 1972; **160** (suppl): 3.
23. Einberger MH, Grim CE, Hollifield JW, *et al*. Primary aldosteronism: diagnosis, localisation, and treatment. *Ann Intern Med* 1974; **90**: 386.
24. Schambelan M. Sebastian A. Hyporeninaemic hypoaldosteronism. *Adv Intern Med* 1979; **24**: 385.
25. Smith MG, Byrne AJ. An Addisonian crisis complicating anaesthesia. *Anaesthesia* 1981; **36**: 681
26. Wagner RL, White PF, Kan PB, *et al*. Inhibition of adrenal steroid genesis by the anaesthetic etomidate. *N Engl J Med* 1984; **310**: 1415.
27. Bravo EL. Phaeochromocytoma: new concepts and future trends. *Kidney Int* 1991; **40**: 544.
28. Desmonts JM, Le Houelleur J, Remond P, *et al*. Anaesthetic management of patients with phaeochromocytoma: a review of 102 cases. *Br J Anaesth* 1977; **49**: 991.
29. Roizen MF, Horrigan RW, Koike M, *et al*. A prospective randomised trial of four anaesthetic techniques for resection of phaeochromocytoma. *Anaesthesiology* 1982; **57**: A43.
30. Roizen MF. Anaesthetic implications of concurrent diseases. In: Miller R, ed. *Anaesthesia*, 4th edn. Edinburgh: Churchill Livingstone 1994: 924.
31. Hull CJ. Phaeochromocytoma. Diagnosis, preoperative preparation and anaesthetic management. *Br J Anaesth* 1986; **58**: 1453.
32. Roizen MF, Schreider BD, Hassan SZ. Anesthetics for patients with phaeo-chromocytoma. *Anesthesiol Clin North Am* 1987; **5**: 269.
33. Longnecker M, Roizen MF. Patients with carcinoid syndrome. *Anaesthesiol Clin North Am* 1987; **5**: 313.
34. Quantrini M, Basilisco G, Conte D, *et al*. Effects of Somatostatin infusion in four patients with malignant carcinoid syndrome. *Am J Gastroenterol* 1983; **78**: 149.
35. Quinlivan JR, Roberts WA. Sutraoperative Octreotide for refractory carcinoid induced bronchospasm. *Anaesthes Analges* 1994; **78**(2): 400–2.

16

Ophthalmic surgery

N. Sutcliffe

- Introduction
- Propofol target-controlled infusion
- Clinical studies
- Closed-loop anaesthesia for eye surgery
- Opioid infusion regimens
- Conclusion

Introduction

Ophthalmic surgery is widely performed under general anaesthesia in the UK, although local anaesthesia is also a popular alternative. This chapter is limited to discussing general anaesthetic techniques. Patients requiring ophthalmic surgery tend to be at the extremes of age with all the potential problems associated with this. In optimizing conditions for this type of surgery, the anaesthetist has a crucial role to play, particularly for intra-ocular procedures such as cataract extraction and intra-ocular lens implantation. The aim is to provide an immobile eye with a low intraocular pressure (IOP) and a smooth recovery without coughing, restlessness, nausea or vomiting. While attenuating the rise in IOP at laryngoscopy and intubation may not be important in those with normal IOP, it may be of great relevance in patients with perforated eye injuries and in situations where there is pre-existing high IOP such as in glaucoma.

Intraocular pressure regulation

- External pressure
- Choroidal blood volume (venous pressure, P_aCO_2 and arterial pressure)
- Aqueous and vitreous volumes

The choroidal blood volume is maintained by autoregulation provided the systolic blood pressure is above 90 mmHg. Venous congestion caused by coughing, straining and poor position should be avoided as well as vasodilatation caused by a raised P_aCO_2. Volatile agents and induction agents (apart from ketamine) cause a reduction in IOP. Nitrous oxide (N_2O) has no effect unless air or sulphur hexafluoride are present within the globe. Non-depolarizing muscle relaxants cause a small fall in IOP, while suxamethonium causes a transient increase in IOP due to contraction of the extraocular muscles and muscles of the globe.

The traditional general anaesthetic technique usually includes volatile maintenance with opioid supplementation and a muscle relaxant to facilitate tracheal intubation and artificial ventilation. The advantages of this technique are that the airway is secure, P_aCO_2 can be controlled and thereby avoid the effects of a high P_aCO_2 on IOP. Adequately monitored neuromuscular blockade ensures an immobile eye. Infusions of propofol can simply be substituted for the volatile maintenance using the same basic technique but with the benefits of rapid recovery and reduced nausea and vomiting.

The disadvantages of the traditional technique are that laryngoscopy and tracheal intubation can cause a large increase in IOP, especially if the procedure proves difficult or there are prolonged attempts. The presence of an endotracheal tube frequently causes coughing in the post-operative period (1,2). Volatile anaesthetics have a higher incidence of post-operative nausea and vomiting. These factors may potentially damage the operated eye. In addition, there is inevitably a delay while waiting for spontaneous respiration to return following neuromuscular blockade as well as the need for reversal agents. There is also an increased risk of awareness associated with paralysis.

Propofol target-controlled infusion

Target-controlled infusion (TCI), which offers rapid and fine control over depth of anaesthesia, provides an alternative option to traditional techniques. The airway can be maintained with a laryngeal mask (LMA), provided there are no contraindications. It has been shown that the use of the LMA results in greater haemodynamic stability avoiding the stress response to intubation and the resultant increase in IOP (3,4). Spontaneous respiration may be preserved by finely adjusting the level of hypnosis and analgesia. Anaesthesia can be deepened if desired and respiration assisted by hand or with pressure support mode ventilation, without requiring muscle relaxation.

Propofol has been shown to be an ideal anaesthetic agent for this type of surgery. It is particularly suitable for infusion because of its pharmacokinetic profile with fast onset and offset compared with other available intravenous (IV) agents. In addition, the recognized anti-emetic properties of propofol are of benefit in ophthalmic surgery. It has been shown that a greater post-induction fall in IOP occurs with propofol compared to thiopentone (5). The potentially harmful effects of intubation are also attenuated to a greater extent; an effect enhanced by a supplementary bolus of propofol prior to intubation (6). In circumstances where a rapid sequence induction is indicated, propofol ± alfentanil has been demonstrated to obtund the effect of suxamethonium and intubation on IOP. Moreover, laryngoscopy and intubation have a much greater effect on IOP than suxamethonium itself (7). The 'Diprifusor' TCI system is the most controllable delivery system for propofol.

Analgesia as part of this technique can also be given via a TCI system with the most suitable opioids being alfentanil and remifentanil; however, these systems are not yet commercially available. Alternatively, N_2O and/or bolus opioids can be used.

Clinical studies

There have been several studies describing the use of propofol infusions for ophthalmic surgery using slightly different techniques. Comparisons have been made of the LMA and endotracheal tube to maintain the airway. Methods of opioid administration with artificial or spontaneous ventilation have also been evaluated.

The laryngeal mask airway versus the endotracheal tube

With the advent of the LMA, it has become possible to avoid intubating patients. More anaesthetists are now happy to ventilate patients with a LMA and there have been studies comparing the two techniques for ophthalmic surgery. A modified version of the LMA with an armoured tube to prevent kinking can be helpful and is less bulky around the operation site.

Akhtar *et al.* compared airway maintenance with either an endotracheal tube or LMA (2). All patients were anaesthetized with 'Diprifusor' TCI propofol, paralysed and ventilated. There was no significant difference in a number of parameters including mean arterial pressure (MAP) and IOP but there was a significantly higher incidence of coughing and breath-holding in the intubated group postoperatively. Coughing may increase the IOP to more than 50 mmHg (normal IOP is 16 ± 5 mmHg), which is especially important after intraocular surgery and in patients with perforating eye injuries.

In contrast to this, other studies have shown a significantly greater increase in IOP following intubation compared with LMA insertion (1,4). Volatile agents were used to maintain anaesthesia for these cases rather than propofol infusions. Volatile agents are recognized to be less effective in attenuating the response to intubation compared with propofol and this may be sufficient to account for these differences.

Target-controlled infusion propofol in the elderly

Ophthalmic surgery is often performed on patients at the extremes of age (see Chapter 14). In a comparison by Moffat and Cullen of TCI propofol/LMA/spontaneous respiration group with an etomidate/isoflurane/intermittent positive pressure ventilation (IPPV) group, 40 patients undergoing day case cataract surgery aged 60–88 years were studied (8). There was significant hypotension during induction and maintenance in the propofol group but no haemodynamic response to LMA insertion. In contrast, induction in the etomidate group produced minimal effects on MAP or heart rate but a significant haemodynamic response to intubation. Recovery was smooth in both groups with vomiting occurring in only one patient in the etomidate group. However, no opioids were administered and the patients were given metoclopramide preoperatively. Surprisingly, a slower recovery was demonstrated in the TCI propofol group. The selected blood propofol concentrations of 6 µg/ml for induction reducing to 4 µg/ml for maintenance are quite high relative to the age of this population. Other studies have shown lower propofol requirements in the elderly (3–3.5 µg/ml) (9). The higher incidence of hypotension in the TCI propofol group compared to the etomidate/volatile group suggests a relative overdose and this may account for the differences in recovery. Interestingly, this study also found that despite the high end-tidal CO_2 levels in the TCI propofol group, the IOP remained low and the surgeon found no difference in operating conditions between the two groups.

Supplemental opioids for ophthalmic surgery

A retrospective analysis of 138 patients undergoing eye surgery was carried out in our institution. All patients received TCI propofol as the hypnotic component of their anaesthetic and opioid analgesia via either TCI with a prototype backbar system or bolus injection. Their airway was maintained with a LMA unless they had any contraindication such as reflux oesophagitis or an airway problem, in which case they were intubated and ventilated.

The majority of patients in the TCI group received TCI alfentanil with 52 of them also receiving N_2O. The remainder received oxygen-enriched air. Two patients received TCI remifentanil. Thirty-six patients had bolus opioid and 28 of these breathed spontaneously with a LMA. Five patients had no opioid at all. See Tables 16.1 and 16.2.

There was no difference in alfentanil and propofol requirements with the addition of N_2O in the TCI alfentanil group. This is surprising since other studies have shown a sparing effect on propofol maintenance requirements by both alfentanil and N_2O. We also found that the mean end-tidal CO_2 concentration was not significantly different, suggesting that N_2O had little effect on the depth of anaesthesia in this situation.

The bolus opioid group received fentanyl 1–1.5 µg/kg (24 patients) or alfentanil 3–5 µg/kg (12 patients) prior to insertion of LMA.

The analysis showed that despite different analgesic strategies, there was little difference between the groups in the TCI propofol requirements. In all groups, induction requirements were approximately 25% higher than during maintenance. The difference in induction and

Table 16.1 Propofol and alfentanil requirements in spontaneously breathing patients undergoing eye surgery with and without N_2O supplementation [mean (SD)]

	With N_2O	Without N_2O
No. patients	52	28
Age (years)	62 (21)	57 (22)
Maintenance target concentration		
Propofol ($\mu g/ml$)	3.28 (1.09)	3.38 (0.9)
Alfentanil (ng/ml)	20.4 (8.3)	23.3 (8.28)
Change in MAP		
decrease on induction (%)	13 (15)	9 (11)
increase on LMA insertion (%)	1.31 (17)	3.3(13.5)

maintenance concentrations may be explained by the delay in achieving equilibrium between blood and brain concentrations. The brain or effect site concentration lags behind the blood concentration during the induction phase, but equilibrates during the maintenance phase. Propofol requirement during maintenance of anaesthesia in the paralysed ventilated group was very similar to the spontaneously breathing group, contrasting with the perception that neuromuscular blockade leads to reduced anaesthetic requirements.

The operating conditions were good with all techniques and there was no suggestion of high IOPs in any of the patients despite the fact

Table 16.2 Propofol requirements for spontaneously breathing patients receiving opioids by bolus injection or TCI and for ventilated patients receiving opioid supplementation [mean (SD)]

	Spontaneously breathing		Ventilated
	Bolus injection opioid	*TCI opioid*	*Bolus injection/ TCI opioid*
No. patients	28	82	23
Age (years)	65 (17.5)	57.2 (20)	61.4 (16.6))
End-tidal CO_2 (kPa)	5.8 (0.92)	6.57 (0.96)	4.5 (0.94))
Target blood propofol concentration ($\mu g/ml$)			
induction	4.3 (1.5)	3.8 (1.28)	3.75 (1.09))
LMA	3.3 (1.0)	3.33 (1.2)	3.77 (1.4))
incision	3.16 (0.87)	3.49 (1.09)	3.28 (0.78))
maintenance	2.68 (0.95)	3.32 (1.03)	3.08 (0.95))

that relatively high levels of end-tidal CO_2 were seen in the spontaneously breathing patients. The mean end-tidal CO_2 was 5.8 kPa (SD
0.92) in the bolus injection opioid group and 6.57 kPa (SD 0.96) in the
TCI opioid group. Furthermore, it was found that less than 5% of
patients were nauseated postoperatively and none required an antiemetic. The induction and maintenance requirements in this series of
patients were similar to the propofol requirements described below for
closed-loop anaesthesia.

Closed-loop anaesthesia for eye surgery

Closed-loop anaesthesia requires a measure of depth of anaesthesia as the
input signal. This signal can be used to automatically control the target
blood concentration of propofol. Such a system, therefore, should
maintain a constant depth of anaesthesia and give an unbiased
assessment of anaesthetic requirement. We assessed a series of 10 patients
undergoing eye surgery in our institution with a prototype system of
closed-loop anaesthesia using the auditory evoked potential, as described
by Kenny *et al*. (10). All patients received TCI alfentanil (target blood
concentration 25 ng/ml) and N_2O (60% in oxygen) to supplement
propofol TCI. Mean propofol requirements were 4.5 µg/ml for induction
and 3.26 µg/ml for maintenance. These requirements were similar to
those described above but the system generally made more changes in
the target propofol concentration compared with manually controlled
TCI. This suggests that the anaesthetic requirements vary more than
might be appreciated during changing levels of surgical stimulation or
may simply be a reflection of oscillations inherent in such servo-
controlled systems.

Figure 16.1 shows the propofol target (µg/ml × 10) plotted along with
the auditory evoked potential index (AEPI) and AEPI-Target for one
patient undergoing eye surgery. The system reacts to any lightening of
anaesthesia produced by surgical stimulation by increasing the propofol
target concentration. Inevitably, the target always lags slightly behind
changing depth in anaesthesia as the system can only react to this change,
rather than anticipating surgical stimulation as an anaesthetist would
normally do.

Opioid infusion regimens

Spontaneous respiration

TCI opioids offer the most flexible adjuvant to TCI propofol but
unfortunately this mode of delivery is not as yet commercially available.
As an alternative, a manual infusion regime can be used to approximate
blood concentration. From our experience with a prototype TCI system
for alfentanil, it is suggested a suitable target blood concentration for

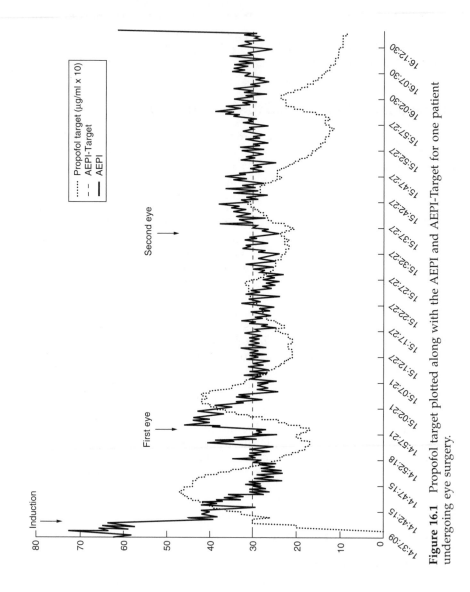

Figure 16.1 Propofol target plotted along with the AEPI and AEPI-Target for one patient undergoing eye surgery.

alfentanil in spontaneously breathing patients of 25 ng/ml for ophthalmic surgery. This target can be achieved by infusing a bolus of 2.5 μg/kg over 1 min followed by an infusion of 0.15 μg/kg/min. However, it is important to be aware that the initial high peak concentration may cause apnoea. Remifentanil can also be used with a manual infusion regime with an equivalent target blood concentration being 1 ng/ml. This can be achieved in approximately 2 min following an infusion of 0.0625 μg/kg/min. The peak blood concentration reached with this infusion rate is 1.5 ng/ml after approximately 20 min.

Remifentanil: ventilating patients during ophthalmic surgery

Following the recent introduction of remifentanil to clinical practice, it is possible to use a high opioid/low hypnotic technique for cases of short duration. There are potential advantages in using such a technique for ophthalmic surgery. As a result, our method of choice now consists of TCI propofol, TCI remifentanil and IPPV with oxygen/air. The LMA is used to maintain the airway unless contraindicated.

Remifentanil, at a high dose, is a potent respiratory depressant and allows artificial ventilation without muscle relaxation. Consequently, P_aCO_2 can be controlled and the possibility of awareness is eliminated since patients are not paralysed. The rapid metabolism of remifentanil results in an exceptionally fast recovery from anaesthesia when used in conjunction with propofol. We find patients are clear-headed early in the postoperative period, thus avoiding unwanted restlessness. Postoperative nausea and vomiting are also very uncommon. Analgesia is provided by the use of local anaesthesia and simple analgesics.

Allowing for the age of the patient, with the elderly generally requiring less, our typical target concentration for propofol would be 2 μg/ml with a remifentanil target concentration of 3–4 ng/ml. Remifentanil has a context-sensitive half-life of 3.5 min, which is constant irrespective of how long the infusion continues. Therefore, simple and rapid control of the depth of anaesthesia is possible to adjust to varying levels of surgical stimulation. It would seem that this technique comes close to providing all the requirements of an ideal anaesthetic for ophthalmic surgery.

Conclusions

Anaesthesia for ophthalmic surgery is optimized with total IV anaesthesia:

◆ Superior perioperative control of IOP
◆ Haemodynamic response to intubation avoided by the use of LMA
◆ TCI opioids allow IPPV without muscle relaxation to control P_aCO_2
◆ Low incidence of nausea and vomiting
◆ Coughing minimized postoperatively
◆ Elderly patients have reduced anaesthetic requirements

References

1. Holden R, Morsman CD, Butler J, Clark GS, Hughes DS, Bacon PJ. Intra-ocular pressure changes using the laryngeal mask airway and tracheal tube [see comments]. *Anaesthesia* 1991; **46**: 922–4.
2. Akhtar TM, McMurray P, Kerr WJ, Kenny GN. A comparison of laryngeal mask airway with tracheal tube for intra-ocular ophthalmic surgery. *Anaesthesia* 1992; **47**: 668–71.
3. Braude N, Clements EA, Hodges UM, Andrews BP. The pressor response and laryngeal mask insertion. A comparison with tracheal intubation. *Anaesthesia* 1989; **44**: 551–4.
4. Whitford AM, Hone SW, O'Hare B, Magner J, Eustace P. Intra-ocular pressure changes following laryngeal mask airway insertion: a comparative study. *Anaesthesia* 1997; **52**: 794–6.
5. Guedes Y, Rakotoseheno JC, Leveque M, Mimouni F, Egreteau JP. Changes in intra-ocular pressure in the elderly during anaesthesia with propofol. *Anaesthesia* 1988; **43** (suppl): 58–60.
6. Mirakhur RK, Shepherd WF, Darrah WC. Propofol or thiopentone: effects on intraocular pressure associated with induction of anaesthesia and tracheal intubation (facilitated with suxamethonium). *Br J Anaesth* 1987; **59**: 431–6.
7. Zimmerman AA, Funk KJ, Tidwell JL. Propofol and alfentanil prevent the increase in intraocular pressure caused by succinylcholine and endotracheal intubation during a rapid sequence induction of anesthesia. *Anesth Analg* 1996; **83**: 814–7.
8. Moffat A, Cullen PM. Comparison of two standard techniques of general anaesthesia for day-case cataract surgery [see comments]. *Br J Anaesth* 1995; **74**: 145–8.
9. Swinhoe CF, Peacock JE, Reilly CS. Evaluation of the accuracy of the 'Diprifusor'. *Eur J Anaesthesiol* 1995; **12** (suppl): 84.
10. Kenny GNC, McFadzean WA, Mantzaridis H, Fisher AC. Closed-loop control of anaesthesia. *Anesthesiology* 1992; **77**: A328.

17

Future developments

S. E. Milne and G. N. C. Kenny

- New drugs and total intravenous anaesthesia
- New methods of drug administration
- Postoperative analgesia, alfentanil and remifentanil
- Closed-loop anaesthesia

Introduction

A successful total intravenous anaesthetic (TIVA) must consist of hypnotic and analgesic components. Propofol is commonly used as the hypnotic and the introduction of a commercially available target-controlled infusion (TCI) pump, the 'Diprifusor', has revolutionized TIVA with propofol.

The analgesic component of TIVA has frequently been provided with alfentanil or sufentanil; however, remifentanil is a recently developed short-acting opioid ideally suited to administration by infusion and has an established role as a component of TIVA.

Although the hypnotic component of TIVA is normally propofol, S-(+)-ketamine may have a use in certain circumstances and may also be employed as the analgesic component along with propofol.

Alfentanil and remifentanil can be used to provide postoperative analgesia, and propofol is useful for patient sedation. These drugs can be administered by constant rate infusions or by TCI. The target concentration can be preset by the anaesthetist or can be controlled by the patient in a manner similar to patient-controlled analgesia (PCA). These methods result in effective and safe analgesia or sedation with a high degree of patient satisfaction.

Concerns about awareness during TIVA are being addressed and new monitors for measuring depth of anaesthesia are being developed. These include the bispectral index (BIS) and the auditory evoked potential index (AEPI). These monitors can be linked to drug administration systems to create closed-loop anaesthesia.

This chapter will look at the new drugs, remifentanil and S-(+)-ketamine, and explore new methods of drug administration including PCA and sedation. Finally, it will look at depth of anaesthesia monitoring with closed-loop anaesthesia.

New drugs and TIVA

Remifentanil

Remifentanil is a recently introduced short-acting opioid. Its rapid onset and short duration of action make it ideally suited to administration by infusion, and it contributes useful analgesia to a TIVA technique.

Pharmacokinetics and pharmacodynamics

The metabolism of remifentanil by non-specific esterases in blood and other tissues ensures that the drug is degraded rapidly and consistently. This novel method of metabolism imparts brevity of action, precise and rapidly titratable effects, non-cumulative opioid effects, and rapid recovery after cessation of administration (1).

The context-sensitive half-time is short at about 3–4 min and is independent of infusion duration, while the measured terminal elimination half-life is 12 to 30 min (2). Central clearance of remifentanil is approximately 3 l/min (3). It is lipophilic and widely distributed in body tissues, with a total volume of distribution of 21.8–30 l (4). Unlike other fentanyl congeners, termination of the therapeutic effect depends mostly on metabolic clearance rather than on redistribution (5).

The pharmacodynamics have been characterized in healthy adult males using a spectral edge encephalogram (EEG) as a measure of opioid effect. Speed of onset is very fast and similar to that of alfentanil with a $t_{1/2}\,k_{eo}$ of approximately 1.4 min for remifentanil (6).

The effect of age and gender on the pharmacokinetics has been studied using EEG as a measure of drug effect. Age and lean body mass both have significant influences on the pharmacokinetic and pharmacodynamic parameters. While gender does not affect these parameters directly, it does affect the calculation of the lean body mass and so must be taken in to account when calculating the relevant parameters for any individual patient. Volume of distribution and clearance decrease by 25 and 33%, respectively, as age increases from 18 to 85 years, while k_{eo} decreases by 50% from age 18 to 85 years (6).

Effect on respiratory and cardiovascular systems

Like other opioids, remifentanil administration results in marked respiratory depression (7). This is reversed by naloxone. However, administration of naloxone is not normally required because termination of the infusion is associated with a prompt recovery of ventilatory response. The beneficial effects of remifentanil including cardiovascular stability occur at blood concentrations greater than that at which spontaneous respiration is depressed. Consequently, most patients require their lungs to be ventilated. This is not usually a problem and can be done via a laryngeal mask airway if intubation is deemed unnecessary. Low-dose infusion regimens during which spontaneous respiration persists can be used but may not confer benefits when compared with other opioids. The postoperative analgesic requirement is often increased and in some circumstances makes postoperative pain control more difficult (see Chapter 2). Heart rate is slowed by remifentanil and there may be a marked bradycardia in some patients. The blood pressure is usually well maintained.

Use with other anaesthetic agents

Remifentanil has a synergistic effect with propofol. In one study the optimum propofol blood concentration for maintenance of anaesthesia in the presence of remifentanil was 2.5–3 μg/ml (8), but will vary with the dose of remifentanil and stimulation from the surgical procedure.

Clinical use

A study of patients receiving propofol has shown that a remifentanil bolus of 1 μg/kg followed by infusion at a rate of 1 μg/kg/min effectively controls responses to tracheal intubation (9). A bolus of 1 μg/kg followed by an infusion of 0.5 μg/kg/min resulted in more hypertension and tachycardia in response to intubation. Recovery from anaesthesia occurred at 3–7 min with both infusion regimens.

In a study of patients undergoing abdominal surgery, a remifentanil 1 μg/kg bolus followed by an infusion of 0.5 μg/kg/min was compared with an alfentanil 25 μg/kg bolus followed by an infusion of 1 μg/kg/ min (10). The study drug infusion rate was reduced by 50% at 5 min after intubation. Responses to intubation and skin incision occurred twice as often in the alfentanil group compared to the remifentanil group. More patients receiving alfentanil had one or more responses to surgery. The times to spontaneous respiration, adequate respiration, response to verbal command and time to recovery room discharge were similar. However, owing to increased variability, the time to extubation was shorter with remifentanil than with alfentanil. There was a similar incidence of adverse events in both groups but the adverse events in the remifentanil group were rapidly controlled by dose reductions.

Remifentanil has been compared to alfentanil for ambulatory laparoscopic surgery (11). Patients received propofol (2 mg/kg bolus followed by an infusion of 150 μg/kg/min) and either remifentanil (1 μg/kg bolus followed by 0.5 μg/kg/min infusion) or alfentanil (20 μg/kg bolus followed by 2 μg/kg/min). Fifty-three percent of remifentanil patients and 71% of alfentanil patients had intraoperative responses or required dose adjustments during maintenance. Awakening times in the two groups were similar, but the remifentanil patients were slower to be discharged from the recovery room and required postoperative analgesia sooner than the alfentanil patients. In the study the delayed discharge from the recovery area was a potential problem since this is a labour intensive, expensive care area.

Remifentanil has also been used in cardiac (see Chapter 9) (12) and neurosurgery (see Chapter 11) (13–15).

Use in patients with hepatic and renal failure

Ninety-five percent of remifentanil is metabolized by hydrolysis of the propanoic methyl ester group to yield the carboxylic acid metabolite, GR90291, which is excreted in the urine. The half-life of this metabolite is longer than that of remifentanil, ranging from 88 to 137 min, but it has a potency 4600 times less than remifentanil, as measured by μ opioid-induced EEG changes.

Patients with chronic, stable, severe hepatic disease awaiting transplantation and healthy matched controls were each given a 4 h infusion of remifentanil at 0.0125 μg/kg/min for 1 h followed by 0.025 μg/kg/min for 3 h or a 4 h infusion at double these rates (16). There were no differences in any of the pharmacokinetic parameters for remifentanil or GR90291 between the two groups. The patients with hepatic failure were more sensitive to the ventilatory depressant effects of the drug, but the clinical significance of this finding is unknown.

Patients with renal failure and matched controls were given remifentanil infusions as described above (17). The clearance and volume of distribution of remifentanil was not affected by renal failure. Patients with renal failure showed a marked reduction in the excretion of GR90291 and its half-life increased from 1.5 h in the controls to over 26 h in the patients with renal failure. The steady-state concentration of GR90291 is 25 times higher in persons with renal failure but simulations suggest that at the end of a 12 h infusion of remifentanil, the metabolite unlikely to produce significant opioid effects.

Summary

Remifentanil is a very useful analgesic drug to use as a component of TIVA. It has applications in most types of surgery and can be administered successfully via a manual infusion or TCI. It can cause problems in recovery. It use would seem to be limited to types of surgery requiring intense analgesia where recovery time is not critical.

S-(+)-Ketamine

The currently available formulation of ketamine contains S-(+) and R-(−) enantiomers mixed in a 1:1 ratio. S-(+)-ketamine is 1.5–4 (18,19) times as potent a hypnotic and analgesic when compared with the racemic mixture. It has also been reported that the recovery time is faster and there are fewer emergence reactions when the S-(+)-isomer is used.

The pharmacokinetic–pharmacodynamic data comparing racemic ketamine and S-(+)-ketamine suggest that S-(+)-ketamine will make control of anaesthesia easier because it has a higher clearance and steeper concentration–response curve than the racemic mixture (20). This ensures that a small change in infusion rate will exert its affect rapidly while a decrease in infusion rate will result in a rapid reduction in effect. The pharmacokinetics of the racemic mixture are less favourable than of the S-(+) isomer not only because of the presence of the R-(−) isomer, but also because there appears to be some intrinsic S-(+) and R-(−) interaction and the presence of the R-(−) isomer may slow the metabolism of the S-(+) isomer.

The clinical usefulness of ketamine has been limited by its cardiovascular stimulating properties and high incidence of psychomimetic emergence reactions.

Cardiovascular stimulation is similar with the S-(+) isomer and the racemic mixture (21). The increased heart rate and blood pressure are due to the sympathomimetic effect of ketamine and are reduced slightly by the concurrent administration of midazolam. Propofol counteracts the sympathomimetic effects and stable haemodynamic conditions result from a combination of propofol and S-(+)-ketamine.

The hoped for reduction in psychomimetic emergence reactions with S-(+)-ketamine has not occurred in practice and the ketamine requires to be combined with another hypnotic drug such as propofol or midazolam (22), although time spent at concentrations likely to cause these effects should be less.

S-(+)-ketamine is likely to replace the use of racemic ketamine but it is unlikely to find a widespread use in anaesthesia. Among its indications are induction of anaesthesia in patients with shock or asthma. It can also be used in combination with propofol for induction and maintenance of anaesthesia for cardiac surgery, particularly in patients with critically occluded coronary arteries in who any reduction in perfusion pressure is undesirable. Other indications for the drug may include repeated anaesthesia in patients with burns or who require dressing changes for other reasons.

New methods of drug administration

The analgesic and hypnotic drugs used for TIVA also have applications outside the operating theatre. Alfentanil and remifentanil have both been used successfully to provide postoperative analgesia and propofol can be administered for patient sedation.

Postoperative analgesia

When opioids are used for postoperative analgesia it is normal to use a long-acting drug such as morphine or diamorphine. These drugs can be given as a bolus dose or as a constant rate infusion.

Several problems exist with these methods of administration. The drugs have a slow onset of action and initially take considerable time to achieve satisfactory analgesia. In order to prevent the need for frequent repeat bolus doses the drug should have a slow offset time, but this results in the risk of drug accumulation, especially in patients with impaired renal or hepatic function.

The speed of onset of analgesia can be improved by using a drug with faster blood–brain equilibration, such as alfentanil or remifentanil. These drugs both have a short duration of action and need to be administered by infusion. If they are administered by a constant rate infusion there is a delay until the onset of peak effect. However, the use of TCI overcomes the problem of the slow onset of analgesia since the drug is administered to attain the desired blood concentration very rapidly.

Alfentanil

The first reported study of TCI for postoperative analgesia involved the administration of alfentanil to 14 patients recovering from major aortic surgery (23). The patients all received TCI alfentanil intraoperatively. Postoperatively an alfentanil concentration was chosen to provide good analgesia with minimal respiratory depression. Nursing staff were then allowed to increase or decrease the concentration by 5 ng/ml if required. The system was used for a mean of 39 h and for 96% of the time the patients experienced little or no pain. The median target blood concentration of alfentanil was 71 ng/ml (range 34–150 ng/ml).

TCI alfentanil has also been used for postoperative analgesia in 20 patients who had undergone major orthopaedic surgery (24). The minimum effective analgesic concentrations ranged from less than 1 to 175 ng/ml and showed substantial inter-individual variability.

The same group of investigators compared TCI alfentanil with patient-controlled morphine for postoperative analgesia in 20 patients (25). The onset of satisfactory analgesia was faster in the TCI alfentanil group with a median time of 20 min compared to 50 min in the morphine group.

An interesting application of TCI is its use to provide PCA. PCA is normally provided by bolus administration of opioid with a lockout period programmed into the pump to prevent overdose. Several pumps are available which provide these functions. Most pumps also have the ability to provide a background infusion of opioid, although in practice the use of a background has not been found to improve pain control in adults.

Patients have been allowed to control the target concentration of alfentanil by using a push-button hand set (26). A successful request from the patient increased the blood concentration by 5 ng/ml. The system provided excellent analgesia in 20 patients recovering from cardiac surgery and compared favourably with a conventional morphine PCA. The patients who received alfentanil were extubated faster than the group who received morphine.

This study was repeated on 120 patients and the TCI alfentanil compared with conventional morphine PCA (27). Morphine was administered in 1 mg bolus doses with a lockout of 3 min to one group of patients and alfentanil was administered using a TCI system to another group. Patient demand increased the target concentration of alfentanil by 5 ng/ml with a lockout of 2 min. If analgesia was not requested in 15 min the target concentration automatically reduced by 5 ng/ml. The minimum target concentration permitted was 15 ng/ml and the maximum was 150 ng/ml. The overall mean visual analogue pain scores in patients using the alfentanil system were significantly lower than those using the morphine system. The patients receiving alfentanil in this study were also extubated sooner. There were no significant differences between overall sedation scores, incidence of postoperative nausea and vomiting, haemodynamic instability or hypoxia.

Another study compared patient-controlled TCI alfentanil with PCA morphine in patients undergoing major spinal surgery (28). Both methods provided equally effective analgesia. In both the previous studies, there was a suggestion that the alfentanil patients were less sedated but statistical analysis of sedation scores failed to confirm this.

Alfentanil has been administered by TCI and the patient allowed to control the target concentration, to provide analgesia for extracorporeal shock wave lithotripsy (ESWL) (29). The rapid offset of action, following infusions of short duration, makes alfentanil well suited to this procedure since pain diminishes rapidly with the termination of the shocks and patients wish to return home with minimal residual drug effects. There is also considerable inter-individual variation in analgesic requirements for ESWL. The median maximum target alfentanil concentration was 45 ng/ml (range 30–110 ng/ml). All of the patients who used the technique expressed a high degree of satisfaction with it.

Remifentanil

Manually controlled infusions of remifentanil have been used for postoperative analgesia with a little degree of success.

In one study 157 patients undergoing abdominal, spine, orthopaedic or thoracic surgery were anaesthetized with propofol and remifentanil (30). Postoperatively the remifentanil infusion was continued at a rate of 0.05 µg/kg/min. The remifentanil was titrated with bolus doses of 0.5 µg/kg and infusion rate changes of 0.05 or 0.1 µg/kg/min. After 46 patients had been treated the protocol was changed. The initial infusion rate was increased to 0.1 µg/kg/min because of unsatisfactory pain control immediately upon emergence from anaesthesia. Seventy-eight percent of patients required infusion rates of 0.05–0.15 µg/kg/min, while 5% were less than 0.05 µg/kg/min and 17% were greater than 0.15 µg/kg/min. Respiratory adverse events occurred in 29% of patients and included low S_aO_2, apnoea or ventilatory depression. Two patients were treated with naloxone in the recovery room. The administration of a bolus dose of remifentanil preceded the onset of respiratory depression in 19 out of 45 patients.

In another study a total of 116 patients were anaesthetized with remifentanil and propofol intraoperatively (12). Remifentanil was continued into the postoperative period at a reduced infusion rate. Initially, the investigators used a rate of 0.05 µg/kg/min of remifentanil. If the patient reported moderate or severe pain a bolus dose of 0.5 µg/kg was administered and the infusion rate doubled. However, as in the previous study, this regimen led to a high incidence of adverse events. The protocol was altered and the initial infusion rate increased to 0.1 µg/kg/min. Mild pain was treated by a 25% increase in infusion rate, while moderate or severe pain was treated with a 25–100% increase in infusion rate and a bolus dose of 0.5 µg/kg. If the patient was pain-free for 10 min the infusion rate was reduced by 25%.

Eighty-three patients received an initial infusion rate of 0.05 µg/kg/min and 33 patients an initial infusion rate of 0.1 µg/kg/min.

During the course of the study 10 patients suffered a total of 22 adverse events deemed by the anaesthetist to be life threatening. These included apnoea, thoracic muscle rigidity, respiratory depression and hypotension. All of these events occurred while receiving remifentanil for postoperative analgesia. Eighteen events occurred with the 0.05 µg/kg/min initial infusion regimen and four events when receiving the 0.1 µg/kg/min initial infusion regimen. The adverse events were attributed to rapid changes in the remifentanil blood concentration. Patients were treated either by reducing or discontinuing the remifentanil infusion.

The authors conclude that an initial remifentanil infusion rate of 0.1 µg/kg/min titrated to individual need can provide effective postoperative pain relief in the presence of adequate respiration. They recommend that it should only be used in the presence of adequate patient supervision and monitoring, and also recommend that bolus dose administration should be avoided.

Remifentanil has recently been administered via a patient-controlled TCI system (31). Thirty patients received remifentanil intraoperatively for orthopaedic surgery. At the end of surgery the remifentanil concentration was reduced until the patients breathed spontaneously. This occurred at a mean blood target concentration of 1.05 ng/ml. The patients were then able to increase the target concentration via a push button handset. A successful demand increased the target concentration by 0.2 ng/ml with a 2 min lockout. If there were no demands within 30 min, the target concentration was reduced by 0.2 ng/ml. Satisfactory analgesia, as judged by a visual analog score of less than 3, was achieved in a mean time of 18.9 min from the start of PCA remifentanil. The mean remifentanil target concentration was 2.02 ng/ml. There were no episodes of hypoxia or apnoea. This study demonstrated that patient-controlled TCI remifentanil can be used safely in the postoperative period and overcomes the transition to alternative analgesia following the termination of a remifentanil infusion which has been used intraoperatively. Unlike in the previous studies, the use of TCI prevented rapid changes in the blood concentration of remifentanil which are thought to be associated with ventilatory depression and chest wall rigidity.

The advantages of TCI for analgesia include:

◆ Rapid onset of analgesic blood concentrations of drug
◆ Ability to use drugs with short blood–brain equilibration half-lives ensuring rapid onset of analgesia
◆ Ability to use drugs with a short duration of action and prevent accumulation but yet ensure long-lasting analgesia by maintaining the target concentration over time
◆ Ability to alter rapidly the level of analgesia
◆ Rational continuation of the analgesic used intraoperatively into the postoperative phase
◆ Possibly less patient sedation
◆ High degree of patient satisfaction with the technique

TIVA with closed-loop control of anaesthesia

Closed-loop control requires that the measured response is used as the input signal of a control system. The system is then able to alter its output to keep the measured variable within preset limits. The concept has been used to control blood pressure and muscle relaxation.

When applied to depth of anaesthesia, the system should be able to detect the level of consciousness and then alter the administration of anaesthetic agent to ensure that the patient remains unconscious.

The benefits of closed-loop control are:

◆ The system titrates the level of anaesthesia directly to the needs of the individual patient
◆ Overcomes inter-individual differences in pharmacokinetics and pharmacodynamics
◆ Targets patient response rather than a pre-defined concentration
◆ Improves patient care by relating the drug delivery directly to the patient's requirements
◆ Avoids under- or overdosing
◆ Removal of observer bias, which can assist research

Satisfactory anaesthesia requires adequate cardiovascular and respiratory stability, no patient movement, and no patient recall of events during the procedure. The ultimate test of a closed-loop system for anaesthesia is that the system should be capable of delivering an anaesthetic agent to a spontaneously breathing patient during surgery.

TIVA provides a very convenient method of administering the anaesthetic agent. Alterations in the blood concentration of anaesthetic drug can readily be achieved by altering the infusion rate of the drug.

A closed-loop system based on BIS has recently been developed (32,33). This system has been reported in patients undergoing lower extremity surgery under locoregional anaesthesia. Propofol was administered by feedback control to maintain the BIS value at 50 and a mean arterial pressure of 70–85 mmHg. During the control period insertion of the laryngeal mask airway caused movement in 11 patients and subsequent movement occurred at a rate of 1.8 (SD 1.7) movements per hour. There were no significant haemodynamic changes and no patients reported awareness during the postoperative interview.

A closed-loop anaesthesia system based on the AEPI has been developed in Glasgow by Kenny and colleagues and has been named CLAN (Closed Loop ANaesthesia) (34,35). The AEPI is entered into a controller which calculates the target blood concentration of propofol needed to maintain the AEPI at a predetermined value. Propofol is administered by a TCI. See Figure 17.1.

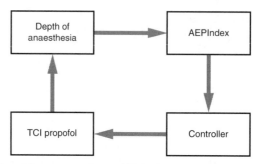

Figure 17.1   Closed-loop anaesthesia (CLAN) system using the AEPI as the measure of depth of anaesthesia and controlling a TCI of propofol.

CLAN has been used for body surface surgery, cardiac surgery and partial hepatic resections. It functions well in all situations with the exception of ENT surgery where electrode placement for the recording of AEP can be difficult. This is currently the only system which operates satisfactorily in non-paralysed patients breathing spontaneously.

The initial reports described 27 patients who received an alfentanil infusion and 66% N_2O in addition to the TCI propofol (34). There were no instances of patient awareness and all the patients would be happy to have the same anaesthetic again. Three of the patients moved but the movements were slight and did not interfere with surgery.

Another study reported the propofol requirements in 12 patients receiving TCI alfentanil at a target of 15 ng/ml and breathing 66% N_2O (35). The median target concentration of propofol used to maintain anaesthesia was 3.5 μg/ml with a minimum and maximum concentration of 2.4 and 4.0 μg/ml, respectively. The median intra-patient pharmacodynamic variation in propofol requirements during surgery was 6 to 7 times greater than the median inter-patient pharmacokinetic variability.

Conclusions

TIVA introduces the possibility of many exciting developments in patient care. Propofol, remifentanil and alfentanil are the drugs with the best profiles for administration by infusion. They are likely to see increased use in anaesthesia and sedation when administered by manual infusions or TCI. S-(+)-Ketamine may also have a role in certain circumstances.

PCA using a TCI pump has been shown to be a safe and effective technique with alfentanil and remifentanil. Although TCI pumps capable of altering their infusion rates in response to patient demand are not yet commercially available, the technology is well established. The development of remifentanil, a potent opioid ideally suited to administration by TCI, means that the technique may be used more widely.

References

1. Patel SS, Spencer CM. Remifentanil. *Drugs* 1996; **52**: 417–27.
2. Kapila A, Glass PS, Jacobs JR, *et al*. Measured context-sensitive half-times of remifentanil and alfentanil. *Anesthesiology* 1995; **83**: 968–75.
3. Egan TD, Lemmens HJ, Fiset P, *et al*. The pharmacokinetics of the new short-acting opioid remifentanil (GI87084B) in healthy adult male volunteers. *Anesthesiology* 1993; **79**: 881–92.
4. Egan TD, Minto CF, Hermann DJ, Barr J, Muir KT, Shafer SL. Remifentanil versus alfentanil: comparative pharmacokinetics and pharmacodynamics in healthy adult male volunteers. *Anesthesiology* 1996; **84**: 821–33.
5. Egan TD. Remifentanil pharmacokinetics and pharmacodynamics. A preliminary appraisal. *Clin Pharmacokinet* 1995; **29**: 80–94.
6. Minto CF, Schnider TW, Egan TD, *et al*. Influence of age and gender on the pharmacokinetics and pharmacodynamics of remifentanil. I. Model development. *Anesthesiology* 1997; **86**: 10–23.
7. Amin HM, Sopchak AM, Esposito BF, *et al*. Naloxone-induced and spontaneous reversal of depressed ventilatory responses to hypoxia during and after continuous infusion of remifentanil or alfentanil. *J Pharmacol Exp Ther* 1995; **274**: 34–9.
8. Vuyk J. Pharmacokinetic and pharmacodynamic interactions between opioids and propofol. *J Clin Anesthesia* 1997; **9** (suppl 6): S23–6.
9. Hogue CW Jr, Bowdle TA, O'Leary C, *et al*. A multicenter evaluation of total intravenous anesthesia with remifentanil and propofol for elective inpatient surgery. *Anesth Analg* 1996; **83**: 279–85.
10. Schuttler J, Albrecht S, Breivik H, *et al*. A comparison of remifentanil and alfentanil in patients undergoing major abdominal surgery. *Anaesthesia* 1997; **52**: 307–17.
11. Philip BK, Scuderi PE, Chung F, *et al*. Remifentanil compared with alfentanil for ambulatory surgery using total intravenous anesthesia. *Anesth Analg* 1997; **84**: 515–21.
12. Russel D, Royston D, Rees PH, Gupta SK, Kenny GNC. Effect of temperature and cardiopulmonary bypass on the pharmacokinetics of remifentanil. *Br J Anaesth* 1997; **79**: 456–9.
13. Baker KZ, Ostapkovich N, Sisti MB, Warner DS, Young WL. Intact cerebral blood flow reactivity during remifentanil/nitrous oxide anesthesia. *J Neurosurg Anesthesiol* 1997; **9**: 134–40.
14. Guy J, Hindman BJ, Baker KZ, *et al*. Comparison of remifentanil and fentanyl in patients undergoing craniotomy for supratentorial space-occupying lesions. *Anesthesiology* 1997; **86**: 514–24.

15. Warner DS, Hindman BJ, Todd MM, *et al.* Intracranial pressure and hemodynamic effects of remifentanil versus alfentanil in patients undergoing supratentorial craniotomy. *Anesth Analg* 1996; **83**: 348–53.
16. Dershwitz M, Hoke JF, Rosow CE, *et al.* Pharmacokinetics and pharmacodynamics of remifentanil in volunteer subjects with severe liver disease. *Anesthesiology* 1996; **84**: 812–20.
17. Hoke JF, Shlugman D, Dershwitz M, *et al.* Pharmacokinetics and pharmacodynamics of remifentanil in persons with renal failure compared with healthy volunteers. *Anesthesiology* 1997; **87**: 533–41.
18. Pfenninger E, Baier C, Claws S, Hege C. Psychometric changes as well as analgesic action and cardiovascular adverse effects of ketamine racemate uses S-(+)-ketamine in sub anaesthetic doses. *Anaesthetist* 1994; **43** (suppl): S68–75.
19. Mathisen LC, Sjelbred P, Skoglund LA, Oye I. Effect of ketamine on NMDA receptor inhibitor in acute and chronic orofacial pain. *Pain* 1995; **61**: 215–20.
20. Adams HA, Werner C. From the racemate to the eutomer: (S)-ketamine. Renaissance of a substance? *Anaesthesist* 1997; **46**: 1026–42.
21. Adams HA. S-(+)-ketamine. Circulatory interactions during total intravenous anesthesia and analgesia-sedation. *Anaesthesist* 1997; **46**: 1081–7.
22. Engelhardt W. Recovery and psychomimetic reactions following S-(+)-ketamine. *Anaesthesist* 1997; **46** (suppl 1): S38–42.
23. Davies FW, White M, Kenny GN. Postoperative analgesia using a computerised infusion of alfentanil following aortic bifurcation graft surgery. *Int J Clin Monit Comput* 1992; **9**: 207–12.
24. Van den Nieuwenhuyzen MC, Engbers FH, Burm AG, *et al.* Computer-controlled infusion of alfentanil for postoperative analgesia. A pharmacokinetic and pharmacodynamic evaluation. *Anesthesiology* 1993; **79**: 481–92.
25. Van den Nieuwenhuyzen MC, Engbers FH, Burm AG, Vletter AA, Van Kleef, JW, Bovill JG. Computer-controlled infusion of alfentanil versus patient-controlled administration of morphine for postoperative analgesia: a double-blind randomized trial. *Anesth Analg* 1995; **81**: 671–9.
26. Checketts MR, Gilhooly CJ, Kenny GNC. Patient-maintained analgesia with alfentanil after cardiac surgery: a comparison with morphine PCA. *Br J Anaesth* 1995; **74** (suppl 1): A439.
27. Checketts MR, Gilhooly CJ, Kenny GNC. Patient maintained analgesia with target-controlled alfentanil infusion after cardiac surgery: a comparison with morphine PCA. *Br J Anaesth* 1998; **80**: 748–51.
28. Irwin MG, Jones RD, Visram AR, Kenny GN. Patient-controlled alfentanil. Target-controlled infusion for postoperative analgesia. *Anaesthesia* 1996; **51**: 427–30.
29. Irwin MG, Campbell RC, Lun TS, Yang JC. Patient maintained alfentanil target-controlled infusion for analgesia during extracorporeal shock wave lithotripsy. *Can J Anaesth* 1996; **43**: 919–24.
30. Bowdle TA, Camporesi EN, Maysick L, *et al.* A multicentre evaluation of remifentanil for early postoperative analgesia. *Anesth Analg* 1996; **83**: 1292–7.
31. Schragg S, Kenny GNC, Mohl U, Georgieff M. Patient-maintained target-controlled remifentanil for the transition to early postoperative analgesia. *Br J Anaesth* 1998; **81**: 365.
32. Struys M, De Smet S, Audenaert S, Versichelen L, Mortier E, Rolly G. Development of a closed loop system for propofol using bispectral analysis and a patient-individual pharmacokinetic-dynamic (PK-PD) model. Preliminary results. *Br J Anaesth* 1997; **78** (suppl 1): A76.

33. Mortier E, Struys M, De Smet S, Versichelen L, Rolly G. Closed-loop administration of propofol using bispectral analysis. *Anaesthesia* 1998; **53**: 749–54.
34. Kenny GNC, McFadzean W, Mantzaridis H, Fisher AC. Closed-loop control of anaesthesia. *Anesthesiology* 1992; **77**: A328.
35. Kenny GNC, McFadzean W, Mantzaridis H, Fisher AC. Propofol requirements during closed-loop anesthesia. *Anesthesiology* 1993; **79**: A329.

Index

Acromegaly, 263–4
Acupuncture, 131
Addison's syndrome, 270, 271
Adrenal cortex, 270–1
Adrenal medulla, 272
Age, 37, 149, *see also* Elderly
Airway:
  compression, 188
  reactivity, 176–7
Alfentanil, 7, 26
  cardiac anaesthesia, 167–8
  cardiovascular effects, 30
  clearance, 20
  co-induction with propofol, 74
  day surgery, 154–5
  elderly patients, 240
  elimination half-time, 20
  neurophysiological effects, 213
  pharmacokinetics, 28–9, 42
  postoperative analgesia, 290–1
  postoperative nausea and
     vomiting, 125
  respiratory effects, 31
Althesin, 6
Amnesia, 88
Anaesthetic drug action, 13–14
Analgesia, 155, 251, 289–93, *see
   also* Patient-controlled
   analgesia

Antidiuretic hormone, 264
Antiemetics, 33–4, 127–32
Antihistamines, 129–30
'Apneic' high-flow oxygenation,
  182
ASA fitness levels, 149
Aspirin, 7
Atmospheric pollution, 11
Atracurium, 170
  elderly patients, 241
Auditory evoked potentials, 97–8,
  105–12
  coherent frequency, 109–11
Autoregulation, 207–8
'Awake' procedures, 218–19
Awakening time, 62–3
Awareness, 87–115
  incidence, 91, 101
  long-term effects, 114
  medico-legal aspects, 112–114
  patient complaint of, 113–14
  with total intravenous
     anaesthesia, 98, 101

'Balanced' analgesia, 155
Barbiturates, 16–18
  cardiac anaesthesia, 165–6
  cardiovascular effects, 18

Barbiturates – *continued*
  cerebral protection, 208–9
  neurological effects, 18
  pharmacokinetics, 16–17, 40
  respiratory effects, 18
Benzodiazepines, 6, 18–21
  cardiac anaesthesia, 164–5
  cardiovascular effects, 20
  neurological effects, 19
  neurosurgery, 215–16
  pharmacokinetics, 19, 40
  postoperative nausea and
      vomiting, 121
  respiratory effects, 20
Bilirubin, 38
Bispectral index, 9, 103–5
Blood–brain equilibration, 61–2
Blood concentration, 45–9
Body mass index, 149
Body surface area, 57
Body weight, 57
Bolus plus manual infusion, 70
Bristol technique, 71
British Society for Intravenous
    Anaesthesia (SIVA), 5, 12
Bronchoscopy, 180–3, 185–6
Bronchospasm, 176–7
Burns, 227–8
Burrhole biopsies, 219

Carcinoid tumours, 273
Cardiac disease, 179–80
Cardiac output, 234–5
Cardiac surgery, 158–75
  minimally invasive, 172
  muscle relaxation, 169–70
  postoperative sedation, 170–1
  total intravenous anaesthesia,
      162–70
Cardiopulmonary bypass, 39,
    159–62
Cerebral blood flow, 205–6
Cerebral metabolic rate for
    oxygen, 205
Cerebral metabolism, 205
Cerebral perfusion pressure, 207
Cerebral protection, 208–9

Cerebral steal, 208
Chemoreceptor trigger zone, 126
Children, 57
Chloral hydrate, 6
Chlordiazepoxide, 18
Chloroform, 122
Cholecystectomy, 78–9
Choroidal blood volume, 276
Chronic disease, 149, 159, 179–80,
    241–2
CLAN, 294
Clearance, 20, 45
Clonidine, 251
Closed-loop control, 112, 281,
    293–4
Cognition, 90–3, 103, 105
Co-induction, 69, 74–6, 244, 245–6
Complement system, 161
Computer simulations, 50–2, 157
Connectors, 67
Conn's syndrome, 270, 271
Consciousness, 87–8
Context-sensitive half-time, 16,
    58–9
Corpus callosum, 88
Cost factors:
  day surgery, 156
  postoperative nausea and
      vomiting, 118
  propofol use, 156, 171, 211–12
Craniotomies, 218–19
Cushing's syndrome, 270
Cyclizine, 129–30

Day surgery, 78–82, 147–57
  anaesthesia, 150–4
  analgesia, , 154–6
  economic benefits, 156
  intravenous fluid
      administration, 67
  patient selection, 148–9
  postoperative nausea and
      vomiting, 117, 123
  suitable operations, 148
  target-controlled infusion, 76–7
Dead space, 67, 177

Depth of anaesthesia, 8–9,
    101–102
Desflurane:
    neurosurgery, 213, 217
    postoperative nausea and
        vomiting, 122
Dexamethasone, 131
Diabetes insipidus, 264
Diabetes mellitus, 268–9
Diamorphine, 7
Diazemuls, 19
Diazepam, 6, 18, 19
    clearance, 20
    elimination half-time, 20
Diisopropyl phenol, 6
Diprifusor, 8, 55, 60, 76–7
Dissociative anaesthesia, 22
Dose, 36, 45–9, 57, 70, 71
Droperidol, 33, 128–9
    cardiovascular effects, 33
    clearance, 20
    dose, 128
    elimination half-time, 20
    neurological effects, 33
    side-effects, 128

Ear surgery, 133, 231
Economic factors:
    day surgery, 156
    postoperative nausea and
        vomiting, 118
    propofol use, 156, 171, 211–12
Elderly, 233–48
    anaesthesia for , 242–6
    cardiovascular changes, 234–5
    co-induction, 244, 245–6
    elderly elderly, 233
    hepatic function, 235–6
    hypotension, 243
    muscle relaxation, 241, 246
    neurological changes, 235
    pharmacodynamics, 237
    pharmacokinetics, 236–7
    physiological changes, 234–6
    regional anaesthesia, 254
    renal function, 235–6
    target-controlled infusion, 244,
        278–9

Electroencephalogram, 102, 112
    bispectral index, 9, 103–5
    power spectrum, 102–3
Elimination half-time, 14–15, 20,
    57–8
Emergence reactions, 6, 22, 41
Endocrine pancreas, 268–70
Endocrine surgery, 263–75
Endoscopy, 180–3
Endotracheal intubation, 8, 223
Enflurane, 213, 217
Ephedrine, 131
Equipment, 8, 67
Ether, 122
Etomidate, 6, 23–4
    adverse effects, 198
    cardiac anaesthesia, 166
    cardiovascular effects, 24
    clearance, 20
    day surgery, 153, 154
    dose, 23
    elderly patients, 238
    elimination half-time, 20
    endocrine effects, 24
    neurological effects, 23–4
    neurosurgery, 213, 215
    pharmacokinetics, 23, 41
    postoperative nausea and
        vomiting, 121
    respiratory effects, 24
    thoracic surgery, 198
Explicit memory, 88, 90

Facial injuries, 224–5
Fentanyl, 7, 26
    cardiac anaesthesia, 166–7
    cardiovascular effects, 30
    clearance, 20
    day surgery, 154
    elderly patients, 240
    elimination half-time, 20
    neurophysiological effects, 213
    pharmacokinetics, 28, 42
    postoperative nausea and
        vomiting, 125
    respiratory effects, 31
Fitness, 149

'Flash' bolus, 68
Flumazenil, 21

Ginger root, 131
Glossopharyngeal nerve block, 222
GR90291, 288

Haemodynamic response, 183–5
Half-times, 14–16, 53, 55, 57
Halothane, 213
Head and neck surgery, 223–4
Hepatic blood flow, 37–8
Hepatic disease, 38, 288
Hepatic function in elderly, 235–6
Hyperglycaemia, 269
Hyperparathyroidism, 267–8
Hyperthyroidism, 266–7
Hypocalcaemia, 268
Hypoparathyroidism, 268
Hypothalamus, 264
Hypothermia, 208
Hypothyroidism, 266, 267
Hypoxic pulmonary
     vasoconstrictor response
     (HPV), 179, 195

Implicit memory, 88, 90, 95–6
Induction, 68–71
  bolus plus manual infusion, 70
  'flash' bolus, 68
  infusion rate, 70–1
  intermittent bolus, 68–9
Infusion devices, 67
Infusion rate, 72–4
  induction, 70–1
  maintenance, 71–2
Inguinal hernia repair, 79–80
Inhalation anaesthetics:
  memory effects, 93–4
  neurosurgery, 213, 217
  postoperative nausea and
     vomiting, 122
Insulinoma, 270
Intermittent bolus, 68–9

Intermittent positive pressure
     ventilation, 182
Intracranial pressure, 203–4
Intraocular pressure, 276–7
Intraoral surgery, 225
Intravenous fluids, 67, 131
Intubation, 8, 223
Inverse steal, 208
Isoflurane:
  memory effects, 93–4
  neurosurgery, 213, 217
  postoperative nausea and
     vomiting, 122

Jet ventilation, 183, 228

Ketamine, 6, 21–3
  cardiac anaesthesia, 166
  cardiovascular effects, 23
  cerebral protection, 209
  clearance, 20
  co-induction with propofol, 75
  dose, 22
  elderly patients, 239
  elimination half-time, 20
  emergence reactions, 6, 22, 41
  neurological effects, 22
  neurosurgery, 213, 215
  pharmacokinetics, 22, 41
  postoperative nausea and
     vomiting, 121
  respiratory effects, 22
  S–(+) form, 21, 288–9
  thoracic surgery, 198–9
Ketorolac, 7
Kidney:
  age-related changes, 235–6
  disease, 39, 288

Laparoscopy, 287
  postoperative nausea and
     vomiting, 120, 132
Laryngeal masks, 8, 278
Laryngeal nerve block, 222

Larynx, 221–2
  local anaesthesia, 222
  microlaryngoscopy, 228
Laser surgery, 228–9
Lateral decubitus position, 177–9
Legal aspects, 112–114
Liver:
  age-related changes, 235–6
  blood flow, 37–8
  disease, 38, 288
Local anaesthetic blocks, 222
Lungs, 177

MAC, 98–100
Malignant neuroleptic syndrome,
  33
Mannitol, 209
Manual infusion, 66–8, 72–4
  changing with surgical
    stimulus, 76
  plus bolus, 70
Mediastinoscopy/mediastinotomy,
  186–8
Mediastinum tumours, 188–90
Medico-legal aspects, 112–114
Memory, 87–91, 93–6
Methadone, 7
Methohexitone, 6, 18
  cardiac anaesthesia, 165–6
  clearance, 20
  day surgery, 153, 154
  elderly patients, 238
  elimination half-time, 20
  postoperative nausea and
    vomiting, 121
  thoracic surgery, 197–8
Metoclopramide, 129
Meyer–Overton rule, 13
Microlaryngoscopy, 228
Midazolam, 6, 18, 19
  clearance, 20
  elderly patients, 238–9
  elimination half-time, 20
  neurophysiological effects, 213
Middle ear surgery, 133
Migraine, 119–20
Mineralocorticoid deficiency, 271

Minimum alveolar concentration,
  98–100
Mivacurium, 170
Morphine, 6–7, 26
  cardiovascular effects, 30
  clearance, 20
  elderly patients, 239–40
  elimination half-time, 20
  neurophysiological effects, 213
  pharmacokinetics, 27, 42
  postoperative nausea and
    vomiting, 123, 125, 127
Movement under anaesthesia, 103
Muscle relaxants:
  cardiac anaesthesia, 169–70
  elderly patients, 241, 246
  neurosurgery, 217
  postoperative nausea and
    vomiting, 125
Myasthenia gravis, 190–3
Myasthenic syndrome, 193

Nabilone, 131
Naloxone, 32
Neurohumoral 'stress' response,
  250–1
Neurokinin 1 antagonists, 132
Neuroleptanalgesia, 258
Neuromuscular block, *see* Muscle
  relaxants
Neurophysiology, 203–8
  age-related changes, 235
Neurosurgery, 210–19
  'awake' procedures, 218–19
  muscle relaxation, 217
  total intravenous anaesthesia,
    217–19
Nitric oxide, 206
Nitrous oxide, 9
  atmospheric pollution, 11
  cardiovascular effects, 162
  neurosurgery, 213, 217
  postoperative nausea and
    vomiting, 122–3
Non-steroidal anti-inflammatory
  drugs (NSAIDs), 7, 155
Norpethidine, 28, 30

Obesity, 39, 119, 149
Old age, *see* Elderly
Ondansetron, 33–4, 129
One-lung anaesthesia, 194–5
Open-loop control, 112
Ophthalmic surgery, 276–84
  closed-loop anaesthesia, 281
  intraocular pressure regulation,
    276–7
  laryngeal masks, 278
  opioids, 279–81, 283
  target-controlled infusions,
    277–81
Opioids, 6–7, 26–32
  cardiac anaesthesia, 166–9
  cardiovascular effects, 30–1
  day surgery, 154–5
  drug interactions, 42–3
  elderly patients, 239–41
  endocrine effects, 31–2
  gastrointestinal effects, 32
  muscle rigidity, 29
  neurological effects, 29–30
  neurosurgery, 216
  ophthalmic surgery, 279–81, 283
  pharmacokinetics, 27–9, 42–3
  postoperative nausea and
    vomiting, 121, 123, 125, 127
  respiratory effects, 31
  thoracic surgery, 200–1
Opium, 6
Oral surgery, 225
Oré, Pierre, 6

Pancuronium, 169
  elderly patients, 241
Parathormone, 267
Parathyroids, 267–8
Patient-controlled analgesia, 61,
    290–1, 292
  antiemetic addition, 133–4
Patient-controlled sedation, 257
  target-controlled infusion, 257–8
Perception, 91–3
Permissive apnea, 181–2
Pethidine, 7
  cardiovascular effects, 30, 31

clearance, 20
  elimination half-time, 20
  pharmacokinetics, 27–8
pH, 36–7
Phaeochromocytomas, 272
Pharmacodynamics, 44, 52–7
  age-related changes, 237
Pharmacokinetics, 14–16, 20,
    44–65
  age-related changes, 236–7
  factors affecting, 36–43
  models, 50–2
  and pharmacodynamics, 52–7
Pharynx, local anaesthesia, 222
Phenytoin, 209
Pituitary, 263–5
  tumours, 264, 265
Plasma concentration–time curve,
    14
Plasma protein binding, 37
Plastic surgery, 225–6
Porphyria, 18
Postoperative analgesia, 155, 251,
    289–93, *see also* Patient-
    controlled analgesia
Postoperative nausea and
    vomiting, 116–43
  antiemetics, 33–4, 127–32
  causes, 118–26
  cost factors, 118
  day surgery, 117, 123
  drug factors, 121–5
  effects of, 116–18
  obesity, 119
  patient attitude to, 117
  physiology of, 126–7
  prophylaxis, 134
  and recovery, 116–17
  surgical factors, 120–1, 132–3
  susceptibility to, 119–20
Postoperative sedation, 170–1
Post-traumatic stress disorder, 114
Power spectrum, 102–3
Prolactin, 263, 264
Propofol, 24–6
  cardiac anaesthesia, 162–4
  cardiovascular effects, 26
  clearance, 20

co-induction, 69, 74–6
and convulsions, 211
cost factors, 156, 171, 211–12
day surgery, 150, 154, 156
dose, 25
drug interactions, 42
elderly patients, 239
elimination half-time, 20
hypotensive effects, 163
interaction with monitoring
    equipment, 214
memory effects, 95
neurological effects, 25
neurosurgery, 211–12, 213,
    214–15, 218
ophthalmic surgery, 277–81
pain on injection, 150
pharmacokinetics, 25, 41–2, 212
postoperative nausea and
    vomiting, 121–2, 130–1
postoperative sedation, 170–1
regional anaesthesia, 252–4
respiratory effects, 25–6
thoracic surgery, 199–200
Propranidid, 6
Prostaglandins, 125
PRST index, 101–2
Pseudo steady state, 51
Pulmonary artery compression,
    189

Redistribution half-time, 14–15
Regional anaesthesia, 249–62
benefits of, 249–51
complications, 259–60
in the elderly, 254
patient assessment, 254
postoperative analgesia, 251
suitable surgery, 259
Remifentanil, 7, 26–7, 286–8
cardiac anaesthesia, 168–9
cardiovascular effects, 30, 286–7
clearance, 20
co-induction with propofol,
    74–5
day surgery, 155
elderly patients, 240–1

elimination half-time, 20
with hepatic disease, 288
neurosurgery, 213, 216
ophthalmic surgery, 283
pharmacodynamics, 286
pharmacokinetics, 29, 286
postoperative analgesia, 291–2
postoperative nausea and
    vomiting, 125
with renal failure, 288
respiratory effects, 31, 286
Renal disease, 39, 288
Renal function in elderly, 235–6
Robinson Crusoe experiment,
    97–8, 108

Salience, 96–7
Sedation, 255–6
patient-controlled, 257
patient-controlled/target-
    controlled infusion, 257–8
Sevoflurane:
neurosurgery, 213, 217
postoperative nausea and
    vomiting, 122
Sheehan's syndrome, 264
SIVA, 5, 12
Skin grafts, 226–7
Somatostatin, 273
Sterilization, 80, 82
Sternotomy, 186, 190
Steroids, 209
Strabismus surgery, 121, 123,
    132–3
Stress response, 250–1
Sufentanil, 7, 26
cardiac anaesthesia, 168
clearance, 20
elimination half-time, 20
neurophysiological effects, 213
pharmacokinetics, 28, 42
respiratory effects, 31
Superior vena cava obstruction,
    186–7, 189–90
Supratentorial tumour surgery,
    218
Suxamethonium, 213, 217

Sympathetic response, 249–50
Syringes, 8
  drivers, 8
Systemic disease, 149, 159, 179–80,
    241–2

T3 and T4, 265–6
Target-controlled infusions (TCI),
    4–5, 59–63, 100
  awakening time, 62–3
  blood–brain equilibration, 61–2
  compared to manual infusion,
    100–1
  day surgery, 76–7
  elderly patients, 244, 278–9
  ophthalmic surgery, 277–81
Tenoxicam, 7
Thiopentone, 6, 16
  cardiac anaesthesia, 165
  clearance, 20
  day surgery, 150, 153, 154
  elderly patients, 238
  elimination half-time, 20
  neurosurgery, 213, 215
  pharmacokinetics, 16–17, 40
  postoperative nausea and
    vomiting, 121
  thoracic surgery, 196–7
Thoracic surgery, 176–202
  cardiac disease, 179–80
  total intravenous anaesthesia,
    196–201
Thoracoscopy, 193

Thoracotomy, 193–5
Thymectomy, 191–3
Thyroid, 265–7
Tissue transfer, 226–7
Tonsil surgery, 229–30
  bleeding tonsil, 230
  peritonsillar abscess, 230
Total intravenous anaesthesia:
  administration, 66–83
  historical aspects, 4–5, 6–7
  limitations, 10
  merits, 9–10
  non-surgical procedures, 173
Tramadol, 155
Trans myocardial laser
    revascularization, 172–3
Trigeminal rhizotomies, 219

Vagal stimulation, 120–1
Vasoactive substance producing
    tumours, 273–4
Vasodilators, 213
Venous access, 66
Venturi jet injector, 183, 228
Vercuronium, 170
  elderly patients, 241
Volume of distribution, 15
Vomiting centre, 126

Weight, 57
Within-list recognition test, 93
Wren, Sir Christopher, 6